Family Functioning

The General Living Systems Research Model

CRITICAL ISSUES IN PSYCHIATRY
An Educational Series for Residents and Clinicians

A Continuation Order Plan is available for this series. A continuation order will bring delivery of each new volume immediately upon publication. Volumes are billed only upon actual shipment. For further information please contact the publisher.

Family Functioning

The General Living Systems Research Model

John J. Schwab
Helen M. Gray-Ice
Florence R. Prentice

University of Louisville
Louisville, Kentucky

KLUWER ACADEMIC / PLENUM PUBLISHERS
NEW YORK, BOSTON, DORDRECHT, LONDON, MOSCOW

Library of Congress Cataloging-in-Publication Data

Schwab, John J.
    Family functioning: the general living systems research model/John J. Schwab, Helen
M. Gray-Ice, and Florence R. Prentice.
      p.   cm.—(Critical issues in psychiatry)
    Includes bibliographical references and index.
    ISBN 0-306-46396-2
    1. Family assessment.   2. Family—Mental health.   I. Gray-Ice, Helen M.   II. Prentice,
Florence R. III.   Title.   IV. Series.

RC488.53 .S39 2000
616.89—dc21
                                              00-030935

ISBN 0-306-46396-2

©2000 Kluwer Academic / Plenum Publishers, New York
233 Spring Street, New York, N.Y. 10013

http://www.wkap.nl/

10 9 8 7 6 5 4 3 2 1

A C.I.P. record for this book is available from the Library of Congress

All rights reserved

No part of this book may be reproduced, stored in a retrieval system, or transmitted in any form or
by any means, electronic, mechanical, photocopying, microfilming, recording, or otherwise, without
written permission from the Publisher

Printed in the United States of America

FOREWORD

The family, that most fundamental of human groups, is currently perceived to be changing in response to social, biological, cultural and technological developments in our postmodern society. While the observed changes in families have been considered by some sociologists to be evidence of adaptation and, therefore, normal, the authors of this volume, consider them maladaptive. Viewing society from the point of view of clinical psychiatry, they point to greatly increased numbers of children born to single mothers, soaring rates of divorce, a statistically confirmed increase in mental disorders, increase in reported incest, high rates of depression in younger people and escalation of the amount of reported family violence as evidence that the family, as a social institution, is in crisis and can either move toward renewed vitality or continued deterioration.

Perceiving a need to obtain information about family functioning that might lead to the increased stability and well-being of this critically important type of system, Dr. John Schwab and his associates designed and carried out a research program that began with a thorough review of relevant literature beginning with LePlay's study of 300 families in the 1850's and including important recent statistical studies. They found that although these studies represent advances in understanding the family system, some serious problems with the research remain, one of which is confounding variables such as family function and mental or substance abuse disorders so that if a family member has a problem, such as drug abuse, the family is classified as dysfunctional.

The research program reported here began in the early 1980's when so many people with family problems were treated at the clinic that it aroused concern about the well-being of the family as a social institution. Previous studies, although they had supplied valuable data about the frequency, distribution, and correlates of mental disorders, had focused upon individual patients and had not evaluated dynamic group factors. The focus here is on the family group; its mental health and well-being as its members interact in everyday life.

A variety of methodological approaches were used, including a model, the general living systems (GLS) and Assessment Instrument, the Bell and Schwab family functioning instrument (the GLS), which was developed for use in this research. It is based upon our living systems theory, which identifies 19 subsystems essential at each of seven levels of living systems.

Living systems theory has been applied in research, therapy, or planning in many different kinds of living systems including organizations like hospitals and military units and in individual psychotherapy. In this research, the GLS instrument was found to be effective in identifying patterns of family interaction, helping family members to think about aspects of their relationship that they had not considered pertinent and stimulating thoughts about problem solving. It proved to be nonthreatening, to aid in identifying strengths as well as problems in families and to be liked by family members. It also avoided the circularity of the functioning-illness tautology that often limits approaches to the serious problem of the association between family functioning and mental illness or substance abuse.

This book should interest not only psychiatrists and other clinical personnel working with families, but academic psychologists and sociologists, social workers, systems theorists and researchers, and others concerned with problems at the levels of the family, and the community, and the society.

James Grier Miller and
Jessie Luthi Miller

PREFACE

About 2300 years ago, Aristotle (1952) defined the family as the basic social unit and described its social functions. Two millennia later Rousseau (1763) declared that it was the only natural institution, and through the ages, the pivotal importance of the family in society has been confirmed by the reciprocal effects of individual--family--community interactions. Those interactions determine the soundness or malaise of each of the three levels of biosocial organization and thus influence individuals' character formation and personality development, the integrity of the family unit and its functioning, and societal well-being.

The major reasons for our studying the family stem from the need to obtain information about its functioning that might lead to its increased stability and well-being. For almost 75 years, from the time of Ogburn, Burgess, Locke and their colleagues' work in the 1920s-1940s to Skolnick's in 1991, the debilitating effects of the increasing marital and family instability throughout this century have often been both discounted and rationalized despite the cries of distress from family members in broken homes, some schoolteachers, a few of the clergy, and a handful of family scholars.

We cannot regard the changes occurring in the family as just being in accord with the rapid rate of social change during the past century, as many have argued. Instead of seeing the changes as adaptive, we think they are maladaptive. For five reasons, we need to acknowledge that the family is now in a crisis, at a turning point toward either vitality or debilitation.

The first is that the status and fate of the family are inextricably tied to the health of the state and the well-being of its citizens. That fundamental truth was observed by the philosophers of ancient Greece, confirmed by political philosophers and other scholars many times since, and reaffirmed since LePlay's (Silver, 1982) pioneering investigations during the mid-19th century (see Chapter II). The record of history reveals that changes in the family, such as those that have been taking place in the USA in this century, are painfully analogous and, in many ways, similar to those that occurred in classical Greece after the Peloponnesian War and continued during the two centuries of its decline from about 400 BC to 200 BC. Also, before the "Fall of Rome", the centuries-old Roman family became increasingly decadent. During the 2nd and 4th centuries AD, multiple divorces and various forms of marriage (traditional marriage dignitas, the less binding marriage concubinitas, etc.) became common, similar to what is now occurring in the USA (conventional marriage, covenant marriages, domestic partners, etc.). What do those parallel situations signify?

The second is the extent of suffering so often produced by divorce and the pathologies associated with broken homes, especially the plight of the children who receive inadequate parenting and care. Perhaps most important, we do not know the long-term effects of the extensive family disruption on character formation and personality development. Already, the wide-scale blaming of others, litigation, and unwillingness to assume responsibility that threaten to become national characteristics ("the nation of cry-babies") reflect changes in ideals and character in the 150 years since Emerson's "Self-Reliance" (1844).

Third, the antifamilism of the past few decades has become extreme. On June 1, 1999, newspapers reported that "US quits gathering marriage, divorce stats" (Peterson, 1999). Budget cuts have led the National Center for Health Statistics (NCHS) to discontinue gathering detailed data annually on marriages and divorces. Moreover, the short form of the 2000 Census that 80% of Americans will receive will not even ask about marital status.

Family researchers, demographers, sociologists, and others are reacting with alarm to this dramatic development. Although a selected 16 million Americans will receive the long census form that requests detailed information, projections from that 20% of the population are bound to be inadequate, especially in view of the unprecedented extent of marital and family flux. Diane Solles, a family therapist who emphasizes "smart marriages, happy families," responded: "the message is that nobody cares anymore" (Peterson, 1999, "Defenders", A4)

The demographer Andrew Cherlin at Johns Hopkins University stated that this change "handicaps my ability to give useful information", and Theodora Ooms from the Resource Center on Couples and Marriage Policy stated that "the feds are cutting back on what they tell us, and it is frustrating to those of us who are trying to understand what is happening." A University of Chicago sociologist asked how social scientists can tell "What divorce means to kids if you don't know how many kids (affected by divorce) there are, the ages and education of their parents, income, the very most fundamental pieces of information" (Peterson, 1999, A4).

David Blankenhorn, founder of the Institute for American Values, declared that the budgetary cutbacks "tell us something about the values in our society." Governor Frank Keating who has been trying to reduce the Oklahoma divorce rate by one-third by 2010, stated: "In my state it is easier to get out of a marriage contract with kids than a Tupperware contract" (Peterson, 1999, "Defenders", A4).

Although anti-government groups look at the reduction of data as a step that helps to ensure "privacy" for families, the issues of values are obviously paramount. At this time, limiting information about marriage and divorce can only be harmful to families. Its consequences are bound to be antifamilistic, and "giving up" the need for the data appears to be sending a "giving up" message about family stability and well-being. Columnist Mike Manius responded: "There are federal employees counting the number of California red-legged frogs, and coffin cave mold beetles--two endangered species--but no one counts divorce." (Peterson, 1999, A4)

The fourth is concern about the apparent increased frequency of mental disorders, many of which, genetically and socially, are products of family life. They need to be seen in a social psychiatric perspective. Will borderline personality disorder become epidemic? What does the efflorescence of multiple personality disorder and addictive disorders represent? Portend? Is their prominence during the past few decades reflecting our "borderline" society with the relative neglect of its children and unwillingness to accept that "the health of nations is more important than the wealth of nations" (Durant, 1990)? Although the meaning and the consequences of the prevalent marital and family disruption are being variously interpreted, the harsh statistics about its related pathologies-- medical, psychiatric, and social--cannot be rationalized or dismissed.

Finally, "the mental health function" of marriage and family life cannot be ignored. Although the family is being subjected to immense stress, especially the all-too-pressing financial problems, the weakening of supports associated with the disintegration of the community, and the shifting ideals and practices inherent to a consumer-driven society, as an institution the family has had remarkable endurance. For most persons it gives life meaning and purpose and has often sustained its members "for better or for worse, in sickness and in health." Its mental health functions have long promoted well-being and hope and have been a refuge against despair. Studies of family functioning, therefore, need to focus on family health and well-being as well as dysfunctions and pathologies in order to learn more about how the mental hygiene functions of marriage and family can be enhanced.

In Chapter 1, we discuss the extreme instability of the family and concern about the prevalence of pathologies and problems in our rapidly changing society. Many family scholars and therapists and some social critics blame them on our so-called dysfunctional families, but seldom define function/dysfunction even while they castigate the "dysfunctional family" of the mentally ill, the alcohol and drug abusers, and the delinquent and criminal. Moreover, tautologies are commonplace; for example, one's having an "alcohol problem" is irrefutable evidence per se that his or her family was dysfunctional. Therefore, we have focused our research on the controversial concept of family function/dysfunction.

In Chapter 2, we review the history of family function/dysfunction and cite related research from the English studies of a century ago and the early USA studies up to the present. We emphasize the need for definitions, if not rigor, and then, in Chapter 3, we supply a summary of the theoretical background for the development of our General Living Systems (GLS) Family Functioning Model and theory-based assessment instrument.

In Chapter 4, after presenting a brief summary of our previous, but related, epidemiologic research with families in the community, we describe our current study. In Chapter 5, we discuss the results of our comprehensive interviews in the homes of a systematically selected random sample of 19 families from the community (Study I). We look carefully at the associations between family functioning and mental health/illness symptomatology and behaviors. Our evaluations clarified some of the associations between levels of family functioning and both sociodemographic factors and family members' symptomatic/asymptomatic statuses. Also, we identified the critical subsystems involved with family function/dysfunction.

In Chapter 6, we report the extended use of the GLS Family Functioning Assessment Instrument with two more groups of families: 7 families with a child or adolescent in treatment at our Bingham Child Guidance Clinic and 8 matched neighborhood controls (Study II). Then, we pool the pertinent data on Study I and Study II and, in Chapter 7, summarize the results and present an example of the clinical analysis of each subsystem's functioning as an independent variable and family health and well-being as the dependent variable.

Our evaluations of the families included data on stressful life events, chronic stressors, and families' scores on the Moos and Moos (1981) self-report Family Environment Scale (FES). We were especially interested in the comparisons of the self-report data on the FES with our observer-based data gathered while rating the videotapes of the families as they were being given the new GLS Family Functioning Assessment Instrument.

In Chapter 8, we conclude with a critique of the research, include notes about the observers' ratings, and offer some suggestions for shortening and, we hope, improving the Assessment Instrument. We discuss the clinical utility of the research, especially the use of the assessment instrument, and add a few suggestions for future research.

We consider ourselves fortunate to have had valuable and, at times, seemingly indefatigable assistance from a number of friends and colleagues. Ms. Heddy Rubin and Ms. Anne Bickel devoted many "work and overwork" hours to the numerous preliminary drafts of the manuscript. During the past few years, Ms. Linda Johnson has helped us with both the tedious library and reference work and the preparation of the final draft. We extend our heartfelt gratitude to them.

Two of our colleagues were especially helpful. Professor Roger A. Bell worked closely with us in the early phases of the research and is a co-developer of the GLS Family Functioning Assessment Instrument. Professor David Teller gave us important necessary methodological and statistical advice and, at times, did a lot of the burdensome "hands-on" analytic work. We thank them.

Two more persons gave indispensable help. Ms. Ruby Schwab did much of the editing and Ms. Mariclaire Cloutier from Kluwer Academic/Plenum Publishers both encouraged and tolerated our lengthy, tardy--if not compulsive--"reworking" of the data and manuscripts that resulted in unforeseen delays. We acknowledge our obligation to both of them.

REFERENCES

Aristotle (1952). *Politics*, vol. 2. In R.M. Hutchins (Ed.), *Great Books of the Western World vol. 9*. Chicago, IL:Encyclopedia Brittanica.

Burgess, E.W. & Locke, H.J. (1945). *The Family: From institution to companionship*. New York: American.

Durant, W. (1980). From *What Is Civilization?*, cited in *Bartlett's Familiar Quotations*, p 789. Little Brown and Company. Boston.

Emerson, RW (1844). *Self-Reliance*. Dover Publications, Inc. (1993) Mineola, NY.

Moos, R. H., & Moos, B. S. (1981). *Family Environment Scale Manual*. Palo Alto, California: Consulting Psychologists Press.

Ogburn, W. F. (1922). *Social change with respect to culture and original nature*. New York: Viking.

Peterson, K. S. (6/1/99). *US quits gathering marriage and divorce stats*. U.S.A. TODAY pp. A1&A4.

Peterson, K.S. (6/1/99). *Defenders of marriage feel undercut by loss of stats*. U.S.A. TODAY p.A4.

Rousseau, J.J. (1763). *The Social Contract*. In R.M. Hutchins (Ed.), *Great Books of the Western World*, Vol. 38. (1952) Chicago, IL. Encyclopedia Brittanica: pp. 357-439.

Silver, C. B. (Ed. & Trans.) (1982). *Frederick LePlay: On family, work, and social change*. Chicago: University of Chicago Press.

Skolnick, A. (1991). *Embattled paradise: The American family in an age of uncertainty*. New York: Basic Books.

CONTENTS

INDEX OF TABLES
CHAPTER 5

CHAPTER 6

CHAPTER 7

CHAPTER 8

CHAPTER 1
The Traditional Family in State of Flux

Until the mid-1960's, it appeared that the modern nuclear family had been adapting to the changing needs of urban industrialized societies. However, the extensive changes in families that have been occurring are producing concerns about the loss of the traditional nuclear family. Scholars have differing opinions about the meaning of the changes taking place. As early as 1937, and especially in 1947, in The Family and Civilization, Carle Zimmerman expressed fears that the rapid change in the family "from institution to companionship" signaled an anti-familistic trend and decadence similar to that seen during the decline of Greece and, later, Rome. His forebodings were dismissed by such noted sociologists as Burgess and Locke (1945) and, in the 1950s and 1960s, his ideas were regarded as passé by those of the functional school led by Talcott Parsons (1962), who dominated the social sciences after World War II. Parsons insisted that the changes in the family were adaptive, that the family was not in jeopardy, but was only changing to the companionate type based on affection that was more in accord with modern 20th century life than the outmoded institutionalized marriage and family of the past. Zimmerman (1972), however, predicted that unless countervailing forces developed, the family would be in a crisis by the 1990s. But, he expressed hope for reform and stabilization of the family.

Currently, many family scholars are pessimistic about the fate of the family. In Embattled Paradise, Arlene Skolnick (1991) cited Lasch's (1978) Culture of Narcissism, Bellah and his colleagues' (1985) Habits of the Heart, and Popenoe's (1989) Disturbing the Nest: Family change and decline as presenting bleak views of the family and its future. Skolnick acknowledged that changes were occurring but maintained that those mourning the passing of the traditional family were too often comparing the American family of the 1980s and 1990s with idealized images of traditional, often romanticized Victorian families. She insisted that the 1950s "model of a family "was an aberration.... (Early marriage and having children young) is not compatible with a high-tech, post-industrial society, where the trend worldwide is toward more education."

A CENTURY OF CHANGE

In retrospect, the 20th century has been marked by tumultuous changes--biological, cultural, social, and technological--that included the family. Whether, to what extent, and how the sweeping changes of the century produced such drastic changes in the ancient institution, the family, cannot be determined, but undoubtedly they are associated, and the changes in the traditional family lead to concerns about its state and fate. From a societal perspective, the quintupling of the divorce rate from 0.7/1,000 persons in 1900 to 4.6/1,000 in 1995 (World Almanac, 1996) is evidence of a level of marital and family instability that is unprecedented in Western history. From an individual's point of view, the breakup of relatives and friends' marriages and the consequent destabilization and adverse effects on children have led to tentativeness about interpersonal commitments.

Biological Factors

Biological factors, especially the younger age of puberty and the longer life expectancy than in the past, as well as sociocultural factors, are influencing marriage and family life. The early age of sexual maturity, along with advances in contraception, the legalization of abortion, and such cultural influences as the destigmatization of pregnancy and childbirth without marriage have been accompanied by changes in sexual behavior. In their "Review of Sexual Behavior in the United States", Seidman and Reider (1994) reported that the proportion of 15 to 19 year old females who had premarital sexual intercourse doubled from about one-fourth in 1970 to one-half in 1990. By age 15, about one-third of males and one-fourth of females had been sexually active. Those who initiated sexual activity at a young age were more likely than others to be at a high risk for emotional and behavioral problems as well as AIDS and other sexually transmitted diseases, teenage pregnancies, and having single-parent families.

The preadolescents and adolescents' rampant sexuality is distressing parents and teachers. The following is an illustrative case vignette.

Recently, a 40-year-old Caucasion middle-school teacher sought psychiatric help for the first time because of symptoms of mixed anxiety and depression that had become steadily worse during the school year and had intensified to the point that she was not sure she would "make it one more month until summer vacation began." She was restless, irritable, sleeping poorly, easily startled, worried, sad, and felt as if "my energy had been drained." She had begun quarreling with her husband and also feared that she was alienating her 16-year-old daughter by attempting to over-control her peer activities. The problem was simply "too much stress at work.... their (the students) *raging hormones* are making every class a living hell." (italics ours).

Sexual activity started in early adolescence often is continued with multiple partners into adult life. Most of the young adults, ages 18-24 years, studied by Seidman and Reider (1994) had multiple sex partners, whereas the adults age 25 and older, who were married or cohabiting, were monogamous ("at least for a while"). However, the proportion of adults in committed relationships had been decreasing as a result of "postponed marriage and increased separation and divorce." In 1988, only one-half of 15-44 year old females were married.

The tremendous increase in sexual freedom made possible by advances in contraception, especially "the pill" in 1961, and by the younger age of puberty than in the past have influenced marriage and family. For centuries, virginity was a prerequisite for marriage, especially among the fiercely familistic Anglo-Saxons, who were known for their unusually strong family and kin networks. In the first century AD, Tacitus (1911) praised the chastity of Teutonic youth as a contrast to the license of the Romans. The early Anglo-Saxon marriage contract stipulated that the husband should give his bride a substantial gift on the morning after the wedding in return for her virginity. Also, among staunchly religious Southern Europeans and Hispanic Americans, virginity has long been a *sine qua non* for marriage. Strict chaperonage often was in force until the disruptions of World Wars I and II. Thus, in the past, the desire for sexual activity was a stimulus to marriage and to familism in Western Society but, in recent decades, with the loosening of restrictions, it appears to have become relatively uninfluential.

The lengthened life expectancy, from 50 years in 1900 to 75.7 years in 1994, also is associated with marital stability/instability.(World Almanac 1996). Until the 1960s, the divorce rate could be "explained" as being equivalent to the breakup of families in the past by the death of spouses, often the mother during childbirth, or by the father's desertion. But, with increased life expectancy, marriages can last for many more years than in the past and, in accord with the liberation movements and the freedom of expression during the "do your own thing" decade of the 1960s, divorce rates soared and the USA was on "The Road to Polygamy" described by Lawrence Stone (1989). Serial monogamy had become commonplace. Many of the nation's elite have been divorced. Ronald Reagan was the first divorced President. In "The CEO's Second Wife," Julie Connelly (1989) wrote about business leaders having new, young "trophy" wives. Divorce occurring after 20 or 30 years of marriage was once a rarity but, nowadays, we hear increasingly about one of the partners, usually the man, wanting a new wife and life after three or more decades of marriage. Thus, such biological factors as early puberty and the lengthened life expectancy influence marriage and family and are associated with problems of the many children of divorce and the burden of extended care of elderly parents. Consequently, new approaches to the study of family functioning are needed in order to find ways that prevent or palliate marital and family distress.

Cultural Factors

The influence of cultural factors on changes in the family have been accentuated by the dawning of the new postmodern era during the past few decades. Anderson (1990) emphasized that the relativism, pluralism, and utility-based values of postmodernism lead to a breakdown of "systems of social roles and the concepts of personal identity that go with them.... The collapse of old ways of belief and the coming into being of a new world view threaten all existing constructions of reality and all power structures. (The New Age)... is one of the most psychologically threatening events in all of human history." In this early postmodern era, we can already see the cultural revolutions and the rise of spiritual and psychological cults that result from or lead to increased concern about identity, the self, and the almost epidemic spread of such mental disorders as borderline personality disorder (BPD) and multiple personality disorder (MPD)—illnesses with names and symptoms that depict the instability of our era.

Already, the postmodern climate of opinion has influenced the family both indirectly and directly. The multiplicity of views and behaviors provide cultural acceptance of the variety of interpersonal and marital relationships that have become so common in recent years. Obviously, the relativism and loss of faith in institutions both contribute to and reflect the prevalent marital and family instability. In addition, postmodernism is affecting the family directly, for example, by revolutionizing family therapy. In "Constructing Realities: An Art of Lenses," Lynn Hoffman (1990) described her "move away from a cybernetic-biologic analogy for family-systems theory" to family therapy which has many of its roots in social construction theory. "In therapy, we now listen to a story and then we collaborate with the persons we are seeing to invent other stories or other meanings for the stories that are told.....(This co-constructing accepts the) intersubjective influence of language, family, and culture."

In "Family Therapy goes Postmodern," Doherty (1991) stated that structural theories of family therapy and multi-level theories of family structure and function are now outdated. Even the concept of family systems, sacrosanct for more than half a century, is considered to be "a by-product of mid-20th-century modernist culture. What Freud did for the individual mind, systems theory did for the family."

Postmodern critics maintain that conventional family therapies like the psychoanalytic often disregarded social and cultural influences on the family, neglected such important issues as gender and race, and were reductionistic. In contrast, postmodern family therapy is distrustful of theory and certainty, broadly eclectic, and emphasizes gender, language, interpretation, evaluation, meaning and family stories. Postmodern family therapists use pluralistic and blended approaches that embody, for example, both cognitive and psychoeducation models and also allow for the 'diversity, skepticism, relativism and discourse" described by Doherty(1991). Postmodern therapists insist that it is necessary for families to recognize the societal forces impinging on them, and they often help the family externalize problems. Developing a family narrative is now a key feature of postmodern family therapy, much of which is pragmatic family therapy that emphasizes utility and coping as well as meaning.

Social Factors

Two of the prominent social factors influencing changes in the family are individualism and antifamilism. The importance of the self and of individualism, rather than familism, is exemplified by the drastic steady increase in the number of births to unwed mothers which, in 1995, reached an hitherto unbelievable 30.4% of all births (Boorstein, M., 1998). Further, that negation of the family is coupled with its derogation, both implicitly and explicitly, by the promiscuous use of the rarely defined term "dysfunctional family." Since the mid-1980s, when the cult of victimhood and its blame mentality became prominent, such organized groups as children of alcoholic parents and others who maintain that their addictions, mental disorders, and/or behavioral difficulties are evidence that they came from dysfunctional families, loudly blame their parents and others for neglect and abuse--verbal, physical, emotional, and/or sexual--that caused their problems.

The culture of victimhood and the blame mentality are indicators of subjectivity, evidenced, for example, by the increasing emphasis on the "self" and on individuals and groups' rights in everyday life, the rise of self-psychology as the current conceptual basis of psychoanalysis, and The Culture of Narcissism (Lasch, 1978). Such developments reflect a change in the character of our era from the emphasis on interpersonal relations in the immediate post-World War II decades to a focus on the self since the early 1970s. We need to bear in mind that Goethe (1930) once pointed out that, historically, eras marked by intense subjectivity tended to be regressive in character whereas those characterized by social and cultural objectivity have been known for their productivity and achievement.

Historically, antifamilism is such an unusual phenomenon that one must be concerned about its origin and consequences. Is it a cause or a result of the extreme family instability of the past 30 years? Is it the bitter fruit of the companionate marriage that has no institutional basis?

We cannot discount the possibility that antifamilism is an indicator of the decline of our vitality as a society but hope that such a decline is only cyclic, not indicative of a collapse. The return of interest in modifying the unlimited no-fault divorce laws, which were   first initiated in California by Governor Reagan in the 1960s, and the recent introduction in Louisiana of covenant (greater commitment-limited divorce) marriages signal steps toward buttressing marriage and increasing family stability.

Technological Factors

The massive technological developments of the 20th century are fundamentals of the rapid social change that is occurring. The geographic mobility and the fantastic speed of communication have combined to contribute to the near dissolution of traditional community life.

In his superb essay, "The Fall of the Community, the Ruins of Sex", the poet, Wendell Berry (1992), linked "community disintegration" with sexual, marital and family problems and with the lack of well-being in our society. He defined community as a "commonwealth and common interest.... of people living together in a place, and wishing to do so, a locally understood interdependence of local people, local culture, local economy, and local nature that is able to raise the the standards of local health." Also, the community is a set of arrangements that include "forms of courtship, marriage, family structure, divisions of work and authority, and responsibility for the instruction of children and young people."

Berry sees community life as disintegrating in many parts of the USA as a result of "external predation" by economic interests and also of "internal disaffection" produced by institutional damage, social injustice, and other factors that lead to alienation and anomie. The consequences are mistrust, excessive litigation, and the degeneration of "public dialogue", all of which have a corrupting influence on sexuality, marriage, and the family. Berry warned against the economic aggression that has been devitalizing communities and producing a loss of standards, devaluation of sexual love, loss of connectedness, and, ultimately, lack of meaning in life. The economic brutality in disintegrated communities is accompanied by sexual brutality, and marriage and family life are strained and splintered.

Viable communities usually involve some degree of bonding and caring between families. Also, they have meaningful behavioral and interpersonal as well as geographic boundaries. Neighborliness involves controls and sanctions that limit family violence and provide for mutual security, interests, and social activities that enhance the quality of life throughout the community. Consequently, as postmodern family therapists insist, it is imperative that studies of marriage and family assess the impact of economic and cultural influences on communities as well as on families.

CONSEQUENCES

The changes in the family that have taken place since the 1960s are bound to have both immediate and long-term consequences. Foremost are the high rates of mental disorder, the apparent increase in family violence and possibly incest, and, in particular, the plight of children.

Mental Disorders

During the past few decades, epidemiologic studies have reported significantly higher rates of mental disorder, especially depression in the young, age 15 to 44 years, than in older persons and in the never married, divorced, widowed, and separated than in the married. The Epidemiologic Catchment Area (ECA) Study (Robbins & Regier, 1991) of about 19,000 adults in 5 centers conducted in the early 1980s found that the 6 month prevalence rate of diagnosable mental disorders was about 20%. Fears about the already high prevalence of mental illness and substance abuse were recently heightened by the results of the National Comorbidity Survey (NCS) (Kessler, et al, 1994) of a random sample of 8,098 persons, age 16 to 55, in the 48 contiguous states which found that the one-year prevalence rate was almost 30%, much higher than the rate reported just 10 years earlier. The ominous finding was that the highest rates of mental disorder were in younger respondents, those aged 25-44 years in the ECA study, and those aged 16-20 years in the NCS--the years of courtship, marriage, and parenting.

In 1970, the senior author (Schwab, 1970) discussed the early indicators of a probable increase in depressive illness and, in 1973, he and his colleagues reported the results of their Florida Health Study of 1,645 persons, age 16 to 93 years, which showed that a disproportionately large number of those age 16-22 years had high levels of depressive symptomotogy. Since than, other investigators have confirmed that the mean age of onset of depression has become significantly younger, 16-17 years for bipolar disorder and 22-23 years for major depressive disorder (Klerman, 1988), and also that there has been a significant increase in depressive illness, especially in the young.

In "The Current Age of Youthful Melancholia", Klerman (1988) postulated imaginatively that "agent blue" was responsible for the increasing rates of depression in young people. He conceptualized "agent blue" as a complex set of gene-environment interactions that includes such possible biological factors as pollutants, toxins, and nutritional deficiencies and such psychosocial ones as high divorce rates, changes in family structure, and stressful interpersonal relationships. Weissman (1991) reported that an affirmative response to just a single question about whether an individual had been having increased arguments with his or her spouse or partner in the past year was an indicator (about 45%of the time) that one member was at high risk for depressive illness.

Significant evidence shows that depression has negative effects on families, and that the association between depression and family functioning appears to be interactive, not linear (Keitner, 1990) . The impairments of depression include such marital and family problems as difficulties with communication, problem solving, and affective expression along with deleterious effects on the children and days missed from work, loss of income, and failure to advance occupationally (Wells et al, 1988). A series of English studies have documented the significant dissatisfaction and disharmony that accompany depression in the family and the negative effects on family members of interactions between spouses when one was depressed. (Kreitman et al, 1971 and Hinchliffe 1975).

Probably more seriously, studies have shown that a depressed parent, especially the mother, has deleterious effects on young children in the home. Weissman et al (1972) and Keitner (1990) reported that the children of a depressed parent continued to function poorly even after the parent's condition improved. Thus, in view of the association between increased mental disorder and increased marital and family instability since the mid-1960s, concern about the effects of depression on the family is a major reason for studying family mental health and family functioning.

Family Violence

Family violence--child abuse, spousal abuse, elder abuse, and sexual abuse--is a fiery problem that inflames concerns about marriage and the family. In its 1992 report, "No Boundaries: The physical and mental effects of family violence are seemingly limitless," writers for the American Medical Association (AMA) asserted: "Family Violence is a simple phrase, but it encompasses a horrifying list of abusive behaviors, both physical and psychological. There is seemingly no end to the horrors that some human beings can inflict on those whom society calls "their loved ones".

Family violence has become a public health problem. In 1991, from 2 to 4 million children were abused and neglected, 1.8 million women were battered, and 1 million seniors were mistreated. The total was roughly equivalent to the 6 million cases of coronary heart disease or all types of cancer. Survivors of abuse sometimes have chronic physical impairments; however, the psychological toll seems to be the most widespread, long-term effect (Skelly, 1992). Psychological complications include lowered self-esteem, anxiety, depression, suicidality, substance abuse, psychosomatic symptoms, and the "inability to trust or develop intimate relationships." Skelly emphasized that the long-term consequences for children were especially severe, just witnessing violence in the home has been associated with children's psychosomatic complaints and post-traumatic stress disorder. (Schwab-Stone, et al, 1995).

The AMA Report (1992) declared that a "particularly chilling" result of family violence was that it leads to cycles of abuse. In the report, Ziegler and Kaufman found that about 30% of children from violent households had become abusive parents, a rate 10 times greater than the 3% for the general population. Thus, an abused child grows up to be an abusing parent.

In view of the marked increase in stepfamilies and nontraditional family forms, sociobiological concepts are applicable to the widespread family violence. Concepts of sociobiology hold that emotions, thoughts, and behaviors have evolved nepotistically, that parents have an investment in their own offspring, in the perpetuation of their own genes. Thus, parental bonding is more easily established with one's progeny than with another's offspring. Consequently, a genetic relationship is associated with "mitigation of conflict and violence." In the English speaking nations, a much larger number of stepchildren than biological children in families have been victims of neglect, abuse, and murder. In the USA, the probability of a child living with one or more stepparents being fatally abused was 100 times greater for a stepchild than for a child living with two genetic parents. In Canada, that probability was 62.5 and in England and Wales 15 to 20. Daly, Singh, and Wilson (1993) concluded: "living with a stepparent is the single most powerful risk factor for child abuse that has yet been identified." Moreover, "mutual progeny contribute to spousal harmony, whereas, children of former unions contribute to spousal conflict... (and) children of former unions elevate divorce rates, whereas children of the present union reduce them." Also, stepfamilies "tend to be in more emotional turmoil and more of them have financial difficulties than genetic families"; thus, there is a high stress level in their households. Unfortunately, the steadily increasing number of stepfamilies heightens alarm about the tragic findings on family violence presented by the AMA (1992) and the significance of those reported by Daly, Singh, and Wilson (1993).

Incest

The disturbing problem of incest is receiving attention. Judith Herman (1981) cited Finkelhor's conclusion that 1,000,000 American women had been involved in incestuous relations with their fathers—16,000 new cases each year. But her 1981 and 1985 studies of father-daughter incest indicated that the reported rate probably was too low because most samples consisted mainly of middle-class respondents.

Many family health professionals maintain that the problem of incest is increasing, probably as a result of the efflorescence of stepfamilies. In accord with sociobiological hypotheses, (Daly and Wilson 1998) the lessened blood ties in stepfamilies are associated with increased sexual activity within the family. In "The Normality of Incest," (Gordon and O'Keefe, 1985) reported that biological fathers were more likely to be "non-sexual assailants" who abused their wives and beat their children than to be sexual offenders, whereas social (step-, foster-, and adoptive) fathers "were more likely to be sexual than non-sexual assailants of family members."

The almost universal incest taboo is considered to be essential to social organization and also is at the core of the psychoanalytic theory of personality development and of mental illness. Freud (1927) viewed the horror of incest as equivalent to that of cannibalism, as "abrogating one of those sexual restrictions necessary for the maintenance of civilization." He pointed out that such a powerful prohibition as the incest taboo is ageless, that it has prehistoric roots. In this respect, we can recall that Aristotle considered Sophocles' early 550 BC "Oedipus Rex," to be the masterpiece of Greek Tragedy.

Herman's (1985) studies reported that incestuous families had a conventional appearance and a structure characterized by a "pathological exaggeration of generally acceptable patriarchal norms". The fathers were "good providers," the wives were financially dependent, and the families were semi-isolated and had few social contacts. Fathers enforced discipline through violence, and were "accustomed to the use of force in having their way sexually." The coercive behavior became compulsive, if not addictive, and when the eldest daughter left home, he then violated the next oldest. Clinically, the fathers appeared "pathetic and ingratiating" and attempted to rationalize their behavior. Diagnostically, they showed "a kind of circumscribed sociopathy," an ill-defined personality disorder. Herman cited Gordon's finding that this description of the incestuous father has been stable for more than a century. The mothers were helpless, fragile, and often physically or emotionally disabled. Also, they had more children than non-incestuous families, and were burdened, isolated and dependent.

In the long-term, daughters who were incest victims usually suffered from low self-esteem, poor sense of identity, anxiety and depression, sexual problems, and difficulties in relationships. Other common results are sexual promiscuity, prostitution, mental illness (e.g. BPD, MPD) and/or suicidality. But, Herman found that some incest victims could become well adjusted later in life if they had a supporting, nurturing relationship with a mother surrogate.

In our psychiatric services, many female patients report that they were sexually abused by an older teenage brother, fathers or uncles. In Davis and her colleagues' (1999) study of 118 generally middle-class, female psychiatric inpatients, age 20 to 45 years, 66 (56%) reported a history of sexual abuse before age 18. Also, the sexually abused reported almost 3 times more lifetime suicide events than the nonabused.

In addition to the sharp increase in the number of stepfamilies and the consequent lowering of the incest barrier, incest may become a greater problem than it is currently because of the rise in the number of working mothers and dual-career families. The absence of the mother from the home diminishes control of the children and adolescents' behavior and increases the likelihood that young girls will be sexually molested. In 1960, about one-fourth of married women living with their husbands worked outside the home but by 1990 two-thirds did so, including more than half of all mothers of young children. "Lack of protection by mother" is a centuries-old cry of daughters who became incest victims. Consequently, we hope that studies of family function/dysfunction will show to what extent and in what ways it may be associated with such pathologies as abuse and incest.

Family and Community

The rapid changes that have been occurring in families in the final third of this century seem to be paralleled by changes in their communities. Aries (1962) and Berry (1992) related the increasing loss of the traditional community with the transformation, isolation, and alienation felt by many families, as illustrated by the following case vignette.

Recently, a 60 year old minister resigned as the pastor of a small traditional suburban community church because of stress and depressive symptomatology. In discussing what had been happening to him, he stated in a disillusioned manner that the "business mind-set" had infiltrated the community and Church and that "the pastor was now expected mainly to be a CEO who raised money to move the Church forward, to become a mega-church that would grow at the expense of other small churches." Concurrently, the "consumer mentality" was triumphing and "the day of the small town church is gone--it is a casualty of our mobile society, and there is a loss of neighborly accountability--the loss of the front porch and the addition of a rear deck."

The ongoing disintegration of the traditional community contributes to and reflects the antifamilism that has become so manifest in recent decades. Moreover, the difficulties with relationships and the family problems permeating our society are associated with, if not adversely affecting, character formation and attitudes toward the family and community as evidenced, for example, by the lack of civility and disregard of the rules and regulations needed for responsible, healthful living.

Inasmuch as changes in character stem primarily from family life, especially parenting, and secondarily, but increasingly, from peer influences, the quality of community life requires consideration in family study and therapy. The widespread everyday concern about job security and stress are compounded by businesses and corporations' loss of loyalty to employees, the community, and even their own identity (which often disappears with mergers and take-overs). These changes appear, painfully, to be analogous to the many diverse changes in the family: the fragility of interpersonal relationships, "epidemic divorce," and the plethora of new family structural and living arrangements. Consequently, as postmodern family therapists insist, it is imperative for studies of marriage and the family and how it functions to assess the impact of economic and cultural influences on communities as well as families.

Family/Community and Children

The plight of children in the USA is the most urgent and certainly the most tragic aspect of the family crisis of the 1990s and is a compelling reason for studying family function/dysfunction. The Children's Defense Fund (Ross 1992) reported that 14.3 million children, one of five in the USA, lived in poverty in 1991 and that from 1979 to 1987 the percentage in poverty rose 26.2% (whites 36%). Thus, "America's children grew poorer amid the prosperity of the 1980s." Contrary to popular belief, the "majority were white children living in rural areas or suburbs with at least one employed parent." Median incomes of young families (head of household under age 30) fell 32% between 1973 and 1990 (adjusted for inflation). Children living in poverty (family income less than $13,000 in 1989), often hungry, lacking parenting and nurturance, in poor health, and poorly educated have become the deprived and forgotten in modern America.

In Today's Children: Creating a Future for a Generation in Crisis, David Hamburg (1991) declared: "Today's children are in crisis because today's families are in crisis. Most American children spend part of their childhood in a single-parent family. By age sixteen, close to half the children of married parents will see their parents divorced. Close to half of all white children whose parents remarry will see the second marriage dissolve during their adolescence." Thus, there is a revolving-door pattern in marriage that is stressful for children and adolescents. Remarriage brings a complex set of relationships that include: "The children having full siblings, half siblings, and step-siblings; the children having multiple sets of grandparents; and children of single mothers who do not remarry having fewer active family relationships than children with two parents."

Hamburg (1991) maintained that there is "a broad trend toward the decreasing commitment of parents to their children. Two-thirds of parents now report that they are less willing to make sacrifices for their children than their own parents would have been." Children are less likely to see their parents than in the past, and only 5% see a grandparent regularly. Young children spend a great deal of their time with television. Adolescents become involved in a separate "teen culture and live in highly ambiguous circumstances...They are likely to engage at an early age in such adult activities as smoking, drinking, and sex".

Adolescents have a host of major problems that include educational failure, delinquency, suicide, fatal accidents and homicides, sexually transmitted diseases, and hormonal changes at earlier ages that are exploited by the prevailing consumerism. Our fears about adolescents are steadily increasing as teen sex and violence frequently dominate the headlines. The forebodings so tragically expressed by Friedenberg in his neglected 1964 "The Vanishing Adolescent" unfortunately have materialized. He foresaw not only the younger age of adolescence but also the loss of adolescence as a distinctive, necessary transitional phase of the life cycle: "Homo sapiens is undergoing a fundamental model change (that).... involves a great alteration in the process of personality development. A different kind of adult is being produced.... The change... (is) a weakening in the relationship on the one hand, and stability of identity on the other." Thus, Friedenburg's" views supported Galdston's 1958 contention about a general increase in character pathology resulting from instability of the family and the ascendancy of the consumer culture. That question brings to mind the political cry about "family values" and raises concern about the increasing number of working poor families that is painfully reminiscent of the terrible poverty in England in the 1880s and 1890s that was documented by the pioneering research of Charles Booth in London and Rowntree in York (see Chapter II). Thus, the alarming situation for children and adolescents, attributable to distorted societal values and the family crisis, is all the more reason why further studies of family functioning are needed.

The Mental Hygiene Function of Marriage and Family

It is important for studies of family function/dysfunction to include consideration of the mental hygiene function of marriage and the family as well as the many critical problems that we have mentioned. Both marriage and family have many physical and mental health benefits. Mortality data have shown consistently that married people live longer than the unmarried who, generally, have higher death rates from accidents, disease, or self-inflicted wounds. Also, for many years, community and clinical studies have found that rates of mental, emotional, and addictive disorders were significantly lower among the married than the never-married, divorced, and especially, separated persons. For example, in our study of a random sample of 1645 adults in a north Florida county, significantly more of the divorced, widowed, and separated respondents showed evidence of impairment than did the married. (Schwab, et al., 1979) On subscales that measured specific symptom patterns, significantly more of the separated, widowed, and divorced (and occasionally the never married) reported anxiety, depression, depersonalization, paranoid ideation, and alcoholism than the married. Almost all of the group of 188 (11.4%) of the respondents who were in excellent physical and mental health, the supernormal, were in the top socioeconomic quintile and married; surprisingly few were separated, divorced, widowed, or never-married respondents.

Two competing hypotheses have been advanced to explain why the married are usually found to be in better health than the unmarried. The protective-support hypothesis postulates that the companionship, status, and sense of purpose provided by marriage and family life buffer the members against both stressful life events and the chronic stressors or "hassles" of everyday life. Also, in satisfying marriages, the emotional and cognitive spousal interactions are neuro-physiologically salutary. In contrast, the social selection hypothesis postulates that in choosing a person for marriage, the healthier persons will be selected and those with the symptoms and impairments of mental disorders are less likely to be considered for marriage or to have stable marriages.

In his review of 130 empirical studies of marital status and personal well-being, Coombs (1991) concluded that the evidence supported the protection/support hypothesis. He emphasized that "the therapeutic benefit of marriage remains relatively unrecognized by most youths, the media, and some helping professionals who, preoccupied by the accelerating divorce rates and the variant family forms, question the value of marriage in contemporary society".

In discussing the "mental hygiene" function of marriage, Burke and Weir (1977) examined the helping-relationship in 189 middle and upper-middle class husband-wife pairs, specifically, how husbands and wives help "one another deal with problems and tensions." Previous studies reported that marital satisfaction was associated with greater emphasis on the relational than the situational (children, social life, home) aspects of the marriage. Burke and Weir found that the wives generally initiated the helping process, and that "wives set the stage for the alleviation and the resolution of anxieties and tensions". Older couples showed less helping activity than the younger; it was postulated that they belonged to a generation that placed more emphasis on the situational than the relational aspects of marriage. Children reduced the energies the partners had for each other; working wives wanted their husbands to be more active helpers; husbands' job pressures increased demands for wives to be active helpers with anxieties and tensions; but, working wives seemed not to be as effective helpers as their husbands wished. Severe pressures--work, finances, family illness, children's problems--were associated with each partner's seeing him or herself as the less effectual helper and also with dissatisfaction about the help each received from the other. As a result, with increasing stress, there was an expressed "need for closer relationships with others who could act as helpers."

Burke and Weir concluded that living in a marriage in which there is prolonged tension affects the person's self-concept and views of the world negatively and leads to dysfunctional emotional and behavioral responses to the environment. But a helping marital relationship can set a coping process in motion by acknowledging distress explicitly, by providing validation and comfort, by allowing ventilation of feelings, and by clarifying perceptions and choices and thus reducing the likelihood that accumulated tensions will become pathological. Although the husband-wife helping relationship "often remains undeveloped or at best is left to evolve haphazardly", it can significantly influence the marital partners' quality of life.

Thus, as we have seen, there are many reasons for developing new methods for conducting family research at this time when the family is considered to be in a crisis and when new and a relatively large number and variety of "living arrangements" for gays, heterosexuals, and single parents and their children are becoming common. In view of the variety of domestic relationships and arrangements and responsibilities for children, we have focused our research on family function/dysfunction and on reporting the results of the use of our newly developed, "neutral" Family Functioning Assessment Instrument" with three groups of families from the community and our Bingham Child Guidance Clinic. Consequently, to heed the great Claude Bernard's famous statement: "We call it research because it has been previously searched", we are devoting the next Chapter to a comprehensive review of the topic, Family Function.

REFERENCES

Anderson, W. T., (1990). *Reality Isn't What It Used to Be.* San Francisco: Harper and Row.

Aries, P., (1962). *Centuries of childhood: A social history of family life.* (R. Baldick, Trans.). New York: Knopf.

Bellah, R., Madsen, R., Sullivan, W., et al., (1865). *Habits of the heart: Individualism and commitment in American life.* Berkeley: University of California Press. Bernard, C. Introduction of the Study of Experimental Medicine.

Berry, W., (1992 April 26). The fall of the community, the ruins of sex. *Louisville Courier Journal,* p. D 1,4.

Boorstein, M., (Aug. 8, 1998). Society in transition rethinks legitimacy. *Louisville Courier Journal,* p. C-3.

Booth, C., (1892). *Life and labour of the people in London, Vol. 1.* London: Macmillan.

Burgess, A., (1985). *Rape and sexual assault.* Garland Publishing Co., New York.

Burgess, E. W. & Locke, H. J., (1945). *The family: From institution to companionship.* New York: American.

Burke, R. J. & Weir, T., (1977). Husband-wife helping relationships. The mental hygiene function in marriage. *Psychological Reports,* 40, 911-925.

Connelly, J., (1989). The CEO's second wife. *Fortune Mag.* pp. 52-66.

Coombs, R. H., (1991). Marital status and personal well-being: A literature review. *Family Relations,* Vol. 48, No. 1, 97-102.

Daly, M., Singh, L., & Wilson, M. (1993). Children fathered by previous partners: A risk factor for violence against women. *Canadian J Pub. Health,* pp. 209-210.

Daly, V. M. & Wilson, M., (October 28, 1988). Evolutionary social pathology and family homicide. *Science,* 242.

Davis, M. H., et al., (1999). Personal Communication.

Doherty, W., (1991). Family therapy goes postmodern. *The Family Networker,* Sept/Oct. pp 32-47.

Durant, W., (1980). From *What is civilization,* cited in Bartlett's *Familiar quotations,* p 789. Little Brown and Company. Boston.

Emerson, R. W., (1844). *Self-reliance.* Dover Publications, Inc., Mineola, NY (1993).

Friedenburg, E. Z., (1964). *The Vanishing Adolescent.* Boston: Beacon.

Freud, S. *Totem and Taboo.* New York: New Republic.

Galdston, I., (1927). The American family in crisis. *Mental Hygiene, 42, 229-236.* 1958.

Goethe, J. W., Eckerman, J. P. Oxenford, J., et al., (1930). *Conversations with Goethe <by>Eckerman.* London, J.M. Dent & Sons, Ltd. New York, E.P. Dutton & Co. Inc.

Gordon, L., & O'Keefe, P. ,(1985). The normality of incest: Father-daughter incest as a form of family violence. In Burgess, A. (Ed) (1985) *Rape and Sexual Assault: A Research Handbook.* New York: Garland.

Hamburg, D., (1992). *Today's children: Creating a future for a generation in crisis.* New York: New York Times Books.

Herman, J. L., (1981). *Father-daughter incest.* Harvard University Press.

Hinchliffe, M. K., Hooper, D., Roberts, F. J., et al., (1975). A study of interactions between depressed patients and their spouses. *British Journal of Psychiatry,* 126, pp.164-172.

Hoffman, L., (1990). Constructing realities: An art of lenses. *Family Process,* 29, 1-12.

Keitner, G. I., (Ed.). (1990). *Depression and families: Impact and treatment.* Washington: American Psychiatric Press.

Kessler, R. C., McGonagle, K. A., Zhao, S., et al., (1994). Lifetime and 12-month prevalence of DSM-III-X Psychiatric Disorders in the United States: Results from National Comorbidity Survey. *Arch Gen. Psychiatry,* 51(1): pp.8-19.

Klerman, G. L., (1988). The current age of youthful melancholia: Evidence for increase in depression among adolescents and young adults. *British Journal of Psychiatry,* 152, 4-14.

Kreitman, N., Collins, J., Nelson, B., & Troop, J., (1973). Neurosis and marital interaction:IV. Manifest psychological interaction. *British Journal of Psychiatry. 119.243-252.*

Lasch, C., (1978). *The Culture of Narcissism.* W. W. Norton & Co. Inc. New York.

Parsons, T. (1962). *Youth in the context of American society.* Daedalus, 91 (1), 97-123.

Peterson, K. S., (1999). Defenders. *USA TODAY.* A1, pp. 1, 4.

Popenoe, D., (1988). *Disturbing the nest: Family change and decline in modern societies.* Aldine De Gruyter, N, p 67.

Robins, L. N., Regier, D. A., (Eds) (1991). *Psychiatric disorders in America: The Epidemiologic Catchment Area Study.* New York: Free Press.

Ross, S., (Aug. 12, 1992). The Children's Defense Fund Report. *Louisville Courier Journal.* p. B, 4.

Ross, S., (Dec. 1992). Children's Defense Fund Report. *Charlotte Observer,* p. A-8.

Rowntree, B.S. ,(1903). *Poverty: A study of town life.* London:Macmillan.

Schwab, J. J., (1970). Coming in the 70s: An epidemic of depression. *Attitude,* (2):p. 2-6.

Schwab, J. J., Holzer, C. E., Warheit, G. J., (1973). Depressive symptomotology and age. *Psychosomatics,* 14(3): 135-141.

Schwab, J. J., Bell, R. A., Warheit, G. J., & Schwab, R. B., (1979). *Social order and mental health: The Florida Health Study.* New York: Brunner/Mazel.

Schwab, J. J., Stephenson, J., Ice, J. F., (1993). *Family mental health: History, epidemiology, clinical issues.* New York: Plenum Press, Inc.

Schwab-Stone, M. E., Ayres, T. S., Kasprow, W., et al. (1995). No safe haven: A study of violence exposure in an urban community. *J. Am. Acad.Child and Adolesc. Psychiatry,* 34: 10, pp 1343-1352.

Seidman, S. N. & Reider, R. O., (1994). Review of sexual behavior in the United States. *Am. J. Psychiat.,* pp. 333.

Skelly, F. J., (Jan 6,1992). Violence spurs never-ending circle of pain. *AMA News Report,* p 6.

Skolnick, A., (1991). *Embattled paradise: The American family in an age of uncertainty.* New York: Basic Books.

Stone, L., (1989). *The road to polygamy.* The New York Review of Books, 36(3) pp.12-15.

Tacitus, (1911). *The Works of Tacitus: The History, Germany, and Agricola, A Dialogue on orators, vol.11* (H. Mattingly, Trans.). London: G. Bell & Sons.

U.S. National Center for Health Statistics: Statistical Abstracts of the United States. Washington, D.C. 1997.

Weissman, M. M., Paykel, E. S., & Klerman, G. L., (1972). The depressed woman as a mother. *Soc. Psychiat.* 7, 98-108.

Weissman, M. M., (1991). The Epidemiology of Depression: Update. Paper presented at the Paroxetine Investigator's Update. Scottsdale, AZ.

Wells, K. B., Stewart, A., Hays, R. D., Burnham, A., Rogers, W., et al., (1989). The functioning and well-being of depressed patients. Results from the medical outcomes study. *JAMA,* 262(7), 914-919.

The World Almanac and Book of facts. (1996). Farmighetti, R. (Ed.) (Funk and Wagnalls) Mahwah, N.J. World Almanac Books, p. 974.

Ziegler, E. & Kaufman, J., (Jan. 6, 1992). Violence spurs never-ending circle of pain. *Am Med Assn News Report,* p. 6.

Zimmerman, C. C., (1947). *The Family and Civilization.* New York: Harper and Roe.

CHAPTER 2
Family Function: An Historical and Research Review

Introduction and Definitions

We focused our research on the functions of the family and its functioning because they are essential to each individual's personality development and character formation as well as to the family, the quality of life in the community, and the wider society. In the USA, changing family functions has been a topic of concern throughout this century for many researchers and an array of professionals and semi-professionals, some of whom apply the term, dysfunctional, indiscriminately to families in distress. Confusion about family function/dysfunction is increased by the common failure to specify what the terms mean, how they are associated with the functioning of the family, and their often being equated with the degree of family well-being/distress--an obvious tautology. Therefore, we conceptualized and defined family functions and functioning for our research on family mental health, and have attempted to avoid the function/functioning equals health/illness tautology. We began with a summary of our extensive review of family function research.

The two traditional family functions have been, first, to rear children to become autonomous members of society and, second, to meet the adults' sexual and emotional needs. Lidz (1980) added a third, enculturating its members so that they could carry out the society's vital activities. We specified five essential family functions: (a) the maintenance of the group; (b) the perpetuation of the group; (c) the regulation of the adults' sexuality; (d) the provision of emotional support for family members; and (e) learning and enculturation--the inculcation of values, beliefs, and skills (Schwab, Bell, & Stephenson 1987). The sociologists, Smith & Preston (1977), maintain that in the USA in the latter part of the 20th century there are 7 major family functions: (a) the economic; (b) the reproductive; (c) the regulation of sexual activity; (d) socialization, especially the transmission of the culture to the children; (e) the conferral of status; (f) provision of affection and companionship; and (g) child-rearing.

Earlier in this century, when scholars saw the family as changing, "from institution to companionship," Ogburn and Tibbits (1933), Burgess and Locke (1945), and other family scholars discussed an even longer list of family functions. Also, they maintained that the family was losing many functions, e.g. the educational, security, and the religious, as a result of the rapid social change and the state's assuming more control of persons' daily lives. Consequently, the affectional, companionable, and psychological (personality development) activities were becoming the foremost family functions.

As can be seen, generally the family functions are mainly its purposes. But how the family functions, i.e., its functioning, is a somewhat different concern that is related directly and indirectly to how well it fulfills its functions, and is of importance for the various levels of biosocial integration--e.g. the individual, the group, the community, and the wider society. Thus, research on family mental health and illnesses needs to look at both how the family is functioning and also at how well it fulfills its functions. Either an emotionally healthy family or one in which there is mental illness may or may not fulfill its purposes as a biosocial unit, and its quality of functioning may or may not be directly associated with the mental health/illness of its members.

Many of the functions mentioned have been essential to family life, probably since families were first formed thousands of years ago. However, the importance of one or another of them changes at different times in accord with sociocultural events and historical developments, and they also vary from culture to culture. For example, prior to the urbanization of Western society, the family was primarily an economic unit, especially in rural areas. In contrast, in such Eastern cultures as in India, reproduction often has been the chief function despite dire poverty.

Early Social Studies Associated With Family Functioning

During the first half of the 19th century, increasing concern about existing institutions and the structure of society following the American and French Revolutions, along with industrialization, urbanization, and secularization, aroused interest in associations between the level of family well-being and the vitality of the community/society. Frederic LePlay (Silver, 1982), a French mining engineer and political scientist, started his pioneering studies of family functioning in the 1850s. He hypothesized that members of families that functioned well would be healthy, maintain themselves effectively, and be committed to the well-being of the family. Such families would most likely be found in vital, integrated societies, whereas families that were unstable and not meeting their members' basic material, interpersonal, and spiritual needs would be common in fragmented or decadent societies.

LePlay's research tool was the family budget. He maintained that information about all family income and expenditures would enable researchers to draw conclusions about family life, especially family functioning, as we think of it nowadays. His emphasis on the importance of the family budget is age-old; the root of our word "economy" is the Greek "oikanomia"--household management.

LePlay studied about 300 Western European and Russian workers' families by compiling sociodemographic data and detailed accounts of family income and expenditures into family monographs. Each contained: (a) descriptions of the family; (b) the family budget, the heart of the study; and (c) a short account of the laws, history, and geography of the community.

LePlay used the data to develop a three family typology. The first was the large patriarchal or traditional family consisting of the dominant male, his wife, the unmarried children, and the married sons' families. All of them often lived under one roof or the married sons lived nearby. In those families, found mostly in Eastern and Central Europe, the father was the ultimate authority.

The second, the stem family, consisted of the parents, their unmarried children, and the married son who had been chosen by his father to continue his work and to inherit the family property. It was the major type in stable societies. LePlay attributed the success of the English and American societies to the predominance of the stem type of family structure.

The third was the unstable family type. Such families started with the marriage of two adults who were relatively free of extended family ties, grew with the birth of children, shrank with the successive departures of the members of the new generation, and dissolved after the deaths of abandoned partners, often leaving no trace. Unstable families were found mainly in Western industrialized urban centers.

LePlay linked the stability of both the family and society to a firm family structure, parental authority, the family's ability to save money to buy necessities and to acquire additional property, definite religious beliefs, and good worker-employer relationships. His precise methods and detailed reporting of the data supplied an excellent example for future research on family functions and functioning, as did his finding associations between the various family types and the degree of integration-disintegration of the community and society.

Despite that auspicious beginning, LePlay's studies received only limited attention, and family research developed slowly. However, in the latter decades of the 19th century, the changing social structure, inequities, and distress following the Political and the Industrial Revolutions stimulated controversy about the "nature of man and society" and social justice. A few researchers saw that the family's economic status was fundamental to its functioning, well-being, and fulfilling its functions. As LePlay had foreseen, the economic function of the family in Western society was a burgeoning concern; his family budget was used as the database for other investigators' surveys of families' economic status.

In England, reformers concentrated on the problems of poverty and crowding accompanying industrialization and urbanization. As early as 1846, Friedrich Engels (1972) emphasized that in the 18th century, the invention of the steam engine and machines for spinning and weaving cotton, along with the increasing use of machinery, changed the conditions of life for workers and their families; the Industrial Revolution turned workers into mere machines and degraded family life.

"Family life for the workers was almost impossible under the existing social system. All he has is a dirty and comfortless hovel, which is barely adequate as sleeping quarters. The various members of the family only see each other in the mornings and the evenings. In this circumstance how can family life exist? There are endless domestic troubles and family quarrels which are highly demoralizing for the children and parents" (p. 12).

Engels deplored the widespread child labor: "Obviously a girl who has been an operative since the age of nine has never had a chance to acquire a skill in household duties. Consequently, factory girls are ignorant of housewifery and quite unfitted to become wives and mothers" (pp. 165-166). Also, there were widespread "moral evils." Factory girls had "to grant to their employers the jus primae noctis. In this respect, too, the factory owner wields complete power over the persons and charms of the girls working for him. In ninety-nine cases out of a hundred, the threat of dismissal is sufficient to break down the resistance of girls. The 1833 Report of the Factories Inquiry Commission stated: 'The factory is also his harem'. Most of the prostitutes in Leicester had the factories to thank for their present degradation." (pp. 167-168.)

Thus, we can see the interacting influences of the -- societal (e.g. the factory) -- family -- individual levels which, in such instances, have far-reaching, tragic consequences, especially the demoralization of family life and its pernicious effects on the children and their character development. "When they grow up and have families of their own they feel out of place because their own early experience has been that of a lonely life. Such parents foster the universal decadence of family life among the workers. Similar evil consequences for the family follow from child labor" (p. 161). Engels foresaw the cycles of disadvantage described by Rutter and Madge (1976), and we can see that many of the questions raised about "family values" in the USA in the 1990s were formulated by Engels in 1846. In the USA and other rapidly industrialized/urbanized nations, the problems associated with the drastic socioeconomic changes were having negative effects on traditional family life and functions. In "Middletown Families," Caplow and his associates (1982) described the changes that took place in the 1880s in a middle-sized Indiana city. The introduction of factories and immigrant labor led to a sharp increase in population, the accumulation of wealth, glaring social inequities, and family distress.

The surprisingly large number of divorces in the 1880s and 1890s shocked early family scholars. Carol D. Wright, Commissioner of Labor, reported that they increased from 10,000 in 1867 to 25,000 in 1886, a disproportionate 157% compared to the population increase of 100% from 1870-1890 (Goodsell, 1915).

In England, poverty and the increase in family problems stimulated investigators to study the family's economic functions by conducting surveys to gather data on income, expenditures, and savings in relation to poverty and well-being. In the early 1890s, Charles Booth (1892), a well-to-do English businessman, launched his pioneering studies which found that poverty in London was even more extensive than "the socialists' propaganda" indicated. His surveys revealed that 30.7% of families in lower class districts were living in dire poverty. In 85% of them, poverty was caused by unemployment, large families, and/or sickness; in only about 15%, the causes were idleness, drunkenness, and thriftlessness. Thus, his data contradicted the myth that poverty resulted mainly from personal failure and/or vice.

Booth's major contributions are the still meaningful results of his comprehensive surveys and his classification of the poor into: a) the working poor who, nevertheless, were living in poverty, and b) the underclass. A century later, Bane and Ellwood's (1989) study of children revealed that Booth's 1890 findings were applicable to American families; poverty was attributable mainly to the increasing number of the working poor and was not just a problem in single-parent families or the underclass.

In 1899, Rowntree (1903) started his classic study of all the households in York by conducting a "house-to-house visitation" to obtain information about income and expenditures, as LePlay had done 50 years earlier. Rowntree reported that 27.8% of the total population was in poverty and, of those, 10% did not have the bare necessities of life. After comparing his results with Booth's, he concluded "(that)...in this land of abounding wealth during a time of perhaps unexampled prosperity, probably more than one-fourth of the population are living in poverty, is a fact which may well cause great searchings of the Heart." Unfortunately, his words about the deleterious effects of poverty on family life and functioning in England in the late 1890s are applicable to the demoralization, distress, and desertion in the USA a century later.

The results of those surveys were corroborated by Jack London, who, in 1904, put on worker's clothes and lived for a month in the streets of East-End London. His neglected field study, the description of The People of the Abyss, revealed that the deplorable conditions and wretched family life described by Dickens and Engels in the 1840s and 1850s were commonplace a half century later.

In the USA, the increasing number of families with problems led to studies of family functions related to family finances and well-being. Byington's (1910) study of families in the small community, Homestead, PA, was part of the comprehensive 1905-1910 Pittsburgh Survey. In the Preface to Byington's report, Kellogg (1910, p. v) explained that Byington, who had studied tenement conditions in New York and Boston, portrayed the adverse effects of industrialization on the traditional social institutions and the town as well as the family. Kellogg asked: "Have we not Goldsmith's Deserted Village of late 18th century England but a more serious antithetical problem in an overcrowded, overwrought aggregate of households" (p. v).

Byington obtained detailed family budgets for her "intimate case study of 90 households" (p. vi) and supplemented those data with her observations of the families and the town, much as LePlay had done in the 1850s. In Homestead, the steel industry dominated all aspects of life. The 12 or more hour shifts, weekly wages of about $9.90 for most families, and the conditions of work limited "the fulfillment of family ideals" (p. 171). (See Illustration 1.)

The influences of work and poverty on family functioning have seldom been expressed more meaningfully than by Byington's insistence that "It is through the households themselves that the industrial situation impressed itself indelibly upon the life of the people" (p. 179). The home environment was subject to the smoke and "depressing fumes," and family life was disrupted by "the irregular succession of long hours.... (with) the subordination of household life to industrial life" (p. 174). She concluded that the low wages and long work hours adversely affected family life and that the industrialization had weakened family solidarity.[1]

In 1913, Louise More described family functioning in her report on The Cost of Living for a Wage-Earner's Family in New York City. She studied 200 working-class families on The Lower West Side over a two-year period by making regular home visits and urging them to keep household budgets. About one-fourth (55 families) had annual income deficits for the year; about half "came out even;" and only one-fourth had any surplus--average $104.37 per year. Thus, 75% had no money for emergencies and no savings. More considered the average income needed for a family of 5-6

[1] Homestead has a tragic place in American history. In 1892, the newly organized union struck for higher wages. There was active battling with the hundreds of company Pinkertons who had been employed to protect the scabs. Eventually, the Pennsylvania National Guard broke the strike. The bitterness over the battles persisted for years and even today the strikers' songs are sung in the taverns of that Pittsburgh suburb.

persons to be $850.00 per year or $16.50 per week. Her results revealed only slightly less distress than that reported by Rowntree in York a decade earlier.

More emphasized that "the standards of a working man's neighborhood recognize the wife as the financier of the family" (p. 104). The husband and younger children gave her their weekly wages, and the older children paid $4.00-$8.00 per week for room and board. The husband was given $1.00-$2.00 per week spending money.

By thrift, the average housewife could salvage about $20.00 per year for such contingencies as temporary unemployment and unforeseen expenses, but More did not recommend that degree of thrift because it came at the cost of malnutrition/crowding. She quoted Rowntree: "There is frequently no margin for thrift, money saved means necessary food foregone" (p. 110). More found that "malnutrition is very prevalent in the wage-earner's family.... (and that) truly, the destruction of the poor is their poverty" (p. 106-107). They could not buy in quantity or take advantage of sales because of lack of funds and storage space. Thus, "most families must live from week-to-week" (p. 118).

More concluded with a plea for higher wages and emphasized that the wife/mother was the "manager and dispenser of the household income.... the comfort of the entire family depends on her character and ability" (p. 104). She called for women's systematic and universal instruction "(because) in education for household efficiency lies one of the most important means of bettering the social and economic conditions of our city wage-earners" (p. 111). In this respect, we note that in Ancient Greece, the wife was responsible for the household.

In 1913, in the Utilization of Family Income, Martha Bruére and her husband collected several hundred budgets from middle-class families "all over the United States." Their analyses showed that "the spending of the middle class is standardizing itself" (p. 117). A family of five--father, mother, and three children under age 14--could live efficiently on about $1,200 per year (p. 117). Her middle-class budget allocated per year for rent $144, food $447, clothing $100, operation of the home and utilities $150.00, "advancement" (school costs, insurance, recreation, savings) $312.00, and miscellaneous expenses $46.00.

The major concern was that many families did not have the $1200 per year income required for healthful living. Bruére advocated legislation that would establish an adequate minimum wage or else "we must reorganize business and industry so that people can get what now costs $1200 per year." Another concern was that it was difficult for working people to "provide individually for old age." She recommended that each family allocate the $300 currently used for insurance and savings to a national old age pension program (p. 120).

These pioneering studies of family functioning supported LePlay's emphasis on the overriding importance of the economic function--of employment, income, and the management of family finances. Economic sufficiency was associated directly with family well-being and stability, as it is now strongly associated with the level of an individual's physical and mental health. Those studies also disclosed the deleterious effects of industrialization and urbanization on families.

In discussing the influences of industrialization and urbanization on the increasing prevalence of chronic schizophrenia, Cooper and Sartorius (1977) pointed out that industrialization and urbanization in 19th and 20th century Europe led to such social losses as crowding, and *"negative effects on the size and structure of communities and families"* (p. 55) (Italics ours). The changed interpersonal relationships progressively over several generations affected schizophrenic persons' psychological structures and social interactions adversely and lessened the likelihood of recovery from acute episodes of the illness. An acute form of schizophrenia has probably always existed, but the social and medical changes that transformed Western society in the latter part of the 19th century led to its becoming a severe, chronic illness with a poor prognosis in industrialized urban societies.

In non-industrialized societies, however, conditions favorable to a relatively benign course for schizophrenia include the large family size and integrated community life that encourage favorable relationships and stable roles and obligations and provide social support. In contrast, young persons in industrialized urban cultures develop in small families with sharply focused, often intense interpersonal relationships, and little outside social help or support. To those developments we add the deleterious influence of the rationalization of Western society that, in the early 1920s, Max Weber (1958) foresaw would be pervasive by the end of the 20th century. In a highly rationalized technologically-driven society, mentally ill persons are out of place and are even frightening to "the system", especially when their delusions and hallucinations mirror aspects of the already stress-afflicted bureaucratized wider society.

How to ameliorate the negative, illness-producing influences of highly industrialized, technical, and bureaucratized cultures on the family is a question that has been ignored by most family scholars. Reconstructing communities and community life is a necessary approach, especially when accompanied by adequate economic, political, and other civic support for the family. But that reconstruction cannot take place until there is a national policy that strengthens rather than blames the family for the ills that pervade our society. Programs need to include adequate housing, secure jobs, neighborhood safety, parks, and the aesthetic and spiritual elements that give beauty, purpose, and meaning to families and communities.

In Chapter 1, we discussed the high, increasing prevalence of depression and its adverse effects on family functioning, marital satisfaction, and children's well-being. There is no doubt that depression is inextricably linked to many family factors and that it is an intergenerational mental disorder. Schizophrenia, too, is associated with family factors and, as Cooper and Sartorious (1977) pointed out, the nature and course of schizophrenia are linked to community and societal processes. Thus, studies of family functioning and well-being need to consider the reciprocal individual--family--community interactions, not just the family as an independent entity.

As we have seen, early studies of family functioning focused on the family's economic function during the era of rapid industrialization and urbanization that was transforming early Western society. Researchers emphasized the need to strengthen the family's economic function by a number of measures ranging from educational programs in home economics (household management) for wives and mothers to early pleas for old-age social security programs as Byington, More, and Bruére advocated.

Early Hereditary and Genetic Factors Studies Associated with Family Functioning

After the 1859 publication of Darwin's Origin of the Species (1909) and Spencer's (1908) Evolution, some family research focused on hereditary influences on mental health and illness--the procreative and socialization functions of the family. Darwin's cousin, Sir Francis Galton's 1874 study of Hereditary Genius showed that most successful men in England had ancestors who had distinguished themselves in government, various professions, or the military.

In 1876, Robert L. Dugdale (1910) presented the first comprehensive family study in the USA, The Jukes: A study in crime, pauperism, disease, and heredity. Elisha Harris stated that the individual and family histories that Dugdale had collected provided a verifiable study of "the natural history of crime and pauperism....(over) ruined generations" (p. 4). Franklin H. Giddings (1910) hailed it as "the best example of scientific method yet applied to sociological investigations" (pp. iii).

Dugdale's study, which has been relegated to a footnote in a few textbooks, testifies to the validity of Pasteur's aphorism: "In the fields of research, chance favors the prepared mind." As a New York prison inspector, Dugdale found six related persons under four family names in one county jail. The oldest was a 55-year-old man awaiting trial for receiving stolen goods. His 18-year-old daughter was being held as a witness against him. Her 42-year-old uncle was charged with first-degree burglary and with the attempted rape of his wife's 12-year-old illegitimate daughter who, later, was sent to a reformatory for vagrancy. The two others were brothers, aged 19 and 14, in another branch of the family who were charged with attempted murder after they pushed a child over a cliff.

The six "belonged to a long lineage" that reached back to the early colonists in upper New York state. Very few had married new immigrants. They were a "strictly American family" ... (whose) family name had come to be used generically as a term of reproach" (p. 8). For 150 years, the Jukes had lived in a remote area "in log or stone shanties similar to slave-hovels, all ages, sexes, relations, and strangers 'bunking indiscriminately'.... During the winter, the inmates lie on the floor strewn with straw or rushes like so many radii to the hearth, the embers of the fire forming a center towards which their feet focus for warmth. This proximity, while not producing illicit relations, must have evolved an atmosphere of suggestiveness fatal to habits of chastity" (p. 13). The family was started between 1720 and 1740 by Max, "a hunter and fisher, a hard drinker, jolly and companionable, averse to steady toil" (p. 14). He had numerous progeny; two sons married illegitimate sisters, and their descendants and those of the sons' three sisters constituted the Juke bloodline. Dugdale's case histories revealed that 17 (33%) of the 49 blood-related Jukes were criminals compared to 5 (16%) of the 32 related only by marriage. A later, six generation analysis of public records on the Jukes showed that of the 162 blood-related women, 84 (52.4%) had been "harlots," and 23.5% of the children were illegitimate (p. 27). Also, the Jukes had a high rate of pauperism.

One illustrative family history was: in generation 7, a 6-year-old illegitimate girl; in generation 6, the mother was an illegitimate prostitute; in generation 5, the mother was a "harlot"; in generation 4, the mother, who was illegitimate, married a man whose father was illegitimate. "The environment in this case stands thus: The child is the offspring of an incestuous relation between her mother, when only 14, with her uncle, who had served in state prison, thus showing the influence of her surroundings. The mother (generation 5) kept a brothel and it was no doubt that within its atmosphere the girl was contaminated. Going back to generation 4, we find that the parents keep a low dram-shop which also serves on occasion as a house of assignation....The environment runs parallel to the heredity."

According to Giddings, Dugdale insisted that: "The factor of 'heredity,' whatever it may be, and whether great or small, always has the coefficient, 'environment,' and if bad personal antecedents are reinforced by neglect, indecent domestic arrangements, isolation from the disturbing and stimulating influences of a vigorous civilization, and, above all, if evil example is forced upon the child from his earliest infancy, the product will inevitably be an extraordinary high percentage of pauperism, vice, and crime" (pp. iv-v).

Research during the past century has confirmed many of Dugdale's observations. Three of the most insightful are: the emphasis on families' cycles of disadvantage described a century later by Rutter and Madge (1976); insistence on the "factor of heredity" always having the coefficient-- environment; and, his stressing that the "family system" could have salutary as well as deleterious effects, as shown by the beneficial effects of grouping the less violent and pathological prisoners and separating them "as families" from the more violent. Unfortunately, Dugdale's case vignettes are not outdated; almost daily, in our clinics, we see cases similar in many ways to those Dugdale described, especially that of the child whose mother had an incestuous relationship at age 14.

Although it was written 35 years after Dugdale's study and after the new science of genetics had a scientific foundation, Goddard's classic 1912 study of the notorious Kallikak family is often coupled with that of "The Jukes." Goddard (1973) who brought the famous Binet intelligence Test to the USA in 1911, traced for 10 generations the ancestry of Deborah Kallikak, a 22-year-old inmate at the Training School for Backward and Feeble Minded Children at Vineland, New Jersey. Caspar K, who died in 1735, had come from England and fathered a "family of good stock" that had a reputation for "honor and respectability" for four generations. But, during the Revolutionary War, Martin K., a soldier in Washington's army, tarried in a New Jersey tavern where he met a young woman who was known to be mentally defective. After being wounded in the War, he "married a woman of quality" and became a respectable businessman. But, nine months after the chance tavern meeting, the young woman had a baby and became the ancestress of a long line of "defectives," mentally ill, alcoholics, and/or criminals. In contrast, Martin Kallikak's descendants from his marriage, the other family line, were remarkably free of psychopathology and social pathology. Goddard described his study of the Kallikaks (Greek kallis--beauty, kak--bad) as a true "natural experiment." It stands as one of the most impressive pedigree studies in all family research.

These early family studies point to the importance of the family's basic reproductive function. In the USA, at the end of the 20th century, the reproduction function is being diffused, and in many ways ignored, as evidenced by the changing sexual mores, the loss of the family's institutional base, and the internicine struggles over abortion, family values (with little attention to economic conditions), and day care. Also, deinstitutionalization and inadequate community mental health programs are associated with a sharp increase in the birth rate of the chronically mentally ill.

In the early 1900's, Mendel's findings stimulated researchers' interests in possible hereditary patterns of mental illness and mental retardation, some of which had already been advanced by Darwinian concepts of adaptation and survival of the fittest. Kraepelin's associates, for example, in the 1890s, Köller (1950) and Jost (1950) reported that mental illness was more frequent in the relatives of mental patients than in the relatives of hospital employees who had served as controls. In Zurich, at the turn of the last century, Eugen Bleuler (1911) developed an enduring interest in the psychopathology manifested by the relatives of his schizophrenic patients. By 1916, Rudin and his colleagues at Munich were conducting fairly sophisticated family studies of their patients with mental disorders, especially a family member's risk of developing schizophrenia or manic-depressive illness. Eugenics became a new topic of concern, and some married couples with family histories of mental disorder decided to be childless, as described in Galsworthy's (1922) "Forsyte Saga".

In psychiatry, during the past 30 years, there has been a flurry of interest in pedigree studies. Some of the best known are Winokur and his colleagues' (1982) Iowa 500 studies of mental illness in families, Egeland and her colleagues' (1983) studies of affective disorders in the Old Order Amish, and Kendler and his associates' (1993) research in Ireland on family patterns of schizophrenia. Their research objectives include the determination of patterns of mental health and illness in pedigrees, the risks for individual family members, and the identification of genes responsible for mental illness.

In recent years, repeated studies have revealed the negative effects of depression or of chronic mental illness on family well-being, For example, Keitner and his colleagues' (1990) study of depressed patients' found significant associations between the quality of family functioning, as measured by the Family Assessment Device (FAD), and the presence or absence of mental illness. In his work as a consultant with the Old Order Amish Study in southeastern Pennsylvania, the senior author (JJS) has been in the homes of families in which there was, for example, manic-depressive illness in three or four generations. Usually, those families and their homes showed evidence of impairment of role functioning even when no family member was acutely ill at the time.

In addition, since the late 1970's, research in behavioral genetics has been showing promise of yielding data that shed light on the age-old question about the relative influence of genetic and of environmental factors on temperament, personality, and behavior. Some of those studies of families, stepfamilies, and twins being conducted by Plomin, D. Reiss, Kendler, and their colleagues are presented later in this Chapter.

Anthropological Studies

A third major area of family function research, "culture and personality," became cultural anthropologists' leading interest early in this century. In accord with Hegel's (Harris, 1968) concept of the folk soul and culture configuration, they studied isolated or so-called "primitive" groups to evaluate associations between family structure, child rearing practices, and personality. Their findings have significance for studies of family functioning in view of the current emphasis on the affectional and personality functions of the companionate family, general living systems concepts of interactions between different levels of biosocial organization, and the results of recent studies in behavioral genetics.

In Patterns of Culture, Ruth Benedict (1934), an anthropological functionalist in the tradition of Franz Boas and Bronislow Malinowski, described her study of four tribal groups with which she had done extensive field work. Each had its ethos or set of organizing principles that epitomized the desired character type and socialization processes, including rites of passage for adolescents, that fostered its development. Benedict associated groups' differing child rearing practices and socialization processes with the various tribal "character types." The Zuni Indians in the southwestern United States were Apollonian; they tended to be cerebral, restrained, orderly, and ritualistic. In contrast, the Kwakiutil in the Pacific Northwest were Dionysian; they tended to be emotional, histrionic, violent, and strove for ecstasy in their often frenzied ceremonies and grandiose potlaching. The third group was the Dobuans of the South Pacific, and the fourth was the Plains Indians, who were known for their aggressiveness. Each group had its distinctive ethos and, in each, the personality traits followed a normal distribution. Benedict emphasized that mental illness in an individual had to be defined according to the specific cultural, not universalistic, norms.

Margaret Mead (1968) tended somewhat more than Ruth Benedict to focus on the influence of a specific culture's rites, child-rearing practices, and adolescent guidance on an individual's mental health and illness. Specifically, with accelerated culture change, "the prefiguration of the future and the consideration of the past are missing". The results of Margaret Mead's studies in the South Pacific, which pointed to a strong association between a particular culture, its child-rearing practices, and the individual's personality characteristics, were generally in accord with Benedict's findings (1930). Mead's study of three small New Guinea tribes provided a basis for her valuable studies of adolescents and the family in the USA in the 1950s and 1960s.

Mead (1978) saw the immense mid-20th century developments (e.g. World War II, the atomic bomb, technology and computers) as transforming society within a few decades from being the traditional postfigured (dominated by the elders) and cofigured to being prefigured in that the young had become the determinants of standards and the culture. Thus, the generation gap of the 1960s and 1970s has been having a profound effect. Her emphases on the disorienting effects of rapid social change on individuals and on ensuing generations have special meaning in view of the instability of the American family during the last few decades. The disorientation affects an individual's cognitive and affective processes adversely and thus lessens bonding and cohesion in families, all of which lead to an obvious blurring and weakening of the interpersonal and intergenerational boundaries needed for mental health and security. Also, the cultural confusion deprives persons of community comforts and constraints. Margaret Mead made a significant contribution to the history of culture and thus to psychiatry, and her sustained interest in childhood and adolescence is a haunting remonstrance to the conscience of our era.

According to Harris (1968), the culture and personality school sired by Franz Boas focused on functionalism and thus gave a needed emphasis to family research in the USA. Its major contributions were the analyses of the means by which the community and the family influenced the personality development and character formation of the young, and thereby fulfilled an essential family function. After World War II, however, the power and predation of Western societies fragmented such previously isolated groups as South Sea Islanders and, along with advances in communications/travel, led to cultural confusion. Medical and social pathologies became hallmarks of the ensuing disintegration. Consequently, since the end of World War II, studies of North American Indian tribes and South Sea Islanders have tended to have mainly historical interest.

Anthropologic family studies in the latter decades of this century have lacked the insights and wisdom of such great modern anthropologists as Margaret Mead (1968) and Oscar Lewis (1966), the brilliant epidemiologic approaches employed by Clyde Kluckhohn (1949) and Alexander Leighton (1959, 1963, 1991) and their colleagues, and the perspectives added by Jules Henry (1965) in his now resurrected classic, Culture Against Man. Oscar Lewis' classics, "Five Families" and "La Vida", portrayed the distressing effects of culture change, poverty, and mobility on family cohesion and vitality. In "La Vida", Lewis described the "culture of poverty" and the semi-demoralized existence of the San Juan--New York "transients. In "Mirror for Man": The relation of anthropology to modern life", Clyde Kluckhohn (1949) defined culture as "a set of blueprints for human relations" that includes a group's (family's) distinctive ways of living. His studies of the Navajo in New Mexico and Arizona were developed by Alexander Leighton and his associates who combined the classic anthropologic and the modern epidemiologic approaches to their studies of groups and communities. Alexander and Dorothea Leighton and their colleagues' (1963) ongoing Stirling County Study in Nova Scotia, started in 1949, evaluated the degree of community integration—disintegration (classified by such indices as frequency of broken homes, number of associations, patterns of recreation, and frequency of hostility, crime, and/or delinquency) in relation to the prevalence of mental disorder in culturally different communities. In the more integrated communities, the women's especially low risk of mental disorder was "due to the exceedingly stable character of the Acadian family and to the clarity and consistency of the sentiments... (along with) little ambiguity as to the roles of women".

In the small community, The Road, which in 1950 was "socially disintegrated and had high levels of broken marriages, inter-parental strife, (and) child neglect", the investigators found significant changes by 1963 (A. Leighton, 1965). Increased economic activity and leadership by an inspiring school teacher led to improved housing, more stable family life, less drunkenness, and family participation in church, school, and other community activities.

In the 1960s, Leighton and his colleagues (1963) replicated their study in Nigeria. Again they found that comparatively high rates of mental and substance abuse disorders were associated with family instability and other indicators of community disintegration. Leighton and his colleagues, especially D. Leighton and J. Murphy (1972) have combined anthropologic and psychiatric epidemiologic approaches to carry out this most comprehensive set of studies of family life, community integration -- disintegration and mental illness in this century.

Paris (1992) has argued that social disintegration such as that studied by Leighton and colleagues (1962, 1972), along with the anomie, the normlessness and loss of faith in institutions, described by Durkheim (1896) are conducive to the great increase in impulsive personality disorders, such as Borderline Personality Disorder (BPD), since the 1960's. One of A. Leighton's (1971) most poignant studies, "The Cosmos in the Gallup City Dump" described the disintegrating effects of rapid social change and culture conflict on Native American individuals and their families and community.

In the 1950s and 1960s, Jules Henry expressed alarm about American culture becoming "driven on by its achievement, competition, profit, and mobility drives" (p. 45), and deliberately creating need by advertising directed toward the family as the basic unit of consumption. Also, in Culture Against Man (1965), he described "an unhinging of the old impulse controls." Henry saw that the main function of the family was becoming the unending striving for a higher standard of living as evidenced by increasing consumption. He feared that as obsolescence extended from machines to people, anxiety would increase to the point that it jeopardized the security of personal relationships. Ultimately, however, the greatest danger was the effects of the driven, consumer-oriented culture on the family and the personality development of the young. Unfortunately, many of the fears expressed by Henry have materialized, as evidenced by corporate downsizing and the current epidemic of "affluenza". Many of our patients tell depressively that their main recreation is going to shopping malls where they long for the goods and glitter they see and then use multiple charge cards so extensively that they exhaust their credit, must forego necessities, and suffer from increasing anxiety, depression and anomie, all of which are usually associated with some impairment of family functioning.

The emphasis on consumption as one of the foremost family functions is associated with Henry's views of the creation of need and the proliferation of shopping malls. One of the casualties is the loss of Sunday as a day of worship, rest and family life, as it is left in the dust of shopping, overwork and the pace of everyday activities in the USA in the late 1990s. The drastic cultural changes, however, may have their most negative effects on the young, on personality development and character formation. We need to keep in mind the great W. I Thomas' (1923) insistence that a culture is personified in the personality and character of the young.

Sociological Studies of Family Function 1920 - 1940

During the 1920s, family functioning became an explicit concern. The rapid social change accompanying the widespread use of the automobile, the host of inventions for the home, the excitement of the "Roaring 20s," and the increasing divorce rate after World War I stimulated sociologists' studies of changing family structure and functions.

In his classic, Social Change, W. F. Ogburn (1922) developed the concept of culture lag introduced in 1908 by Alfred Vierkandt. Ogburn attributed many of the difficulties in our society in the 1920s to lack of adaptation--the inability of the human being to adapt to the rapid cultural changes--the problem of the "Stone Age man in the skyscraper."

In 1929, President Hoover appointed a committee headed by W.F. Ogburn to analyze "Recent Social Trends in the United States." In their section, "The Family and Its Functions," Ogburn, assisted by C. Tibbitts (1933), reported the changes in the family that had been taking place. Since the 1890s, the family had been losing many of its institutional functions, especially the economic, the protective, the educational, the religious, the recreational, and status functions. Concurrently, those of growing importance were the family's two major personality functions: those relating to the adults' marital adjustment and those pertaining to the children's personality development. Ogburn and Tibbitts insisted: "The family has always been responsible to a large degree for the formation of character" (p. 661).

Changes in the structure of the family accompanied the changes in family functions. The American household in the 1920s was about one-fourth smaller than in Colonial days. Increasingly, more families were not having any children, more married women were working outside the home, and more families were broken by separation and divorce than in the past. The declining size of and changes in the family led to problems, especially greater "pressure" on the marital relationship as many wives did not have children, and many women were devoting only a few years of their lives to child-rearing. Also, some of the family's personality functions had been reduced or diluted by the declining number of children. Despite the increased amount of time the children stayed in school with the teacher ("substitute parent") and the many peers available in urban centers, "the affectional function is still centered in the family circle" (p. 663).

The changes in the structure and functions of the family were accompanied by increasing family disorganization. About 70% of families studied rated their marriages as satisfactory, but "The speed and diversions of city life are a strain on family relations....Transportation and city life weaken the ties of kinship...(and) friendships and group contacts are made somewhat more frequently on an individual and less on a family basis than formerly" (pp. 701-702).

Various studies indicated that about 1 (14.6%) in every 7 or 8 families was "broken": In 1900, the number of homes broken by separation/divorce had equaled those broken by death, but by 1930 there was a 2:1 separation/divorce: broken by death ratio. Also, discontented married couples were not waiting as long to divorce as formerly; 37% of divorces in 1930 occurred within 5 years after marriage compared with 28% in the 1887-1906 period. In Chicago, in 1920, there were 4 separated to every one divorced couple. About one-third of divorced persons remarried. Ogburn and Tibbitts stated that the increasing breakup of families did not mean that marriage was less satisfying than it had been in the past but "only that certain functions and traditions which once operated to hold even an inharmonious family together have now weakened or disappeared" (p. 663).

Ogburn and Tibbitts expressed concern about the effects of changing family functions on the relationships of parents and children, husbands and wives, and the community. Would the decline in the birth rate and the tendency toward having smaller families affect a child's self-reliance and result in there being more "spoiled children?" "The family is thought of much less as an economic institution than as an organization for rearing children and providing happiness. There is thus a greater individualization of the members of the family" (p.661).

Ogburn and Tibbitts concluded that there were 3 groups of emerging family problems: a) housing and income; b) child rearing (a study of 300 married college alumnae reported that they felt themselves least prepared for family life in regard to "child training"); and c) marital difficulties. "The relationship of husband and wife is clearly at the center of the problem of the modern family, since most families have children with them for only a part of married life or not at all and since so many other functions of the family have declined. The stability of the future family is not clearly seen. It rests a good deal on what research will discover, and the wide dissemination of the results.... The future stability of the family will depend much more on the strength of the affectional bonds" than in the past (pp. 707-708). Unfortunately, Ogburn and Tibbitts' (1933) emphasis on the husband-wife relationship and on the significance of the affectional bonds has turned out to be all too prophetic.

Family Function During the Depression

The Great Depression of the 1930s had a major impact on both the family's structural characteristics and functioning. The marriage rate fell from 10.3 per 100,000 population in 1925 to 9.2 in 1930, but rose to 10.4 in 1935. The median age at first marriage fell only slightly to 24.3 for males and 21.3 for females, but the birth rate dropped 22% from 25.1 in 1925 to 18.7 per 100,000 in 1935 (lower than the death rate); it reached a low of 18.4 again only in 1966. The divorce rate doubled from 0.7 per 100,000 in 1900 to 1.5 in 1925, but stabilized at 1.7 in 1935 (4.6 in 1997) (World Almanac, 1998).

The collapse of the American economy and the unemployment, which increased from 1.6 million in 1929 to a massive 12.1 million in 1932, battered families at almost all economic levels. Even the previously well-to-do felt the depression; according to Mintz and Kellogg (1988), "one-third of the Harvard class of 1911 confessed that they were hard-up, on relief, or dependent on relatives" (p. 139). Many middle-class families were impoverished; for example, 40% to 50% of those in the cities in the Midwest could not make their mortgage payments and thus lost their homes. Also, the destructive impact of the depression produced widespread distress in rural America and in villages and small towns. Mintz and Kellogg described the terrible distress in the coal-mining regions of Pennsylvania and West Virginia, and in Harlan County, Kentucky, families subsisted on weeds and berries (p. 133). In New York City, 110 deaths were caused by starvation in 1934, and in rural eastern and southern Kentucky, pellagra was seen for the first time in years in the early and mid-1930s. The drought and dust storms jeopardized even the meager existence of small farmers. As Steinbeck (1939) described in his classic, The Grapes of Wrath, thousands of the poor became migrants who streamed across the country in long lines of jalopies in the hope of finding work and food in California. And hundreds of thousands of hoboes "rode the rails in search of some type of work."

The effects on the families of the many unemployed were often disastrous. In 1932, 28% of households--34,000,000 men, women, and children--were without a wage earner (Mintz and Kellogg, 1988, p. 134). Although the divorce rate did not decline, in part because few could afford it, desertion was common; the percentage of children placed in orphanages rose sharply, and it is estimated that there were at least 200,000 homeless, vagrant children at large. Other families "made it" only by "doubling up", leaving their homes to crowd in with any relative who could provide even minimal food and shelter.

Family functions and functioning changed. The economic function, production, again assumed paramount importance. Any one who could do so, even children as young as age 5 or 6, attempted to work. Families planted small gardens, "canned" food when possible, peddled nickel and dime articles from door to door, sold or pawned jewelry and household goods, and strove desperately to live as frugally as possible in order to survive. President Roosevelt's hastily developed programs alleviated some of the distress, but the unemployment rate remained high until just before the USA entered World War II. In the mid-1930s, attempts were made to move some of the crowded, unemployed poor families to semi-communal farms or to work in experimentally decentralized industry. However, the average urban, industrialized family moved to a rural area was not prepared for rural life, adapted slowly, and could not take advantage of the opportunities offered (Zimmerman and Frampton, 1935, pp 73-85).

Economists proposed such solutions as the sharing of full-time jobs to increase part-time employment so that most families would have wages from two to three days work per week. They would be expected to raise most of their food on small plots of land made available to them. The government sponsored home economic programs; many married women were paid about $20.00 per month to attend classes on cooking, baking, canning and preserving food, sewing, and money management. In her 1913 study of wage earners' families in New York City, Louise More (1913) had called for women's education in money management and "household efficiency," (p. 111) and, even earlier, in the 1880s, in her struggle for women's suffrage, Harriet Beecher Stowe (?) wrote about the need for women to be educated in home economics.

Research on family functioning during the 1930s focused on how families adapted to the depression. For his classic research, (Angell, 1935) studied 50 University of Michigan graduate students' parental families by evaluating the students' written descriptions of the families' daily lives. Angell conceptualized adaptability and cohesion as the two major factors influencing families' abilities to cope with economic adversity: "The effect of the decrease in income on internal family relations...(was the) essence of the problem" families encountered (p. 5). The depression wrecked the poorly integrated and unintegrated families. But, if the family was at least minimally integrated, a high degree of adaptability was more important for effective coping than a high degree of cohesion. Angell's conceptualization of adaptation and cohesion provided a theoretical basis for Reuben Hill's (1949) excellent study of families' adjustments to World War II separations and postwar family reunions and, subsequently, for Olson and his colleagues' (1983) development of their circumplex model of family functioning.

In the late 1930s, Earl Koos (1946) carried out a two-year intensive follow-up study of a random sample of 62 Manhattan tenement families to evaluate family troubles and functioning during the depression. One major finding was the inverse relationship between adequacy of family organization and the financial and interpersonal troubles. Another was the significant change in parental roles; the fathers lost their hitherto dominant positions and the mothers became the foci of family organization and survival. And still another was changed relationships with the outside world, mainly a reduction in the family's social interactions and activities.

Koos concluded that the culture had not been helpful and blamed both the institutions and "our average middle-class ideology" for the prevailing family distress (p. 121). He expressed concern about the disruption of family roles and the loss of paternal authority on the character formation of the young inasmuch as the family supplies the young with intellectual and moral concepts, determines roles and many social relations, and lays the foundation for spiritual life (p. 92). Unfortunately, Koos' excellent study and his emphasis on family organization, function, and well-being have been somewhat neglected.

In the 1970s, Elder (1974) and later Elder and Rockwell (1979) carried out important studies of the effects of economic deprivation during the depression on the children's lives as adults and on their families. In accord with Angell's views, Elder conceptualized family adaptation as the main link between economic hardship in early life, personality, and life course. Following the father's unemployment, financial losses had produced widespread changes in the division of labor in the family; all family members had to work to meet needs for maintenance. The depression-induced social strains included marital tensions, loss of status, and uncertainty that generally led to the children's later achievement-striving and their orientation toward the future. Elder asserted that the one common value became "the centrality of the family and the importance of children in marriage" (282). Others were the importance of work over family and leisure activities, concerns about security, and belief in the power of money, all of which contributed to "the familistic aura of the post-war years" (p. 282).

In the later comparative study of the Berkeley cohort that went through the depression as children and the Oakland cohort that had been adolescents in the 1930s, Elder and Rockwell (1979) reported that mothers' taking jobs outside the home during the depression supplied the young with a model of the working mother. Thus, it provided a background for the development of the women's movements of the 1960s (p. 292).

The Great Depression had manifold effects on families and their functioning over at least two generations. Although family life was battered during the depression, its importance increased--it alone provided some degree of security. The economic function of the family became paramount. Family members' roles and statuses changed, as evidenced mainly by the mothers' adaptability and resilience and the fathers' diminished position as the head. The effects carried over to the children, many of whom became achievement-oriented, and their productivity led, directly and indirectly, to the consumer-oriented society of abundance for many in the post-World War II decades and to women's slowly achieving "liberation" and increasing status and power since the 1960s. Concurrently, husbands and fathers' dominance of the home and family diminished significantly and, increasingly, women have been becoming the heads of the households either explicitly or implicitly. The extent to which those developments, along with declining parental authority and family instability, affected character formation may be seen in the loss of the sense of personal responsibility, the "blame" mentality, and the increased delinquency, crime, gambling, and drug use since the 1960s.

Post-War Family Functioning

After World War II, family researchers and scholars focused attention specifically on family functions. In 1945, Burgess and Locke issued The Family from Institution to Companionship which became "The Bible" in family sociology. They emphasized that there had been "further modification of the American conception of marriage which had been in the process of accelerated change since the landing of the Pilgrims at Plymouth Rock." (702-703). The new companionate family was seen as less stable than the institutional, and Burgess and Locke noted the further destabilizing effects of the increasing social and geographic mobility. But, they presented an organization-disorganization-reorganization model that would lead to a rosy future for the family. The companionship family's essential function would be "that of developing the personalities of its members through intimate association, affectional interdependence, and emotional security" (p. 718).

After the anticipated wave of often hasty or basically unstable marriages in the immediate post-war years, by 1950 the marriage rate was 11.1 per 1,000 population and the divorce rate 2.6. Both rates fell in the 1950s, the marriage rate to 8.4 per 1,000 in 1960, and the divorce rate to the post-war low of 2.1 per 1,000 in 1958. The median age of first marriages dropped to the low of the century in 1955--for men 22.6 and for women 20.2 years (1991--men 26.3, and women 24.1 years). There was widespread optimism about the centrality of the family during the "familistic 50s." Stable employment, distinct age-gender roles, the father as the traditional wage earner, the woman as housewife and mother, and a home in suburbia were "the American way of life."

Burgess and Locke's views received wide support. Talcott Parson's functionalism that dominated American sociology emphasized the interrelationships of personality, culture, and the social structure as systems and specified that the nuclear family was "a differentiated subsystem of the society." (Parsons and Shills 1951; Parsons and Bales, 1955, p. 356). Parsons (1970), emphasized that the two basic, irreducible family functions

-- a) the socialization of the children so that they could "truly become members of the society," (p. 17); and b) the stabilization of the adults' personalities -- were interwoven into the modern (1970) nuclear family's adult, child, male, and female role types. (p. 21) Parsons and Bales (1955) acknowledged that there were some family strains and that the family was undergoing change, but insisted that its continuing differentiation (mainly specialization) was a reorganization process.

In 1955, in Technology and the Changing Family, Ogburn and Nimkoff reached dizzying heights of optimism about the family and its future. They obtained experts' opinions about the changes that were taking place--e.g. birth control/decreasing family size, declining authority of father/husband, increasing extramarital sexual activity, increasing numbers of wives working for pay, and increasing individualism/freedom of the family members--and concluded that they were indicative of a loss of many family functions and greater individualism (p. 15). However, the "intrinsic role of the family is...in shaping character, in inculcating morals, and in providing happiness (and the family is as significant as formerly)" (p. 19). They attributed changes to external forces impinging on the structure and function of the family, especially the decreased economic function of production (pp. 263-264).

Ogburn and Nimkoff's expansive optimism included not only the future family's fulfilling its personality functions--affection, happiness, and companionship--but also the abolition of poverty and higher incomes for the enlarging middle class. (283, 286) Technology would allow for increased leisure time and recreation, and consumption would become an increasingly more important and time-consuming function. They saw the increasing individualism but did not envision the declining familism of the 1960s and the family crisis of the 1980s and 1990s.

At the end of the 20th century, in view of the concern about the instability of the family, the many pregnancies of unwed mothers, the plethora of single-parent families, overworked parents, children's violence, the surfeit of so-called dysfunctional families, and the host of troubles seemingly flying out of Pandora's Box, the family sociologists' work of the mid-1950s seems to be fictional. The editions of Burgess and Locke's (1945, 1960) The Family from Institution to Companionship and Lerner's (1957) America as a Civilization became the standard textbooks (with Parsons and his colleagues' works as references) in sociology and other social sciences. At best, those scholars were culturally myopic; they did not see Michael Harrington's (1963) Other America, the discrimination that extended to children and debased millions, and the individualism, militarism, and greed that were becoming masters of our fate. We ask: To what extent did the false optimism of the 1950s, supported and publicized by many scholars, contribute to the family troubles later in the century?

Only a few scholars recognized the problems of the family and its loss of functions clearly. In his erudite 1947, Family and Civilization, the much neglected Carle Zimmerman presented a comparative historical analysis of the status and condition of the American family. The weakness of the family's institutional base along with its loss of functions and the mounting social and political antifamilism had become so extreme that the future of the family was in jeopardy, much as it had been in the second and third centuries B.C. when classical Greece was in its decadent phase and, later, in the fourth and fifth centuries A.D., during the decline of the Roman Empire. Zimmerman saw the American family as becoming atomistic--small, unstable, fragmented--not integrated into the community and wider society, much like Le Play's unstable family type of a century earlier.

Zimmerman's work was dismissed by most family sociologists, especially those of the functionalist school. However, in 1971, when the instability of the family had become obvious, Zimmerman was given the prestigious Burgess Award. In his Award address (1972a) and subsequent articles, he asserted that "The family has to reestablish itself by the end of the century or it will be too late" (p. 1, 1972b). The 1990s would be the decade in which the family crisis would be resolved. Despite the antifamilism, that pervaded our political and cultural life, exemplified by "open marriages," Zimmerman expressed modest optimism about the family becoming restabilized by the end of the century.

APPROACHES TO THE STUDY OF FAMILY FUNCTIONS

Early Studies

During the 1950s and 1960s, excitement about the cause and course of mental disorder dominated family research. Researchers studied family systems, mainly in families with a schizophrenic member, usually an adolescent. They developed such concepts as that of homeostasis of the family system, sometimes seen as being maintained by the presence of an emotionally ill family member, of the double bind or "mixed message" that could lead to mental disorder, and even of the "schizophrenogenic mother". Family systems therapies sprang into prominence and troubled families as well as couples with problems often turned to family therapy and/or marital counseling.

Only skeletal concepts of family function had been developed. However, a few early studies evaluated family concepts or processes. Also, the Family Categories schema was developed; it became the basis for Epstein's work (1984) and the McMaster Model of Family Functioning (MMFF). Early research focused on assessing family characteristics, the functioning of the family systems, and their associations with members' mental and behavioral disorders.

In 1963, Van der Veen (Novak & Van der Veen, 1969, 1970) presented an example of an early card-sorting method for evaluating family function. He and his colleagues' used their 80-item Family Concept Questionnaire (FCQ) to compare each parent's concepts (perceptions of the family unit) in 10 well-adjusted families with those in 10 families with a lower level of adjustment as evidenced by the children's having behavior problems. Each parent placed the 80 descriptors on separate cards (for example, "We are an affectionate family") in 9 piles ranging from "least like my family" to "most like my family" and another set from "least like my ideal family" to "most like my ideal family" in the same manner to provide a measure of both their real and ideal family concepts. (p. 47). The Family Satisfaction Score (FSS) represented the amount of agreement between the member's real and ideal family concepts, and the Family Adjustment Score (FAS) represented the amount of agreement between a member's real family concepts and professionals' consensus concepts of an ideal family. The general hypothesis was that the parents' concepts affected family adjustment and adequacy in meeting problems and needs.

Compared to the poorly adjusted families, the well-adjusted had significantly higher concept scores and greater agreement between the mothers and fathers' real-family concepts and also between the parents' real-life concepts and professionals' concepts. Thus, parents' perceptions of their families were related to levels of adjustment/functioning; high levels of differential perceptions were associated with family dissatisfaction, less than adequate functioning, and feeling that the family was not meeting its hopes and expectations. Van der Veen and his colleagues stated that their findings had implications for therapy.

In 1970, Novak and Van der Veen (1969, 1970) used the FCQ to compare disturbed adolescents, their siblings, and normal controls' perceptions of their parents' attitudes to ascertain whether and how parental influences were associated with the children's mental health. Their study of 13 clinic families, each with a disturbed adolescent, and 13 matched normal control families showed that the adolescents' mental disorders were related to their: a) perceptions of relative parental lack of positive regard, empathy, and genuineness; b) less coherent perceptions of their parents and families than the normals' perceptions; and c) disparate views of their mothers' and fathers' roles and qualities, especially of the father's having a negative impact on family life. Novak and Van der Veen emphasized that inasmuch as there was no known "one-to-one relationship between family factors and (children's) psychopathology", children's perceptions of family conditions were determinants of adjustment and satisfaction (p. 328, 1970). The results supported Robin's (1966) contention that the influence of parental attitudes and behaviors on the children's emotional adjustment is more dependent on the child's perceptions of them than what they really are.

In the late 1960s, increasing concern about the validity and generalizability of such concepts of family pathology as the double-bind to clinical situations led to dissatisfaction about the extreme reliance on seeing mental illness as being caused by malfunctioning family systems. Also, the early results of family, adoption, and twin studies of schizophrenia, such as those of Rosenthal, Kety, and their colleagues (1968) in Denmark, indicated that genetic and other biological factors were the basic causes of serious mental disorders. Moreover, the everyday family stress and distress associated with a member's mental illness were more often the consequences than a cause of the mental disorder. Concurrently, the increasing family instability, evidenced by the skyrocketing divorce rate in the late 1960's, stimulated research on family functions in the hope that the increased information could be used to stabilize marriages and families as well as shed light on the course and treatment of mental illness.

Westley and Epstein—"The Silent Majority"

In the late 1950s, Westley and Epstein (1969) began their studies of associations between college students' emotional health and the ways their families were organized. After conducting a pilot study they assessed 97 first-year students' degree of psychological health and studied the 10 most and the 10 least "psychologically healthy" of the 59 families that agreed to participate. The major variable, family organization, defined as the durable modes of relationships between family members, had 5 dimensions: (a) power, (b) psychodynamics, (c) roles, (d) status, and (e) work. The results revealed 5 family power patterns: a) father dominant; b) father-led; c) equalitarian; d) mother dominant and; e) mother-led. Children from father-led families had the greatest chance of being psychologically healthy; in contrast, 64% of children from the equalitarian were emotionally disturbed. The findings suggested that when both parents were healthy, the children tended to be healthy, but when both parents were disturbed, the children also would be disturbed. When one parent was healthy and the other disturbed, the children would be healthy when the parents had a warm, supportive relationship. Also, the children's emotional well-being was associated with their sharing household responsibilities, the presence of one strongly accepting parent, and the participation of the opposite-sex parent in their care. Major conclusions were that the quality of the parental relationship was the important determinant of the children's psychological health and that organizational, structural, and transactional patterns determined the family members' behaviors to a much greater degree than intrapsychic variables.

Westley and Epstein's (1969) The Silent Majority is a pioneering family study. Its limitations are that the sample consisted of urban middle and upper-middle class families, and, methodologically, the same judges rated each individual's health and the family's health. But it was a study of psychological health as well as illness that served as a valuable early approach to comprehensive studies of family functions.

The McMaster Model of Family Functioning (MMFF)

The research that began with The Silent Majority led to Epstein and his colleagues' work with 110 nonclinical families and the formulation of a conceptual framework, The Families Categories Schema, which provided a basis for the development of the McMaster Model of Family Functioning (MMFF) and its research and clinical scales (Epstein, Sigal, and Rakoff, 1978; Epstein and Bishop, 1981). The MMFF was not designed to assess all aspects of family functioning; it focused on health/illness factors that the investigators maintained had the greatest influence on family members' emotional and/or physical health. Health was equated with normality, but: "A healthy family is neither necessarily average nor merely lacking in negative characteristics. Rather, it has described positive features".

The MMFF is based on systems theory. The family is "an open system consisting of systems within systems (e.g. individual, marital dyad) that relate to other systems (extended family, school, community)....A primary function of today's family unit is to provide a setting for the development and maintenance of family members on the social, psychological, and biological levels" (Epstein, Bishop, & Baldwin, 1984, p 77).

Families have three basic tasks: 1) The instrumental, such as providing food, money, and transportation; 2) The developmental, which concern "crises of infancy, childhood, adolescence, and middle and old age... "[such as] the beginning of the marriage [and] the first pregnancy" (p. 78); and, 3) The hazardous task area, which involves managing crises produced by illness, loss of income, etc. Families unable to deal with the major tasks were likely to develop clinically significant problems.

The 6 MMFF dimensions of family functioning are:
1. Problem-solving of both instrumental (e.g. money, transportation) and affective (e.g. affectional, hostile) issues;
2. Communication, the instrumental and affective "exchange of information";
3. Family roles, the members' behavior patterns by which they fulfill both instrumental and affective functions (provide resources, emotional support, etc.) (p. 84);
4. Affective responsiveness, the "ability to respond to a given stimulus with the appropriate quality and quantity of feelings" (p. 86);
5. Affective involvement, the extent to which members are interested in each others' interests and activities; and

6. Behavior control, a family's way of handling dangerous situations, expressing psychobiological needs and drives, and socializing within and outside the family.

Two assessment instruments have been developed. The McMaster Family Assessment Device (FAD) is a 53-item self-report questionnaire for each family member over the age of 12. The 7 scores for each of the 6 dimensions of the MMFF and the 1 for overall family functioning reflect members' perceptions of their family functioning. The scores discriminate between families with and without psychiatric problems and measure response to treatment.

The psychometric properties of the FAD were investigated in large nonclinical, psychiatric, and medical samples. "In general, scale reliabilities were favorable... (and) over 90% of FAD items loaded on factors hypothesized by the McMaster Model" (Epstein, Bishop, Ryan et al. 1993, pp. 156-57). The FAD has been used extensively in clinical settings, including Family Practice and Rehabilitation Medicine as well as Psychiatry, a family outcome study, and in the selection of superfunctioning families for a therapeutic foster placement program. For example, a study of stroke patients and their spouses showed that they functioned as couples about as well as a matched medically healthy group and better than couples in which one spouse was a psychiatric patient. However, family role functioning was altered, the family was faced with problems related to the disabilities. Furthermore, the impact of a disabled stroke member on family functioning depended on it's financial circumstances. Bishop (1986) emphasized that the quality of family functioning affects the outcome of rehabilitation for stroke patients. In describing his own post-stroke dysphasia, Buck stated that "a stroke is actually a family illness" (1963, p 37).

During the 1970s, Epstein and his colleagues (1984) carried out innovative patient-therapist studies. In one, they placed emotionally disturbed children in superior-functioning families as assessed by the MMFF. Those families were as effective as residential child treatment centers; however, the disturbed child was seldom completely incorporated into the healthy family, indicating that such families have boundary and membership issues. Also, patient-therapist families that did not belong to a collaborative network of similar families were unable to deal with some disturbed children.

A study with the FAD of the general health and emotional well-being of 178 couples in their 60s revealed that almost two-thirds of the husbands and wives reported optimal family functioning. But, there were some striking husband-wife differences. For husbands, physical health status was more predictive of emotional well-being than either family functioning level or retirement status; in contrast, for wives, family functioning was more predictive of emotional well-being than physical health status and retirement status was unrelated.(Epstein et al., 1993, p. 156).

Epstein, Bishop, and their colleagues' (1981) studies of patients and their families with diverse illnesses are promising. Also, as mentioned in Chapter 1, Keitner and his colleagues (1990) have used the FAD to identify the negative effects of depression on family function during the acute phase and after remission. More recently, Friedmann, McDermut, Solomon and their colleagues (1997) reported that their study of family function with the FAD in families of 296 psychiatric patients with various major disorders (e.g. major depression – N=111, schizophrenia spectrum – N=61, bipolar disorder – N=60, anxiety disorder – N=15, substance abuse disorder – N-48) and 353 controls showed that, compared to the controls, "having a family member in an acute phase of psychiatric illness was a risk factor for poor family functioning" (p.357). In particular, high percentages, 80% of the families of those with anxiety disorders and 74.8% of those with major depression, had "unhealthy functioning" on communication, and from 57% to 80% of the various patient groups had impaired general function. Psychiatric status explained a significantly higher percentage of the variance in the family functioning scores than such sociodemographic factors as SES. The investigators concluded that family therapy in conjunction with other psychiatric interventions should be "part of a comprehensive approach to the treatment of acute mental illness... and that the importance of family interviewing (was supported by the finding that) although such sociodemographic characteristics as husband' age and SES were associated with levels of family functioning, "having a family member with a psychiatric illness was... a much stronger predictor of poor family functioning" (p. 365).

The second instrument, the McMaster Clinical Rating Scale (MCRS), is completed by therapists after a clinical assessment; it also consists of 7 scales, 1 for each of the 6 dimensions of the MMFF and 1 for overall family functioning (I. Miller, et al., 1994). On each dimension, the family is rated on a 7-point scale ranging from very disturbed to superior. Studies of the reliability, validity, and clinical utility of the MCRS found that: 1) naive as well as advanced family therapist raters could rate the dimensions; 2) there were acceptable interrater reliabilities overall, but some difficulties with the ratings of the affective dimensions; 3) there was a moderate correlation among the scales -- scores for the 6 dimensions correlated (mean r=.73) with the General Functioning Scale scores; 4) tests for concurrent validity with 93 depressed psychiatric inpatients, 41 adults with mixed psychiatric diagnoses and 28 day hospital children revealed significant correlations between FAD scores and MCRS ratings except for Behavior Control in the depressed and Affective Responsiveness (.31) in the mixed psychiatric group; 5) discriminative validity was shown by the significant differences between 25 depressed inpatients' MCR's ratings on Affective Involvement when admitted to the hospital and following recovery. Thus, improved functioning after treatment for depression could be assessed by the MCRS. Also, assessments of predictive validity in children of dysfunctional families showed that on the MCRS Behavior Control scale, 5-year old children in families with dysfunctional ratings had a higher rate of clinical disorders both at age 12 and again at age 16 than children of families with healthy ratings (Maziade et al., 1990). Also, 4-month old infants of families with dysfunctional ratings on the Behavior Control and Communication Scales had lower levels of intellectual functioning at age 4.7 years than those from families with healthy ratings.

I. Miller, Kabacoff, and colleagues (1994) concluded that overall the MCRS had "acceptable psychometric properties for continued research use and development" (62,63). The various dimensions of family functioning showed some intercorrelations because they should be related to one another; "when families have difficulty in one dimension it usually creates problems in the other dimensions as well" (p. 62). The investigators emphasized that their model of family functioning "is highly defined and behaviorally based" (63); thus, the constructs have utility in both self-report and observer-based forms. "With the possible exception of the Beavers Systems Model (Beavers and Hampson, 1990), no other family model offers such a complete approach to families". (65)

Members' self-report scores and observers' ratings of families often have not been significantly correlated. Two exceptions are the scales based on the Beavers Systems Model with their .20 to .77 correlations, (Beavers and Hampson 1990) and I. Miller and colleagues (1994) FAD-FCRS correlations. Beavers and Miller and their colleagues attribute the satisfactory correlations between their self-report and observer-rated scales to the scales being based much more on clinical experience than theory.

Olson and McCubbins (1983) considered the usual lack of significant correlations between self-report and observer-rated scales to be the result of differences in perspectives--internal vs. external. Sigafoos, Reiss, Rich, et al., (1985) maintained that the differences have been produced by such contextual factors as the interviewers and/or raters' influence and pointed out that 3 specific factors influence responding: 1) the stimulus provided by the instrument; 2) the language needed to respond; and 3) the interpersonal context in the research setting. In addition to the inherent differences in the two methods, I. Miller et al. (1994) emphasized that the self and the observer have differences in perspective. Ransom and his colleagues (1990) argued that such different methods of family assessment as self-report and observer ratings yielded different types of data and were not interchangeable because the information provided by each method is unique and should be preserved as such.

In view of the strong associations between family dysfunction, marital distress, and family disruption, Stevenson-Hinde and Akister (1995) used the FAD and the CRS to study 100 nonclinical English families, each of which had a four-year-old child. Comparisons of the self-report and observers' ratings of family functioning revealed significantly high correlations between the FAD scores and the CRS ratings, especially for allocation of roles and general functioning; the lowest correlations were for Affective Responsiveness and Behavioral Control. Of the families, 10% were unhealthy according to both the parents' self-reports on the FAD and the observers' CRS ratings, and an additional 13% were unhealthy according to either the FAD scores or the CRS ratings. That 23% total was close to the 25% of mothers whose DAS scores indicated marital distress. Also the mothers' self-reports on the Dyadic Adjustment Scale (DAS) scores correlated well ($p \geq .001$) with all scores on the FAD dimensions, except Behavior Control, and also with the CRS ratings. Stevenson-Hinde and Akister concluded that the FAD scores were significantly related to the CRS ratings, that there was a close relation between family functioning and marital adjustment, and that "one in four families with young children might benefit from intervention (that would prevent) family break-up." (p. 346)

Epstein, Bishop, and Baldwin (1993) maintained that, in contrast to the Beavers-Timberlawn approach, the MMFF focuses on current functioning, "puts less emphasis on the formal structure of the family systems" (134), and deals more with such instrumental issues as role functioning and behavior control issues. They concluded that in "ongoing clinical and research work, we continue to be impressed by the importance of a loving and supportive relationship between the parents.... Strong support, genuine concern, loving care, and the absence of chronically persistent and nagging destructive hostility... serve as a foundation that can bear the weight of much strain inside and outside the family group" (p. 154). They predicted that a family system could not function satisfactorily in the absence of such a parental relationship.

The development of the MMFF and of the FAD and CRS to assess families and measure their response to treatment is a significant forward step in the application of knowledge about the family and the real-life problems encountered by members with chronic physical illnesses, disabilities, and psychiatric illnesses. We have presented a fairly detailed description of the model and instruments and of their use because they are the products of decades of systematic work by Epstein and his colleagues and have proven clinical utility. Although we did not use the FAD in our family study, we are now using it in some clinical studies; patients state voluntarily that they "like it." (Schwab & Humphrey, 1996).

The Beavers' Systems Model

Since the mid-1960s, when Beavers collaborated with Lewis to study family systems at the Timberlawn Hospital, Beavers and Hampson (1993) and their colleagues have been developing measures of family functioning. They established the following "cornerstone criteria for the study of family competence:"

1) *family functioning--largely observable interactions-- "takes precedence over symptoms or typology"; (p. 73)*
2) *family competence is on a continuum ranging from effective, healthy family functioning to dysfunctional patterns;*
3) *families at the same levels of competence may show "different functional and behavioral styles of interacting" (p. 74); highly competent families have the ability to shift functional styles in accord with developmental changes; in contrast, most dysfunctional families display rigidity;*
4) *family assessment requires information from both "outsider" observer/therapist's ratings and "insider" family members' reports (Hampson, et al, 1989); and*
5) *competence in small tasks is related to competence in everyday life, raising children, etc.*

The Beavers' Model of Family Competence with its two constructs -- competence and style -- and its scales have been designed to assess: "How well the family, as an interactional unit, performs the necessary and nurturing tasks of organizing and managing itself" (p. 74). Indicators of competence are: egalitarian leadership, strong parental or other adult coalitions, and established generational boundaries. Their lack is associated with relatively lower levels of system competence. Competence also involves the individual family members developing autonomy.

The Beavers Interactional Competence Scale has a Global score, its subscales have high interrater reliabilities, and the scale has validity; it successfully discriminated clinic from nonclinic families and also specific diagnostic samples of clinic families. It has been used with Anglo, African-American, and Mexican-American families and has "culture-fairness" (p. 75).

Observers rate the scale on: a) the structure of the family (overt power, parental coalitions, and closeness); b) the family mythology and its congruence with reality (very congruent to very incongruent); c) goal-directed negotiation (at 9 levels -- from extremely efficient to extremely inefficient); d) autonomy (clarity of expression, responsibility, and permeability all rated on 9 point positive to negative scales); e) family affect (range of feelings, mood and tone, unresolvable conflict, and empathy rated on 9 point generally positive to negative scales); and f) a Global Health-Pathology Scale rated from 1, healthiest, to 10, most pathological.

Family style was conceptualized as referring "to the (relative) degree of centripetal (CP) or centrifugal (CF) qualities in the family" (p. 75). CP members are oriented toward the family, cohesive, and try to repress or deny negative/hostile feelings about each other as they bind the children to the family. When they develop mental disorders, members become anxious and/or depressive, and do not act-out or become aggressive. In contrast, CF members seek gratification from interactions and activities outside the family and, compared to CP members, are more comfortable with negative feelings about the family, tend to expel children before they have completed individuation, and develop externalizing disorders more often than the internalizing.

Family systems are flexible. Competent families alter their style during various stages of the life cycle in order to meet developmental needs; for example, a young family is "optimally centripetal" and thus can meet the children's needs but, as the family matures, its becoming more centrifugal enables children to leave home successfully. Family Style is measured by observers' ratings of the Beavers' Interactional Style Scale on 5-point positive to negative subscales: a) How families deal with members' dependency needs; b) Adults' conflicts--rated from quite open to covert and hidden; c) The family members spacing of themselves -- from lots of room to members crowding together; d) Families attempts to appear to outsiders as being well-behaved to being unconcerned; e) Members' feelings about being close -- from consistently emphasizing to denying closeness; f) Families ways of dealing with assertive/aggressive qualities, ranging from discouraging to soliciting them; g) Expression of either positive or negative feelings; and h) a Global Centripetal/Centrifugal Family Style Scale that ranges over 9 degrees from having a strong inner to a strong outer-orientation.

The CP family style was found to be more prominent among Mexican-American than among the Anglo or African-American families. The CF style has been associated with lower socioeconomic status (Hampson, et al. 1990).

The Self-Report Family Inventory (SFI) is a 36-item questionnaire designed to assess family members' reported perceptions of family competence and style that can be completed by children as young as age 10. Items are answered on a 1 to 5 scale as fitting the family very well, fitting somewhat, or not fitting. Examples of items are: doing things together; having a say in family plans; arguing a lot; warmth and caring; a sad and blue mood; and, taking responsibility for one's behavior. Two others are: a) "my family functions very well together" rated 1, to -- "my family does not function well together at all, we really need help" – rated 2; and, b) the rating of independence as 1 -- no one is independent", to 5 --"family members usually go their own way" (p. 103).

The SFI yields a Competence score for each member, and a Cohesion score which is "an estimate of Family Style." (p. 77) Thus, it is a brief screening device that can identify "potential family dysfunction," (p. 77) and supplies "insider," self-report information about the family that complements "outsiders'" ratings. Beavers and Hampson emphasized that determining family functioning solely by self-report has been "elusive."

The Beavers Systems Model's axes are Competence and Style. The continuum of Family Competence on the horizontal axis, ranges from optimal functioning to the severely dysfunctional, or from equal-powered and successful interactions to dominance-submission patterns and then to extreme, noninteractive rigidity. The five levels are the healthy, adequate, mid-range, borderline, and severely dysfunctional families.

Family Style on the vertical axis ranges from the highly centripetal (CP) to the highly centrifugal (CF) but is not a continuum. Dysfunctional families are at one of the two extremes whereas the healthier are toward the middle and tend to be mixed and flexible.

Beavers and Hampson have presented unusually comprehensive descriptions of various degrees of family function/dysfunction, and have identified 10 clinical family groupings, for example:

1) The Optimal characterized by a systems orientation, clear boundaries, contextual clarity, relatively equal power, intimacy, autonomy, joy and comfort in relating, skilled negotiation, and significant transcendent values;

2) The Adequate are relatively effective, but, in contrast to the optimal, place greater emphasis on control, conflict is more often resolved through intimidation than negotiation, and emotional needs are somewhat short-changed;

3) The Midrange, the most numerous, have obvious pain and difficulty in functioning. Their emphasis on control limits intimacy, they have boundary problems, and the children are more likely to develop behavioral disturbances than those from either adequate or optimal families.

7) The Borderline families' preoccupation with control issues diminishes satisfaction and intimacy. There are many "you shoulds". Members receive little emotional support from each other, have difficulties with individuation, and have boundary problems. The family mood varies from overt depression to rage;

10) The Severely Dysfunctional have difficulty negotiating conflicts, coping with crises, resolving ambivalence, having coherent interactions, and defining goals. Other characteristics are the lack of a power structure, unclear communication, problems with boundaries, few negotiating skills, depression or cynicism, being unresponsive to others' needs, and being pervaded by frustration, anger, and guilt. The growing child has an incomplete sense of the self and identity problems, and the lack of differentiation of the self makes it difficult to resolve conflicts or to deal with problems: Members have difficulty sharing feelings, developing goals, and dealing with loss. "The system wallows like a rudderless ship." (p.

89) Beavers and Hampson expressed concern about such dysfunctional patterns becoming cyclical: "unmourned loss becomes crippling to the next generation (of families)"[2] (p. 89).

Beavers, Hampson, and their colleagues have carried out many studies. For example, in a study of families with a retarded child, there was a wide range of family competence. The more competent were able to deal openly with their feelings whereas the dysfunctional had "an almost universal taboo on dealing with feelings" of despair. (p. 91).

Ongoing studies, which include evaluations of self-report versus observational assessments, found that parents' SFI scores tended more often toward the more competent direction than the observer-rated scores. Also, often an adolescent was more critical than the parents and gave the family a low SFI rating. Beavers and Hampson (1993) emphasized that the assessment of Competence and Style can guide a therapist's intervention strategies. CP families attend more sessions and are much less likely to drop out of therapy than CF families; the therapist's actively joining in with them and disclosing therapeutic strategies minimizes power differentials and increases the likelihood of a favorable outcome. In contrast, with CF families, it is better for therapists to use lower levels of joining and disclosure and to maintain a greater power differential in therapy sessions (p. 92).

Beavers and his colleagues have gathered information on more than 1,800 families in clinical and nonclinical settings over the past 30 years. Some general findings are:

1) The optimal family is the "ideal" for family functioning but is not the "normal" inasmuch as only about 5% of families overall and 11% of a nonclinical sample have been classified as optimal;

2) Most nonclinic and clinic families were in the adequate to midrange levels of family competence; and

3) Only about 3% of nonclinical and 11% of clinical families were severely dysfunctional. "This finding controverts the speculations of many `dysfunctional family' advocates, who attempted to convince us that the dysfunctional family represents the norm in modern America. Rather, the data suggest a reassuring bell-shaped curve, with extremes of health or incompetence being small parts of the whole, and the bulk of American families doing reasonably well yet with considerable room for improvement" (Beavers and Hampson, 1993, p. 93).

Beavers and his colleagues' work with families from different backgrounds in different settings and with differing health statuses is a

---

[2]The 5 Clinical Groupings not described are: 4) the Midrange Centripetal; 5) the Midrange Centrifugal; 6) the midrange mixed; 8) the Borderline Centripetal; and 9) the borderline Centrifugal.

substantial contribution to our knowledge about families and to our understanding of family functioning. Beavers (1985) has written about Successful Marriage and he and Hampson (1990) have also described Successful Families: Assessment Guides Intervention.

Lewis' and Colleagues' Family Competence

In the 1960s, Jerry Lewis, and his colleagues (1976) began to study healthy families because "little is known systematically about the processes of healthy family systems" (p 117). For a pilot study, they obtained 11 volunteer white, upper-middle class families from a local Protestant church; all had intact marriages and at least one adolescent child. The investigators gathered self-report data by giving scales developed in their work with adolescents and families at the Timberlawn Psychiatric Hospital and also obtained observational data by having the families come to the research setting to be videotaped while carrying out family interactional tasks. The inter-rater reliability of the videotape ratings was established and the observers' ratings and subjects' scale scores correlated significantly with the global health/pathology scale scores (.30 to .79). In addition, the families kept daily logs of each member's physical health, medications, professional medical care, hospital days, and other events for six months.

The researchers developed criteria for ranking the families on a global health-pathology continuum, and then added 33 middle-class families, including some patients' families, to obtain 44 for their ongoing research. The goal was to assess family competence on a continuum ranging from the competent to the dysfunctional. Lewis (1989) defined family competence as "the extent to which a family accomplishes two cardinal tasks: 1) producing psychologically healthy children who can function autonomously and enter into enduring relationships outside the family; and 2) stabilizing the parents' personalities while facilitating their continuing development" (pp. 2-3). As we have seen, for centuries, most family scholars considered those to be the two essential family functions. Family competence has five components: (a) power structure, (b) degree of family individuation, (c) acceptance of separation and loss, (d) perception of reality, and (e) affect. Lewis' (1989) "Continuum of Family Competence" (p. 89) ranges from flexible to rigid to chaotic and consists of: (a) the highly competent, (b) the competent but pained, (c) the dominant-submissive, (d) the conflicted, and (e) the severely dysfunctional. Of the 44 volunteer families, 10-12 were healthy and many more were "adequate." Lewis and his colleagues (1976) emphasized: "We simply do not know the relative proportions of optimal, adequate, or various degrees of dysfunctional families in a general population" (p. 205).

The Highly Competent Family is "the ideal." It is characterized by high levels of closeness, commitment, and psychological intimacy even though each parent is autonomous and there are definite parent-child intergenerational boundaries. The parenting style is authoritative, not authoritarian. Communication is open, spontaneous, and contains a wide variety of feelings. "Overall, there is a warm, caring family mood. Humor is valued" (Lewis, 1989, p. 5).

Characteristics of the Competent but Pained families include "underlying parental conflicts around issues of closeness and intimacy," but the conflicts do not involve the children who probably will be psychologically healthy. The marital pattern is that of the "pursuer-pursued." Husbands and wives are emotionally remote and intimacy-avoiding persons; the family system is not warm and can appear stilted. "Competent but pained families facilitate individuation and autonomy in family members, but do not encourage the development of strong attachments" (Lewis, 1989, p. 6).

Dominant-Submissive marriages are characterized by high levels of commitment, variable levels of closeness, an absence of intimacy, and skewed power. The family system is rigid, controlled by the dominant parent who will not permit the expression of differences of opinion or affect. These families are dysfunctional because of the "increased probability of the development of psychiatric syndromes in either the submissive spouse or the children" (Lewis, 1989, p. 6).

The fourth type, the Conflicted, is characterized by the spouses' chronic conflict. The basic problem is power, but conflicts arise about parenting, money, sex, etc. "The chronic conflict over the relationship structure can be understood as a system mechanism that facilitates contact without closeness or intimacy" and with low levels of commitment (Lewis, 1989, p. 7). In these strife-ridden families, the children become involved and often choose sides, but sometimes they can distance themselves.

The last type, the Severely Dysfunctional, consists of three subtypes: 1) The parents have a symbiotic relationship with fused identities and often poor levels of individuation. Children are either incorporated into the symbiotic system or excluded from it; 2) "One parent dominates the family with his/her psychotic distortions" (Lewis, 1989, p. 7). Many of these families have a paranoid outlook on the world. The children may or may not become involved; and 3) Complete parental alienation with one parent sometimes developing a close relationship with a child.

In their books, No Single Thread and The Long Struggle: Well-Functioning Working-Class Black Families, and their articles, Lewis and his colleagues (1976, 1983) reported the results of their research on the continuum of family competence. Lewis and Looney's (1983) evaluation of a small sample of marginally low income black families revealed that, contrary to their hypotheses, the characteristics of competence in the black families were similar to those found in white middle- and upper-middle class families.

Much of Lewis and his colleagues' early work can be seen as a prelude to their study of how competent family systems develop over time. In <u>The Birth of the Family: An Empirical Inquiry</u>, Lewis (1989) described the background for the research and the theoretical issues, and presented a selective review of literature on "the transition to parenthood." He built on Erikson's (1959) theory of the epigenesis of psychosexual development with its 8 stages from birth to death, a task specific to each stage, and the effects of either resolution or failure of resolution of the task on future development. Lewis noted that Wynne (1984) had adapted Erikson's concept of developmental stages and their specific challenges to the family life cycle, and had postulated, for example, that the development of attachment or mutual caretaking is the couple's initial relational task. Successful attachment enhances effective communication whereas dysfunctional attachments include emotional over-involvement, "flat" detachment, or criticism/withdrawal that leads to communication difficulties. Wynne described four communication patterns--the functional, the amorphous, the guarded, and the fragmented (Lewis, 1989, pp. 24-25).

Thus, Erikson's and Wynne's concepts of epigenesis, along with Bowen's (1984) theories of individuality/togetherness, are fundamental to Lewis' views of the continuum of family competence. The psychological health of the parents and children is dependent largely on the parental balance between individuality and mutuality. The key processes "in negotiating this relational balance" (p. 25) are commitment, power, closeness, intimacy, and autonomy.

Lewis and his colleagues' family development study subjects began with 40 young, volunteer, white, middle-class married couples in which the wives were in the second trimester of their first pregnancy. Only 2 couples (5%) dropped out after the initial interview. The mean duration of marriage was 4 years; 34 husbands and 29 wives worked outside the home.

Data from the ongoing study are available from the Time 1 interviews (second trimester of pregnancy), Time 2 interviews (shortly after the birth of the infant), Time 3 interviews (infant 3 months old), and Time 4 interviews (infant 1 year old). Subsequent interviews have been completed. The subjects were studied as individuals, dyads, and triads in the hospital at the time of the birth, at the Research Foundation, and in their homes (Lewis, 1988a, p. 151). After 5 years, 37 (92.5%) of the 40 couples were still participating, including the 6 that moved away and were interviewed by researchers who traveled to the homes. Lewis emphasized that the distribution of power in the relationship is critical because, when it is not reasonably equal, one spouse plays "a decisive role in the determination of the ways in which other issues are `negotiated'" (Lewis, 1988a, p. 154).

Videotapes of marital interactions were rated in accord with the Beavers-Timberlawn Family Evaluation Scales. The raters were not blinded; they had access to each spouse's semi-structured individual interviews, transcripts of the marital interview, and data from the scales. Subjects were rated for overall level of marital competence on a 10-point scale.

At Time-1 (second trimester of the first pregnancy) of the 38 couples: 8 (21%) were rated highly competent; 13 (34%) competent but pained; 10 (26%) dominant-submissive, complementary; 7 (18%) severely conflicted; and none severely dysfunctional. Lewis stated: "This type of distribution in which 21 (55%) of 38 couples can be understood as either having competent relationships or as manifesting strengths in child-rearing despite marital pain is consistent with our earlier studies of families containing adolescent children" (Lewis, 1988a, p. 159). Greater competence was significantly associated with higher socioeconomic status. Generally, higher socioeconomic status is associated with improved functioning of most types; unfortunately, that finding indicates that lower socioeconomic status is associated with relatively low functioning.

Other Time-1 findings were that individual psychological well-being was associated with a competent relationship whereas lack of well-being, especially a wife's anxiety or depression, was associated with a dominant-submissive or severely conflicted relationship. (Lewis, 1988a, pp. 158-159). Ratings also revealed that in 30 (79%) of the 38 couples, the spouses had equivalent levels of psychological health. Overall, the 24 (63%) couples with average or higher levels of psychological health had significantly higher marital competence scores than the other 14 (37%) couples. Lewis wisely cautioned against "translating clearly dysfunctional dyadic interactional patterns into individual psychopathology" (p. 161). An average or high level of psychological health in one spouse appeared to be a necessary, but not sufficient, condition for a competent marriage. "Although the individual psychological health of the spouses plays a role in the type of relationship that evolves, that role is but a partial explanation of the quality of the relationship" (p. 162).

Ratings from the second trimester of pregnancy evaluations led to the hypothesis that: "Couples who have evolved more competent marital structures prenatally are more likely to incorporate the child successfully into the family" (p. 162). Both dyadic and triadic measures at Time 3 (the infant 3 months old) and also at Time 4 (1 year after the birth) were used to test that hypothesis.

Lewis and his colleagues (1988c) summarized the results of this important study.

1) The findings supported the application of the concepts of epigenesis to family systems inasmuch as resolution of key relationship issues early in marriage "forms a basic template for the characteristics of the evolving triadic system" (pp. 419-420);

2) The continuum of marital competence demonstrated its utility; the prenatal competence of the marriage predicted how well the child

would be incorporated into the family at both three months and one year;

3) Relationship measures were much more important determinants of the incorporation of the infant into the family than individual psychological health measures; consequently, "the data support the system construct that the whole is greater than the sum of its parts" (p. 420);

4) Measures of marital satisfaction had little predictive value;

5) There were few associations between changes in the level of marital competence and incorporation of the child into the family;

6) The findings indicated "the need for more complex models of family development" (p. 420);

7) Families that function well are underrepresented in "current model building" (p. 420);

8) Spouses who had not evolved a mutually satisfactory level of closeness were vulnerable to crises;

9) Couples with traditional, gender-stereotyped marriages may present stable marriages but have difficulty with the transition to parenthood;

10) Highly conflicted couples were relatively unpredictable;

11) Only 2 (5%) of the 38 couples had improved relationships 1 year after the birth of the child.

Lewis and his colleagues (1988c) concluded that there was a need for studies with larger samples and more complex models. Also, they pointed out that the transition to parenthood was difficult even for couples with relatively good educational and economic resources. "It is likely that single parents and couples with fewer educational and economic resources might well experience even greater stress in this important developmental transition" (p. 421).

The ongoing "Birth of the Family" study should be one of the most important family studies in the latter part of this century. Its major limitations are that it consists of middle- and upper-middle class white families in Texas, and the generalizability of the results is limited. Also, tautologies are inherent in studies of family competence and mental health. But, longitudinal studies, such as The Birth of the Family, are needed to establish the characteristics of healthful family functioning and of family competence over time, ascertain changes at different times in the family life cycle, and assess the outcomes for the children.

Lewis and his colleagues' emphasis on the significance of an egalitarian parental relationship is somewhat at variance with Westley and Epstein's (1969) report In The Silent Majority, that the children from their "father-led" families in Rhode Island had a much greater chance of being psychologically healthy than those from the "equalitarian" families. Also, in their controlled study of disturbed adolescents' perceptions of their families,

Novak and Van der Veen (1969, 1970) concluded that the father's effective, warm role in the family was important for the mental health of the adolescent. We think it is possible that the father's assuming a reasonable level of power in the family is more important when there are adolescents than just young children in the family. In view of the strong trend toward individualism in the USA, finding that competent families are characterized by a high degree of autonomy and egalitarianism on the part of the parents raises questions about the stability of those marriages over time. The widespread trend toward individualism could have a destabilizing effect on marriages and families, especially the many without institutional supports.

Recently, Lewis and his colleagues have revised the Beavers-Timberlawn Family Evaluation Scale (BTFES). The new Timberlawn Couple and Family Evaluation Scales (TCFES) consisting of 18 family and 16 couple scales is designed "to evaluate the functioning of family and marital systems" (pg. 4). The BTFES had been a widely used observational measure of family health and dysfunction but had not been designed to measure couples' marital functioning. The TCFES contains added Adult Leadership and Inappropriate Parent-Child Coalition scales, as well as the former scales for assessing structure, autonomy, problem-solving, affect regulation, and disagreement-conflict (2 to 5 subscales each). To evaluate the 18 scales, 63 two-parent and 17 single parent families with a child in a psychiatric inpatient unit were videotaped as part of a treatment outcome study while each discussed tasks, e.g. what they would like to change in the family, plans for a family activity, and the best and worst aspects of their relationship. The tapes were rated by two trained graduate psychology students; mean interrater reliability was 0.68. Also, the TCFES was tested with a nonclinic sample of 28 families that had participated in the "Birth of the Family" project. The internal consistency and other psychometric properties of the scales were satisfactory, and comparisons of both the clinic and non-clinic families' scores with the Georgia Marriage Q-Sort and other widely used scales revealed satisfactory construct validity. The TCFES Couple scores were highly related to self-reported marital satisfaction and marital problems scores were consistent with Hampson and his colleagues' (1988) reports of consistency between self-report and observational measures. The investigators' extensive clinical and research background and their intensive, thorough approach to the development of the TCFES enhance its utility for family studies.

Belsky's Pennsylvania State University Infant and Family Development Project

In 1983, Belsky, Spanier, and Rovine reported the initial results of their longitudinal "The Transition to Parenthood" study of family functioning in 70 volunteer lower-middle and middle income families from the last trimester of pregnancy until the infant was 9 months old. Methods included interviews with the couples, questionnaires given to each spouse individually, and observations of interactions and other behaviors in the home. Spouses and couples that initially scored high on measures of marital adjustment and functioning tended to do so across the 1-year period of study. But, the addition of a first-born or later-born infant had a negative impact on the marital relationship. Cohesion subscale scores dropped significantly for women during the postpartum period and declined for men, but less so. Romance scores also declined, but not significantly. The "honeymoon period" that might extend through the first postpartum month was no longer apparent by the third month postpartum. The addition of the child increased the burden upon the wife who often had to take care of the home as well as the baby. As the marriage became increasingly focused on instrumental functions, it was decreasingly focused on emotional expression. The overall quality of marital interaction was lower for couples with more than one child than for those with only one child.

Belsky and his colleagues concluded that the transition to parenthood, or the addition of another child, affected the marital relationship significantly. The overall level of marital quality declined but the rankings of individual spouses and couples remained relatively unchanged, i.e. those who scored either high or low on marital functioning in the last trimester of pregnancy were at the same level both three and nine months postpartum. The decline in marital quality might be "a function of the increasing instrumental nature of family life associated with child care" (p. 568).

In 1989, Belsky and his colleagues outlined their Pennsylvania State University Infant and Family Development Project. They viewed the family as an entity composed of multiple interrelating elements and subsystems, and emphasized the importance of interdisciplinary studies that look at how children affect marital functioning and how the marriage influences parent-child relationships and child development.

The project is a three-cohort longitudinal study of maritally intact, Caucasian, working and middle-class families bearing and rearing their first child. Total enrollment consisted of 250 families; 173 were in the second and third cohorts. Two-thirds of the 173 fathers were college graduates; 16% had less than a high school education. Average annual income was $24,000; 14% had more than $40,000 per year and 46% less than $20,000 per year. The couples were young, husbands' mean age was 28.6 years and wives' 26.6, and the average length of marriage was 3.9 years. The families were studied in the last trimester and when the infants were three and nine months of age. Parents in the second cohort responded by mail to questionnaires about personality factors when the infants were 15 months of age.

Marriages that functioned well prior to the birth of the child continued to function well after the transition to parenthood although feelings of spousal love declined and ambivalence about the marital relationship increased. Joint leisure activity decreased and the household division of labor became more traditional. Conflict increased while problem-solving communication decreased. The investigators maintained correctly that such changes are reciprocally related and cannot be subjected to linear causal analysis.

Although spousal relationships changed, patterns of parent-infant interaction remained consistent. Generally, mothers assumed primary responsibility for the children; the fathers were secondary parents. The degree of the father's involvement varied with the functioning of the marital relationship; spousal interaction promoted father-infant interaction. Mothers of insecurely attached infants experienced a greater decline in the quality of marital relationships than did mothers of securely attached infants. Also, the degree of security about the infant-mother attachment covaried with changes in the mothers' opinions of themselves. Overall, the quality of the marriage affected the multiply-determined infant-mother attachment bond. Belsky and his colleagues emphasized that the family system is a complex social organization composed of both developing individuals and relationships that cannot be characterized at one point in time. Moreover, only limited evidence indicated that adults change in some fundamental way upon becoming parents.

The results revealed that the two general types of family systems were the engaged, in which high levels of interaction took place in all three dyads and the disengaged in which either low levels of interaction were observed across all three dyads or only the mother-infant subsystem was highly interactive. The mothers' personality characteristics and the spouses' appraisals of each other distinguished the engaged from the disengaged prior to the infant's birth.

The investigators stated candidly that they doubted whether their research was truly systemic even though they had focused on the family as a system, its members as elements of the system, and the subsystems as the interacting elements/relationships. They concluded that studying individuals, relationships, the interdependence of relationships, and family triads was only a beginning, that it was also necessary to study such characteristics of systems as self-stabilization, self-organization, and hierarchical organization.

Such longitudinal research as that of Lewis and colleagues and that of Belsky and his colleagues' is important and is needed. Only long-term follow-up of a large sample of families from the upper, middle, and lower socioeconomic strata can show how changes (births, divorces, remarriages) in the composition and structure of families are associated with the adults and children's well-being and development. In particular, families varied socioeconomic statuses should be associated with differential responses to SLE and to life's transitions. Also, the parents' being in their childbearing and child rearing years will enable investigators to see how the cohorts are affected by historical events and sociocultural processes.

Unfortunately, we have not been able to obtain any recent reports of the results of Belsky and his colleagues exciting project. Belsky's research interests are now focused on infants and children's attachment.

Family Functioning Research Problems – Pless and Satterwhite

As early as 1973, I.B. Pless and B.Satterwhite discussed a persisting research problem: available instruments for measuring family functioning did not deal with similar multi-dimensional concepts of functioning. Also, instruments needed to be tailored for use in clinical settings. They conceptualized family functioning as "the dynamics of everyday life: the way in which the family, as a unit, operates across many dimensions," (619) and developed their self-report Family Functioning Index (FFI). It contains 16 questions pertaining, for example, to intrafamily communication, decision-making, marital satisfaction, and the level of general happiness and closeness of the family unit, each of which was scored 0, 1, 2 according to degree of congruence with optimum functioning. The FFI was tested for validity and reliability and then used with 43 mothers and 39 fathers entering therapy in family counseling agencies and also with a random sample of 399 families taking part in a general health survey. Six counselors assigned to families of children with chronic physical disorders also used it. Pless and Satterwhite urged clinicians, especially those working with physically ill children, to use the FFI inasmuch as many studies have shown that family stress is associated with children's physical illnesses, and that the degree of family integration influenced children's responses to rehabilitation.

The Moos and Moos Family Environment Scale (FES)

As part of the comprehensive development of instruments to assess the social environment in psychiatric hospital units and various correctional and community settings, R. Moos and colleagues (1974) also developed the FES. They based it on their conceptual formulation of three general areas and 10 specific dimensions of family functioning and on the data obtained from testing 200 items indicative of the family environment (Moos and Moos, 1981). Ten subscales (9 items in each) were developed; 3 of them -- cohesion, expressiveness, conflict -- assess the interpersonal dimension; 5 are measures of independence, achievement orientation, intellectual-cultural orientation, active-recreational orientation, and moral-religious emphasis related to the personal growth dimension; and the remaining 2 subscales, organization and control, assess the systems maintenance dimension. A family score is obtained by summing the members' individual subscale scores and dividing by the number of members participating. The scores can be charted as a profile similar to that of the Minnesota Multiphasic Personality Inventory (MMPI) scores, and/or can be used as either raw or standardized scores that measure particular dimensions. Also, a family incongruence score is obtained by summing the differences between members' individual subscales scores and dividing by the number participating.

Moos and Moos built both content and face validity into the FES by defining their constructs (e.g. cohesion, control), selecting items conceptually related to the 10 dimensions, and obtaining data from a study of 285 families representative of the Bay Area population, including a group of Black and Hispanic families. The items met specified criteria for scale construction, and the subscales had acceptable internal consistencies. Moos (1990) maintained that the FES has acceptable levels of construct, concurrent, and predictive validity as evidenced by the results of its use in a wide variety of situations such as adaptation to pregnancy and parenthood, childhood and adolescent adjustment to parental divorce, adjustment among families of psychiatric and medical patients, and treatment outcomes for patients with alcoholism, depression, and other disorders. They have established norms as well as profiles of normal and non-clinical families.

We have used the FES extensively in our research and clinical work (Schwab, et al., 1993). We averaged the individual members' subscale scores to obtain family scores, and determined the family incongruence score by measuring the differences between members' scores. We and Boake and Salmon (1983) have found that Louisville norms were higher on cohesion, much higher on moral-religious emphasis, and lower on conflict and on intellectual-cultural orientation than Moos' Bay Area norms.

Of the random sample of 43 families that entered our epidemiologic study (1993), we designated 3 (7%) as interpersonally effective in view of their high mean scores on the cohesion and expressiveness subscales and also on the intellectual-cultural and active-recreational subscales. In contrast, the apathetic cluster contained 4 (9%) families with low mean scores on 7 of the 10 subscales. Each of those 4 obviously troubled families had at least one member who was symptomatic. The structure-oriented cluster contained 11 (25%) families that had high scores on the organization, cohesion and moral-religious emphasis subscales. The fourth cluster, the moral-religious oriented, contained the 25 (58%) families that had high scores on cohesion, expressiveness, and moral-religious emphasis but were relatively unstructured.

Of the 43 families, at least one person in 25 (58%) of them met the criteria for being symptomatic with a mental or substance abuse disorder. The interpersonal dimension subscale scores reflected their varying levels of distress; the 25 symptomatic families had significantly lower mean cohesion and expressiveness scores and a higher mean incongruence score than the 18 asymptomatic.   The interpersonally effective and the moral-religious clusters contained smaller percentages of symptomatic families than the structure-oriented and, especially, the apathetic clusters with their high percentages (73% and 100% respectively) of symptomatic families.

The FES subscale scores had surprisingly good predictive value. We were able to predict family symptom status from the FES subscale and incongruence scores by using stepwise discriminant function analyses and logistical regressions. At Time 1, the FES subscale scores classified 67.4% of the families correctly as to symptomatic status, 86.1% for depression. High family conflict scores were predictive of drug problems. All of the 17 families with children under the age of 16 were correctly classified as being either symptomatic or asymptomatic; families' low independence subscale scores were significant predictors of the children being symptomatic. Depending on the measure (e.g. CES-D scores, drug use) logistic regressions correctly predicted the specific symptom status of 62.8% to 83.7% of the families on the various measures used. The mean cohesion score was the most powerful predictor of symptomatic status.

Families with certain symptoms had reasonably specific FES profiles. For example, those with high CES-D scores tended to have significantly low mean cohesion, expressiveness, intellectual-cultural orientation, and moral-religious emphasis subscale scores and a higher mean incongruence score than families in which no member was symptomatic on the CES-D. Thus, the FES subscale scores accurately reflected current distress.

The Time-1 FES subscale scores also turned out to be excellent predictors of Time-3 symptom status, 15 to 18 months later; 82% of the families were correctly classified as being either asymptomatic or symptomatic solely by the stepwise discriminant function analyses of their Time-1 FES subscale scores. Thus, the quality of the family environment was associated with symptomatology and predictive of symptom status at a reasonable level of accuracy over a 15 - 18 month period of time even though there had been some changes in various families' symptom status and/or life situations.   A healthful (normal) family environment was associated with a family's not being symptomatic and, conversely, a family environment characterized by relatively low cohesion, expression, independence, and moral-religious emphasis subscale scores and by the members' divergent views of the family was associated with the onset of symptomatology over that time period.

Although the FES is considered to be a rather general measure of family functioning, we found that it is what it purports to be -- a family environment scale. It supplied information on the quality and quantity of family interactions, the family's orientations and values, and features pertaining to organization and control within the family. Also, it provided an overall assessment of family members' attitudes toward each other, a view of their interests and priorities in everyday life, and a glimpse of intrafamily dynamics and differences.

Some concern about the validity of the FES constructs has been expressed by researchers who have used factor analytic approaches to study its psychometric properties. For example, Waldron, Sabatelli, and Anderson (1990) gave the FES to 366 employees and 462 college undergraduates and reported that the FES "is best represented by (only) six factors rather than 10" (p. 269). They concluded that inasmuch as "several of the scales fail to perform reliably, ... the continued use of the FES as an instrument is not warranted" (p. 270). However, Waldron and her colleagues' large sample of only one subject for each middle and upper class family appears to be a poor choice of a study population. That choice and the use of factor analyses neither reflected nor replicated the original work and the bulk of the research with the FES through the years.

Roosa and Beals, (1990), studied the internal consistency of 5 FES subscales by administering the FES to 311 stressed and 74 control "families". But in each "family" only one adult completed the interview and almost all respondents were middle-class females with some college education. Roosa and Beals reported that their reliability coefficients were lower than those Moos had reported. They then attempted to generate scales from the FES items by having 12 psychology graduate students assign the various items to different scales after they had been given the titles and definitions of the scales. The graduate students were able to agree with each other and place the items in the correct original subscale only about 50 to 60% of the time. Consequently, Roosa and Beals (1990) raised questions about the validity of the FES subscales and concluded that their results "illustrate the importance of examining the reliabilities of instruments, even well-known and widely used instruments for each sample studied." (p. 191)

In response, Moos (1990) emphasized that Roosa and Beals had studied a relatively homogeneous population, given the FES to just one family member, and had also used factor analytic techniques in an attempt to develop relatively circumscribed but highly internally consistent dimensions. That approach differed drastically from his insistence that the FES was developed "to create conceptually broad subscales composed of a diverse set of items" (p. 206) that could be used effectively with diverse populations. Also, Moos emphasized that in order to make further advances in family assessment, "Researchers need to use conceptual and psychometric criteria rather than rely too heavily on the pursuit of internal consistency, reliability, and factor analytic approaches to scale construction and validation."

In their "Final Comment," Roosa and Beals (1990) acknowledged many of the points presented by Moos and agreed that their sample consisted mainly of Caucasian females whereas many of Moos' studies were conducted on families from differing ethnic backgrounds in which a number of members were given the FES. However, they insisted that in view of the error variance in the scores of FES scales with low reliability coefficients that they had found, the results might not be interpretable, and that they had decided not to use their already collected FES data.

In contrast, we point out that Bloom (1985) has found the FES to be useful; in fact, much of the FES served as the bulk of his Family Functioning Scale (FFS). Also, recently, Phillips, West, Then, and Zheng (1998) noted that in China there was a lack of measures that could be used to evaluate families' characteristics and functioning. Therefore, they examined the reliability and validity of a revised Chinese Version (CV) of the FES and used four of its scales with 120 respondents from 64 schizophrenic patients' families and 126 respondents from 119 control families. The psychometric properties of the FES Cohesion, Conflict, Intellectural-Cultural Orientation, and the Active-Recreational Orientation scales were satisfactory. (The remaining 6 FES scales need further revision for use in China.) Compared to the controls, the schizophrenic patients' families had higher conflict, lower cohesion, and poorer adaptability and were less likely to be involved in intellectual and recreational activities. Thus, the investigators found the results valid and useful and discussed the need for, and the difficulties of, making the Western instruments culturally meaningful in China.

We (Schwab, et al., 1993) have found the FES to have significant research and clinical applications. In Chapters V and VI, we report the results of its use with a random sample of 19 families in the community and also with 15 clinic and non-clinic families.

Reiss' Problem-Solving "Paradigm Model"

Since the early 1970s, David Reiss and his colleagues at George Washington University have been developing their problem-solving "Paradigm Model" of family functioning in order to provide a classification of families that has clinical utility. Despite the great need for criteria that will predict whether a family continues in therapy, investigators' have outlined only a few predictors of families dropping out of treatment early. Identified predictors have been low socioeconomic status, authoritarianism, and therapy being initiated by only one spouse.

In "The Family Meets the Hospital," Reiss and his colleagues (1980) pointed out that like persons, families can be considered unitary cases, and that classifying them according to their style of adapting to new situations helps to predict their responses to treatments. They viewed the classification as analogous to a character diagnosis or to person's way of responding to problematic events (p. 141).

Reiss and colleagues assessed family members' behaviors in problem-solving situations in the laboratory by procedures that had been tested for reliability and validity. They evaluated two dimensions: (a) configuration, or the extent to which family members use each other's observations and ideas to solve test problems; and (b) coordination, or "the degree to which each family member integrates or dovetails his or her own problem-solving efforts with others" (p. 142). The 2 dimensions have been found to be independent and to provide 4 combinations: (a) those high on both configuration and coordination are the environment-sensitive--family members who work together to explore and understand the environment similar to Wertheim's (1973) "open-integrated" families; (b) those high on configuration but low on coordination are the achievement-sensitive who explore and master laboratory situations but do so in a competitive, not a cooperative, manner like Wertheim's "externally open-integrated" families; (c) those low on configuration but high in coordination are the consensus-sensitive that work so closely with each other that their high level of cooperation interferes with problem-solving because they "thirst for agreement and consensus no matter what the consequences for problem-solving" (p. 142), are frightened by the outside world, and become a self-protection group like Wertheim's "closed-pseudointegrated"; and (d) those low on both coordination and configuration are the distance-sensitive who work separately and ineffectively and are pessimistic about obtaining help from others, similar to Wertheim's "closed-disintegrated" families.

Reiss and colleagues (1980) used their card-sorting procedure (CSP) to compare 32 families with an adolescent on an inpatient unit that had an intensive group-focused treatment program with the other 88 families admitted during that time. There were no significant differences between the groups' sociodemographic characteristics. The families were classified shortly after admission according to their approach to the problem-solving situations that had been carried out in a laboratory. Family members sat in telephone booths in the laboratory and communicated with each other only by telephone as they attempted to solve a 3-phase card-sorting task, first, individually, then as a family while they were permitted to talk to each other, and finally, again individually. Family members' conversations were recorded and their activities videotaped.

Also, families participated in a weekly, one hour multiple-family-staff meeting for program planning. A researcher attended all meetings to obtain data about: (a) who spoke to whom; (b) choices about seating and changes in seating; (c) sociometry or responses to monthly questionnaires asking each person which members of the group he/she liked the most and least; (d) responses to a cohesiveness questionnaire; and (e) attendance.

The cardinal processes studied were: (a) status - the family's conspicuousness and influence in the large group setting; (b) openness of boundaries that referred either to willingness to form new relationships or to the family's clinging together; and (c) cohesion -- both felt cohesion and attendance. Family level data were obtained by summing individual scores and dividing the total by the number in the family to yield a single family score. In reality, such scores are only the average of the individuals' scores, not a family score.

Reiss and colleagues predicted that: (a) members of environment-sensitive families would explore the new environment, work together, and score high on status, openness of boundaries, and cohesion; (b) the achievement-sensitive would score low on status and, because of competitiveness, would pay a great deal of attention to each other, be less open to outside experiences, and have low scores on boundary-openness, but would score high on cohesion because each would feel that he/she was "doing pretty well in this place" (p. 143); (c) the consensus-sensitive would have low scores on status, boundary-openness, and cohesion because the members yearn for agreement and coordination at any price and, inasmuch as the outside world is frightening, would develop firm boundaries and have low morale and feelings of estrangement; and (d) the distance-sensitive would be pessimistic, tend to disperse, and to have open boundaries but would regard themselves as failures and thus exhibit helplessness and have low scores on status, boundary-openness, and cohesion.

The environment-sensitive had high scores on status, boundary openness, and on cohesion. The achievement-sensitive had relatively low scores on boundary openness and on cohesion. The consensus-sensitive had relatively non-distinctive scores. The distance-sensitive had high scores on boundary openness, low scores on status, and very low scores on cohesion.

The results supported the hypotheses about the environment-sensitive and the achievement-sensitive families. The results, for the consensus-sensitive were somewhat mixed; "The danger they most fear may not come from without but from unacknowledged negative feelings within the family itself" (p. 153). As expected, the distance-sensitive families were low on status, openness of boundaries, and cohesion consistent with their relatively poor laboratory performances and suggestive of the members' isolating themselves. But, contrary to expectations, the predictions were significant only for the parents. The adolescents' status in and engagement with the group were unpredictable; each tended to have his/her own norms, make individual choices, and to establish his/her own status.

Reiss and colleagues concluded that the family can be diagnosed or classified as a unitary entity. Also, their family classification system enabled them to make qualitative and quantitative predictions about the risk of treatment failure. Environment-sensitive families turned out to have the least risk of failure to continue the treatment program -- they were conspicuous, had open boundaries, and engaged in the therapeutic community. The risks posed by the achievement-sensitive and the consensus-sensitive families were subtle and qualitative; members were engaged heavily with each other and maintained boundaries around themselves but did not enter freely into the therapeutic community. The distance-sensitive had the greatest risk of failure; they were inconspicuous, felt little cohesion with the group, had poor attendance at group meetings, and were likely to be dropouts. Wertheim had predicted that such "closed-disintegrated" families would be difficult to treat in family therapy (Reiss, et al., 1980, p. 154).

Epstein and his colleagues (1981) compared Reiss' Paradigm Model with the MMFF. In many ways, high configuration reflected empathic involvement and "personal involvement in `roles," and coordination indicated clear communication and assessed "well-handled systems maintenance, management, and roles" (p. 95). But, Epstein and colleagues considered the four-case family typology to be "premature" and, questioned whether it had predictive value because it may be "too gross a measure" and left out important aspects of family functioning. They concluded that the clinical utility of Reiss' model was "questionable" because it required extensive observations of family behavior and was too time consuming for clinical work. Instead of developing a typology, they prefer to identify dimensions of functioning and determine how families are distributed on them.

Despite such criticism, Reiss and his colleagues' (1980) study is an important addition to family research. Although their method is complicated, requires a laboratory, and families have to have reasonably good educational backgrounds to participate, it is directed toward treatment and was the first successful use "of a family classification scheme to predict a family's response to a family-oriented treatment program" (p. 141). Their approach enabled them to make predictions about a family type according to the *way*, not just *whether*, it solved problems (italics ours). Thus, the predictions were not tautological, varying degrees of family function or competence would not necessarily be associated with differential outcomes as is true of most other approaches. Although it has limitations, Reiss and his colleagues' problem-solving model is promising and their research is a major contribution to the field.

Reiss and his colleagues continuing work with their paradigm model is impressive. In "The Family's Conception of Accountability and Competence: A New Approach to the Conceptualization and Assessment of Family Stress", Reiss and Oliveri (1991) used data from the social community to increase understanding and meaning of stressful life events (SLE) research. They pointed out that usually the seriousness of an SLE depends on the family's perceptions of it, their responses, and their own intuitive theory of family stress. Reiss and Oliveri maintained that community level concepts are important, especially the views about family accountability for producing or exacerbating the event, as are the family's competence or ability to protect itself from the disruptive and deleterious effects of SLE.

To test their innovative approach, the investigators defined family stress as "an event that by community standards is high in the capacity to disrupt ordinary family routines" (p. 197). Thus, they avoided or reduced the tautology implicit in the assignment of the meaning of the event by the family and also allowed for a relatively more objective appraisal of the quality and effectiveness of the response to the event than is usually possible. In addition, they emphasized the necessity to distinguish between SLE indicative of psychopathology or relationship difficulties from those which are not. They recruited 45 suburban Washington, D.C. Caucasian, two-parent, step- and non-divorced families, each with a high school student. The parents were in their mid-40's, fathers' mean educational level was 17.4 years, and the mean marital duration was 20.2 years -- they were "middle-class". Each family was interviewed in the research laboratory to elicit information about each SLE that occurred and to undertake the Card-Sort Procedure (CSP) that assesses configuration, coordination, and closure (the family's flexibility when given new information). The group's total SLE were evaluated for consensus and each event was rated by the family for magnitude of its disruptive capacity and for degree of externality (family or other accountability).

The 18 consensus items that had both high magnitude and externality ratings were considered to be the "most secure indicators of the community's conception of families and stress" (205). They were then placed in categories or zones on a high-low magnitude – high-low externality "community map". Examples are: parents have a baby (high on accountability) is in the Family Transformation Subzone on the map; family member attempts suicide (high magnitude but less family accountability) is in the Family Turmoil Subzone; parent loses job is in the third, the Family Crisis Subzone; family home burglarized (low accountability, highly external event) is in the fourth or Family Ravagement Subzone; and, an event such as "relative changes job" (little impact on and family not accountable) is in the fifth or Enviromental Curiosity Subzone. Reiss and Oliveri (1991) concluded that their findings "suggested an intricate concept of family competence and accountability that achieves high levels of consensus within the community" (p. 210).

We think that this is important research and that it has significance for understanding and studying both family functioning and mental illness. Reiss and Oliveri have enlarged the conventional views of family stress, and their conceptualizations and findings highlight such important points as the degree of importance to the family of, e.g. SLE affecting grandparents rather than other blood relatives, the differential gender effects of SLE, and the identification of events as either rare or common. Finally, this research underscores the need for a family – community sociology and the necessity to include community characteristics and processes in studies of family life and function. For example, a child's entering school may burden a family although its community stress rating might be low; in contrast, there would be high family-community agreement about losses following a natural community-wide disaster. Also, the findings can identify alienated family groups that need the support of self-help groups. Reiss and Oliveri maintained that the research approach and the results also have therapeutic implications; for example, families with highly idiosyncratic views about family development and/or family issues are at high risk for dropping out of therapy.

The California Health Project

During the past few years, continuing efforts have been directed toward developing new measures for evaluating family functioning. Fisher, Ransom, and Terry's (1993) California Health Project, is a comprehensive study of health and four domains of family variables--world view, emotional management, structure/organization, and problem solving. The goals were "to explore the structure and pattern of the variables in each family domain in order to assess the relationship between them and the self-reported health of husbands and wives...(and thus create) empirically based models for use in family and health research." (p. 69) Their research sample consisted of 225 Anglo or Hispanic families, each with two heterosexual adults and at least one teenage adolescent, in a suburban central California community. They were interviewed in their homes and also in three-hour laboratory sessions that included a 30-minute videotaped family problem-solving game. Each family was paid $100 at the completion of the protocol.

One group of family variables pertained to both the husbands and the wives' health and a second group to gender-specific associations with health. For each spouse, his or her view of the world was associated with health. Optimism was a shared-spouse attitudinal variable representing a shared disposition. Of the emotion management variables, the couple's avoidance of intimacy and conflict was associated with the wives' negative health scores, whereas expressions of anger and hostility were associated with the husbands' negative health scores.

For both husbands and wives, the structure/organization core family variables associated with health were a) family coherence -- members' beliefs that they could manage their lives and the world about them; b) family religiousness; and c) organized cohesiveness that included clarity of roles and rules in the family and cohesion--closeness of family ties. Organization and cohesion, usually viewed as two distinct dimensions of family functioning, were considered a single, integrated construct.

The major gender differences were that three core family variables--life engagement, role flexibility, and shared roles -- were associated with the husbands' health whereas differentiated sharing, a specific intrafamilial issue, was associated with the wives' health. Satisfaction and productivity, along with not drinking and smoking, were significantly related to the husbands' health, whereas variables reflecting mood and self-appraisal were related to a much greater extent to the wives than to the husbands' health. Fisher and his colleagues considered these gender differences to be consistent with a social role explanation inasmuch as the wives' negative health was more strongly than the husbands' associated with the avoidance of intimacy and conflict, mood and emotional health, and the salience of interpersonal relations.

Fisher and his colleagues' identification of core family variables related to health can increase understanding of family processes. But, currently the findings are correlates of health and are not explanatory. Moreover, the findings relate mainly to the spouses' individual and interpersonal characteristics and thus have a much greater potential for increasing understanding of family members' health-illness than for understanding family function specifically. We have concern about the lack of generalizability of the findings because the sample was composed of relatively stable, semi-urban families. Inasmuch as family instability is one of the hallmarks of our era, there is a pressing need for investigators to take some risks and cast a fairly wide net so that their findings will be applicable to families representative of a cross-section of life and times in the USA as the new century begins. We hope that Fisher and his colleague's follow-up data will enable them to make some explanatory statements and possibly develop a causal model. Then, their task will be to determine its applicability to other segments of our population.

Benson and Colleagues' Family Study

To begin their studies of family functioning—focused specifically on linkages between the mothers, fathers, and adolescents' degree of satisfaction with the family and family system factors--Benson and his colleagues (1995) looked at the limits of self-report measures, in particular the extent to which an individual member's report on the family was a valid indicator of the characteristics of the family system. Also, how could family level data be obtained from individual members' self reports? A common approach has been to sum all the members' scores and average them, but doing so masks individual members' differences. To meet that difficulty, investigators often calculate the differences between members' scores to obtain a discrepancy score; however, that procedure can compound the biases in each member's scores. Still another approach has been to compute the degree of agreement (kappa statistic) among individual family members on the items under consideration.

Benson and his colleagues stated that such approaches do not examine simultaneously "the patterns of convergence and divergence *within* and *across* family members." (p. 324) Therefore, they used a factor analytic approach to obtain family-level data on family functioning. They hypothesized that both individual factors and family system factors would emerge in their study of 360 individuals (father, mother, and adolescent) in 120 intact Caucasian suburban families living near a major metropolitan area in California. Each family member was given Bloom's 1985 Family Functioning Scale (FFS) that had been developed from factor analytic studies of the FES, FCQS, FACES III, and the FAM.

For each family, the members' self-report responses to items were pooled so that all the variables in the pool would be the unit of analysis. The investigators noted that types of factors that emerged would depend upon the individual member's responses, which, in turn, reflected his or her cognitive processes, conceptualized as those referable to both semantic memory (memories and inferences drawn from experience) and to episodic memories (recollections of episodes or singular events).

The first analysis, an individual-only factor model, was based on the assumption that, with the family as the case, the 45 scale scores (15 for each member) measured only three individual factors. It produced a poor fit, indicating that the subscales measured more than individual factors. The second analysis, based on the assumption that the scales measured only the 15 family system constructs in the FFS, also did not fit the data well, indicating that the subscales measured more than the family systems constructs. Further factor analyses led to the deletion of the authoritarian and disengagement scales and to the emergence of 3 individual level and 6 family system level factors. The 3 that reflected a sense of feeling satisfied with the family, being happy with it, and feeling support from family members were termed Individual Satisfaction with the Family and developed as Father Satisfaction, Adolescent Satisfaction, and Mother Satisfaction scales. The remaining 6 were family system level factors-- family religiosity, family cultural orientation, family conflict, family social orientation, family organization, and family enmeshment--from which 6 composite family system scales were constructed.

Regression analyses showed significant but seemingly obvious relationships between higher levels of education and higher family cultural orientation and also between family organization and smaller family size. For the adolescents, mothers, and fathers, both family social orientation and cultural orientation were significant predictors of satisfaction. For both the adolescents and the mothers, conflict was negatively related to satisfaction, and for the mothers, enmeshment was negatively related to satisfaction. Inasmuch as family structure characteristics were unrelated to satisfaction, the investigators stated that structural variables played only a "peripheral role in understanding family system processes" (p. 333).

Benson and his colleagues concluded that neither an individual-only factor model nor a family-only model was sufficient, that both individual and family factors emerge as patterns in family members' self reports as evidenced by convergence within the individual's perceptions and also by divergence from others' perceptions. The presence of individual factors "implies differences in affective perceptions across family members," (p. 331) and points to the importance of understanding individual satisfaction in clinical work with families. Also, valuing individual satisfaction in therapy may reduce some of the "oppressive dynamics in families particularly toward women" (p. 331) described by Jacobson (1983).

Analyses of the six family factors revealed a commonality of perceptions across family members that "contradicts the supposition that self-reports reflect only perception within individuals" (p. 332). Benson and his colleagues maintained "that individuals shared perceptions of family conflict, family organization, or family enmeshment because they used similar inference processes", probably stemming from common standards for evaluating much of what was happening to them. Also, episodic memory processes were contributory inasmuch as many events or episodes usually involve the entire family or occur in a family context and members' share memories of the episodes that lead to similarities in their views of their families' characteristics.

The influence of common family standards for evaluating some dimensions of functioning was relevant for family religiosity, family cultural orientation, and family social orientation, the three family factors that "represented family *mesosystem* characteristics, or the interface between family and other systems" (p. 333). The family's cultural orientation being the strongest predictor of family satisfaction for the parents is important because it can reduce the impact of internal family pressures and "imbue family life with broader cultural meaning." (p. 333) Emphasizing that community-level conceptions influence the interpretation of events in family mesosystems points to the importance of community influences and standards (or the lack thereof) as shown by the results of Reiss and Oliver's (1991) study of family stress. Also, it increases the significance of Benson and his colleagues' important finding that the family's social orientation was the strongest predictor of satisfaction for the adolescents. We think that viable community networks reduce internal family triangulation and potentiate fluidity within the family.

We regard the results pertaining to *mesosystem* factors as being especially important at this time, when downsizing by corporate America and the disintegration associated with suburban-exurban affluenza and technological developments are splintering community life. There is need for increased understanding of the links between individual systems and family systems, and also, of mesosystems and of community influences in accord with principles of GLS theory which hold that all living systems--e.g. cell, individual, family, community--depend on the functioning of 19 analogous subsystems. Benson and his associate's results, however, are limited because they were working with a homogeneous sample of upper middle-class suburban families and findings from such a homogeneous group need to be compared with the results of studies of lower socioeconomic and of heterogeneous groups.

The factor analytic approach to the study of family functioning based on the members' self reports is meaningful and interesting. Such an approach may reduce some of the loss of information and get closer to yielding more valid family-level scores based on the individuals' self-reports than does the more simple averaging of members' scores. The factor analytic approaches used, for example, by Bloom (1985), and by Benson and his colleagues' (1995) are a contribution to the methodology of studies of family functioning. However, as pointed out by R. Moos (199_) factor analytic strategies also have limitations. Moos stated that they include

Behavioral Genetics and Family Functioning

The recent growth of the field of behavioral genetics has added a significant perspective to the understanding of childhood development and sibling relationships and has a potential for increasing understanding of family interactions and functioning. The importance of long accepted genetic influences is illustrated by Scarr and Weinberg;'s (1991) finding that adopted children's IQ scores were more closely correlated with their biological parents' than their adoptive parents' educational levels. Also, the IQ scores of biologically related siblings correlated at .35; in contrast, adopted children who were living in the same family had a .00 correlation. Such findings indicate that the influence of the shared environment is "negligible in the long run" (p. 164), and point to the importance of genetic influences on intelligence. In "Genetic Influences on the Family Process: The Emergence of a New Framework for Family Research," Bussell and Reiss (1993) maintained that inasmuch as an individual is the product of genetic as well as environmental influences, findings from behavioral genetics research "may permanently alter family scientists' measurements and models of the family environment" (p. 162). Therefore, genetic and other biological factors must be given weight, along with the interpersonal and psychosocial, in comprehensive studies of family functioning.

In their Virginia female twin study of childhood parental loss and psychopathology in later life, Kendler and his colleagues (1996) examined both genetic and environmental data. The effects of shared environments were slight; their best fitting model included genetic effects, nonshared environmental effects, and such specific environmental events as a childhood parental loss. Parental loss accounted for 1.5% to 5.1% of the risk for various mental disorders and for 7% to 20.5% of the tendency for disorders to aggregate in siblings. Parental separations tended to be associated with major depression, generalized anxiety disorder, or panic disorder whereas early parental death was associated with phobias or panic disorder. Such findings that quantify environmental risk for various types of mental disorder underscore the importance of studies of family functioning aimed toward determining the multiple, varying family factors associated with health and well-being as well as illness.

In their continuing studies of psychopathology in the Virginia female twins, Kendler and colleagues (1996) have used a genetic-epidemiologic design "to clarify the role of genetic and environmental factors in...parenting behavior." They studied parental warmth, protectiveness, and authoritarianism by administering a modified form of Parker's (1985) Parental Bonding Instrument (PBI) to the 606 fathers, 848 mothers, and both members of the 546 monozygotic and dizygotic twins. Thus, they could obtain reports from four sources: a) fathers and mothers; b) the twins; c) each twin reporting on the quality of the other twin's parenting; and d) twins reporting on their parenting of their own children. Analyses showed that parents and twins' reports varied considerably; parents emphasized that they treated both children the same whereas the twins' responses indicated that their own temperaments elicited the degree of parental warmth each had received. Kendler (1996) concluded that "Parenting is influenced by attitudes derived from one parent's family of origin as well as by genetically influenced parental temperamental characteristics." The eliciting of parenting is influenced by the offspring's temperament which, in turn, is under partial genetic control. Genetic factors in both the parents and children were more important for *warmth* than for *protectiveness* or *authoritarianism*", for which environmental factors were largely responsible. Thus, Kendler's results support R. Q. Bell's 1968 report of "A reinterpretation of the direction of effects in studies of socialization".

Results of studies are pointing to the significant influences of the nonshared family environment on children's mental, emotional and personality development. In 1976, Loehlin and Nichols reported that the nonshared family environment resulting from children's varying experiences in the family, e.g. from their differing ordinal positions, temperaments, ages, and family size/composition, affected their family interactions as well as their development. The nonshared family environment also is a product of differential parenting, siblings' differential experiences with each other and peer groups, and differential exposure to life events. According to Bussell and Reiss (1993), inasmuch as the heritability of behavior rarely exceeds .50; environmental factors explain much of the individual variation observed, and "nonshared environmental influences explain substantially more of the variation in children's personalities, interests, and adjustment levels than the common family environment" (p. 163). Thus, environmental influences operate more on an individual than on a family basis, and it is important to identify specific environmental factors that influence personality and development. Attention is being focused on the children's microenvironments within their families in view of Bussell and Reiss' report that they and other investigators have found that such variables pertaining to the composition and structure of the family as the total number of siblings and their age, gender, and birth order account for only little of the variance in children's abilities, and behaviors.

The influence of parents' differential treatment of children is being studied by Bunn, Stocker, and Plomin (1990) in their Colorado Adoption Project (CAP). Their finding that children who experienced a great deal of maternal control but relatively little maternal affection were more likely than their siblings to be anxious or depressed supports the results of Parker and his colleagues' (1983) series of well-controlled studies of the Parental Bonding Index (PBI) in England. Depressed adolescents and young adults reported that they had received overprotection and control but little warmth and affection from their mothers—Parker's "affectionless control." In contrast, the not depressed reported that they received a great deal of maternal affection. Later reports from the mothers supported the young persons' views of how much overprotection, control and demonstrable affection they had received.

Reiss and his colleagues (1993) have been engaged since the late 1980s in a comprehensive longitudinal study of a nationwide sample of 720 two-parent families with pairs of same sex adolescent siblings that consists of six groups: a) families with monozygotic twins; b) families with dizygotic twins; c) nondivorced families with full siblings; d) stepfamilies with full siblings; e) stepfamilies with half siblings (25% genetic similarity); and f) stepfamilies with unrelated siblings (no genetic relationship). The design of this nonshared environment and adolescent development (NEAD) project reflects three assumptions: a) it is necessary to include more than one child in a family research design; b) environment is "a multidimensional construct which includes common exposure and differential experiences" (p. 171); and c) different genetic mechanisms, family dynamics, and perceptual processes mediate environment effects. Some early results were that "genetic differences between children explained 26% of the variance in environmental measures, and genetic effects explained 51% of the variance in maternal closeness of her children." Ongoing NEAD research is focusing on the effects of nonshared environments.

The results of Reiss' and his colleagues' research have a direct bearing on family function and functioning. Their two-sibling design enables them to study family-level strategies for managing conflict within the family system, children being triangulated in troubled marriages and having traumatic experiences, and even influences between marital conflict and sibling rivalry. Integrating genetic and environmental data provides an opportunity, especially in twins and adoptees, to disentangle the effects of social processes (e.g. divorce) from genetic effects. In this respect, one major hypothesis is that marital instability leads to polarization within the environment and to more nonshared or unique family experiences for one sibling than another. Early findings indicate that there is a great deal of noncomparability in families with differing structures; for example, the correlations for maternal closeness of full siblings in nondivorced families was 0.28 in contrast to .04 in stepfamilies even though the biological mother of the children was the same in both types of families. Such findings indicate that siblings in nondivorced families have more shared experiences than those in stepfamilies (pp. 173-174).

Bussell and Reiss' research that included the use of Strauss' (1979) Conflict Tactics Scale showed that there are substantial nonshared effects in families, specifically, the differential treatment of children in regard to aggression, actual or symbolic (threaten to hit). A child who has more aggressive interactions with parents than the other children in the family is at greater risk for psychological disturbance than the others regardless of the age difference between the siblings. The effects of aggression in the family are not limited to the child who is singled out for it inasmuch as the other children also show signs of disturbance in anticipation of any aggression in the family. In low aggression families, the intimacy between parents and children leads to enhanced sensitivity to each other's actions and reactions. Also, girls are more sensitive than boys to family processes because they "tend to be more emotionally embedded in the family system during adolescence" (p. 176).

This important research, with its emphasis, for example, on the children's personality development and behavior, is obviously of central importance to family functioning. Traditionally, one of the two main family functions has been the development of children to become members of families and to function as the adults in society later in life. Behavioral genetics research indicates that certain relational experiences are "risky for all children across families whereas other patterns of interaction are uniquely risk-producing for children if they are treated differently than their siblings... (for example) close maternal-child relationships seem universally to protect children from suicidal ideation regardless of whether a sibling in the same family receives more or less maternal affection" (p. 177-178). Also, differential parental punitiveness was "more highly correlated with adolescent antisocial and depressive symptoms than the differential receipt of parental warmth and support" (p. 178).

Bussell and Reiss concluded that their multidisciplinary research will enable them to develop several models of human development. We think that genetic behavioral models such as theirs are mini-revolutions in ways to study families. The integration of genetic and environmental data into new models will lead to investigators getting "closer to understanding how families work and function" (p. 178).

CONCLUSIONS

Our overview of studies of family function and functioning shows that the various functions vary in importance in accord with prevailing historical and sociocultural processes. In the nineteenth century, when industrialization and urbanization were transforming Western society and many in the cities were poverty-stricken, the economic function was paramount. In the mid-19th century, LePlay developed a pioneering, in-depth approach to the study of the family and its well-being based on analyses of family budgets. The adequacy of the income and the nature and extent of its expenses, along with its form and structure, were major determinants of family well-being and stability. His family budget and typology of families served as a basis for other studies later in the century, most which focused primarily on assessments of family income and were designed to ascertain the extent of poverty and look at ways to improve family life. Some leading studies emphasized that the wife/mother's role should include functioning as the home economist; also, Social Security programs were needed to ensure family stability and well-being in later life.

During the "Roaring 20's", the family was changing significantly; the affectional and companionate functions were increasing in importance and there was a weakening of the traditional institutional foundation of the family. In the 1930's, the development of the Great Depression racked American society and brought the economic function of the family once again to the fore. The increasing degree of marital instability during the 1920's leveled off as "home and hearth" became essential, often even for survival during the Depression. Early studies by Angell (1935), which focused on adaptation and cohesion as the major variables determining the adequacy of the families' response to extreme stress, revealed that family adaptability was critically necessary for survival and family well-being. And, Koos (1946) found that economic stressors were leading to changes in family roles and probably influencing the children's character development. Also, degree of organization was fundamental to the family's functioning and its integrity as a unit.

The widespread effects of World War II accelerated social change, and the optimism following victory stimulated research on the family as part of the war against mental illness. The major goals of those studies in the 1950's were to increase the understanding of family dynamics in relation to the development and course of mental disorder in a family member, usually an adolescent. That research, often in a hospital or research laboratory, led to increasing interest in the interactions and dynamics of family life and an emphasis on the family group with Ackerman's (1958) three players--father, mother, and index patient.

The development of family system theories in the 1950's and 1960's was in accord with the widespread interest in general systems theories in social sciences and in organizations. Consequently, from the early 1960's to the early 1990's, tremendous power was ascribed to family systems, which usually were undefined but accepted as gospel--the only modern, approved way to understand and work with families with relational problems, mental illness, and/or substance abuse/dependence disorders. The term, family systems, was used so widely, if not promiscuously, that Murray Bowen (1989) declared that it was becoming meaningless.

The studies of family function during the past half century are an impressive group that have both everyday functional meaning and also clinical utility. Also, there is reasonable agreement on some of the characteristics of functional and so-called dysfunctional families in relation to members' mental health/illness. However, often family function/dysfunction have not been defined, the purposes of the family not stipulated, and, sometimes, the aims of the studies not specified.

Since World War II, research on family function has consisted mainly of gathering and analyzing data from one of two sources or from both. The major approach has been to obtain members' self-reports on items about such family characteristics as cohesion, adaptation, affectivity, and satisfaction on instruments tapping various aspects of family function and life. The other has been to obtain observer-based ratings of live and/or videotaped interviews of families performing a specified task in order to evaluate such indicators of family function as problem solving, decision making, and clarity of communication. However, the lack of conceptualization and definition of family function has handicapped much of the research.

Some major, well designed studies have been carried out during the past 50 years. In the late 1950's, Westley and Epstein's (1969) studies of associations between college students' emotional health and the ways their families were organized showed that the quality of the parental relationship was the important determinant of the children's psychological health and that the organizational, structural, and transactional patterns determined the families' behaviors to a much greater extent than intrapsychic variables. Based on that work, Epstein and his colleagues developed the McMaster Model of Family Functioning (MMFF) and its research and clinical scales-- the self-report Family Assessment Device (FAD) and the McMaster Clinical Rating Scale (MCRS)--for rating various dimensions of family functioning. Work during the past few decades with the FAD and, sometimes, the MCRs has included studies of samples of families with various types of physical and mental illness, especially depression, and its usually negative impact on the family. Epstein, Bishop, and their colleagues (1993) concluded from their extensive clinical and research work that "we continue to be impressed by the importance of a loving and supportive relationship between the parents...strong support, genuine concern, loving care and the absence of chronically persistent and nagging destructive hostility...serve as a foundation that can bear the weight of much strain inside and outside the family group" (p. 154).

Since the 1960's, Beavers and his colleagues in Dallas, TX have focused on the measurement of family competence. The Beavers' model of family competence with its two constructs – competence and style – and its scales have been designed to assess: "How well the family as an interactional unit, performs the necessary and nurturing tasks of organizing and managing itself" (p. 74). Their Self-Report Family Inventory (SFI) is a 36 item questionnaire designed to assess members' reported conceptions of family competence and style.

Beavers and colleagues have developed a continuum of family competence ranging from optimal functioning to the borderline and then to the severely dysfunctional, and have gathered information on more than 1,800 families in clinical and non-clinical settings over the past 30 years. Some general findings were that the optimal family is the "ideal" for family functioning but is not the "normal" inasmuch as only about 5% of families overall and 11% of a non-clinical sample have been classified as optimal. However, most clinical and control families were in the adequate to mid-range levels of competence and only about 3% of non-clinical and 11% of clinical families were severely dysfunctional. "This finding controverts the speculations of many dysfunctional family advocates, who attempted to convince us that the dysfunctional family represents the norm in modern America. Rather, the data suggest a reassuring bell-shape curve, with extremes of health or incompetence being small parts of the whole, and the bulk of American families doing reasonably well, yet with considerable room for improvement" (p. 93).

Jerry Lewis and his colleagues also have studied family competence over a period of time. They developed self-report and observer-rater scales and carried out intensive studies of 44 middle-class volunteer and patients' families to develop their "Continuum of Family Competence" which ranges from the flexible to rigid to chaotic families. The Highly Competent Family is the "ideal" (about 25% of families studied) and "many more were 'adequate" (competent but pained, dominant-submissive, or conflicted), but a few were severely dysfunctional because of the "increased probability of the development of psychiatric syndromes in the child or submissive spouse". Lewis discussed the characteristics of the various families but stated that "we do not know the relative proportions of optimal, adequate, or various degrees of dysfunctional families in the general population."

Lewis and Looney (1983) carried out a significant study of small sample of relatively low income African-American families. Contrary to their hypothesis, the characteristics of competence in the families were similar to those of the upper and middle-class Caucasian families they had studied.

Their most important research during the past 15 years has been the ongoing "Birth of the Family" study of 40 families beginning with the mothers' first trimester of pregnancy. Almost 90% of the families have continued to participate. Some early major conclusions are that couples that functioned well prior to the birth of the first child were likely to do so after the birth and were more likely than others to incorporate the child into the family successfully. However, only 2 (5%) of the 38 couples had improved relationships 1 year after the birth of the child. Also, the marital relationship measures were more important determinants of the incorporation of the infant into the family than individual psychological health measures.

The "Birth of the Family" study is one of the most important family studies of this century. Its major limitation is that the sample is composed of upper socioeconomic strata families with unusually stable marriages. Nevertheless, such longitudinal studies can be extremely meaningful, especially when they include studies of the children over time.

Belsky and his colleagues' apparently interrupted longitudinal study of their large heterogeneous sample of Pennsylvania families also found that marriages that functioned well prior to the birth of the first child continued to do so after the transition to parenthood. But, generally, the affectional relationship and marital satisfaction diminished as the instrumental functions increased following the birth of the first child.

The "Circumplex Model of Marital and Family Systems" developed by Olson and his colleagues in the late 1970s was based on Angell's and R. Hill's conceptualization of family adaptation and integration as the significant variables in family function/dysfunction. Different versions of Olson and colleagues' Family Adaptability and Cohesion Evaluation Scales (FACES) have been used during the past 20 years. FACES II was used in Olson and colleagues' (1983) highly publicized National Survey of 1,000 families that turned out to have a host of both conceptual and methodologic problems; for example, almost all of the volunteer families were middle class Lutherans with unusually stable marriages. The Olson Circumplex Model and the FACES have been vigorously criticized; results of studies by Green and his colleagues found that the FACES based on a circumplex model of family function, had "little utility in judging family assessment, practice, or research" (p. 70). They cautioned clinicians and researchers about its use. Olson defended the model and his research but has accepted the validity of the criticisms and joined other researchers in the development of a revised model and assessment instruments.

We think that there is little need for the further development and/or refinement of the commonly used scales that assess family affectivity, attitudes, other characteristics, and members' degree of marital/family satisfaction-dissatisfaction. But, there is a great need for new, innovative approaches to family function research. In addition to the ongoing studies in behavioral genetics that we summarized, other promising research is aimed toward completing a "biopsychosocial" spectrum by evaluating some family-community or mesosystem processes to complement the behavioral-genetics and the many existing, if not redundant, family attitude, satisfaction-dissatisfaction and symptom scales.

One of the new family-community studies is Reiss and his colleagues' SLE research in which they evaluated community standards for the magnitude or disruption produced by an event and also the degree of family accountability or "externality". The significance of a SLE occurring to a family then could be judged more meaningfully than when only an individual or family's evaluations of the event were considered.

The Family Environment Scale (FES) developed by Moos and Moos (1981) has been widely used during the past 20 years. It was especially useful in our longitudinal study of a random sample of 43 families in Louisville, KY. The results correlated with family members' mental health-illness and also had surprisingly good predictive value. The symptomatic families (according to their scores on the Diagnostic Interview Schedule, alcohol/drug measures, the Diagnostic Interview Schedule for Children, and. also the Child Behavior Checklist) had significantly lower mean cohesion and expressive scores and higher mean family incongruence scores than the asymptomatic. Also, at time-1, the FES scores correctly classified 82% of the families' (100% of the children's under age 18) symptomatic status at time-3, about 20-24 months later. (Schwab, Stephenson, Ice, 1993)

Other major family functioning research in the past 15 years includes B. L. Bloom's development of his Family Function Scale (FFS) based on factor analyses of items in the FES, FCQS, FACES, and FAM, and extensive research with large numbers of university students. A few results were that students from intact families were more cohesive and expressive and less conflicted than those from disrupted families. Bloom (1985) concluded that families prized high cohesive and expressiveness, little conflict, a high active recreational orientation, high sociability, an internal locus of control, a democratic life style, and the absence of a laissez-faire approach to life.

D. Reiss and his colleagues "Paradigm Model" of family function is a singular contribution to the study of the family. It was developed to provide a classification of families that has clinical utility, e.g. predictors of dropping out of treatment. The method involves the use of the investigators' card-sorting procedure (CSP); family members sat in "booths" in the laboratory and communicated with each other only by telephone as they worked to solve the card-sorting tasks descriptive of their family characteristics. The results showed that a family could be classified or diagnosed as a unitary entity and the family classification system enabled Reiss and colleagues to make qualitative and quantitative predictions about the risk of treatment failure.

Although the method is laborious, it has special significance in that it is not tautological. Predictions can be made about a family type *according to the way, not just whether*, it solved problems. (Italics ours.) We regard this work as extremely promising. Also, the CSP has recently been used in a study of family stress with sample families from the community.

The relatively new California Health Project is a study of health and four family domains: world-view, emotional management, structure/organization, and problem solving. Fisher and his colleagues' (1993) study of 225 Anglo or Hispanic families in a suburban California community showed that the avoidance of intimacy and conflict was associated with the wives' negative health scores whereas the expression of anger and hostility was associated with the husbands' negative health scores. The identification of family variables related to health can increase understanding of family processes. Currently, however, those findings are correlates and are not explanatory, and the "middle-class" sample was not representative of the poverty, marital instability, and stress battering many families.

The second is Benson and his colleagues research on linkages between family members' degree of satisfaction with the family and family system factors. They have examined the limits of self-report measures, especially the extent to which an individual member's report is a valid indicator of the characteristics of the family system and used a factor analytic approach to obtain family-level data by pooling family members' responses to items on Bloom's FFS for their analyses. Both individual and family factors emerged as patterns in members' self-reports. The investigators concluded that the commonality of members' perceptions "contradicts the supposition that self-reports reflect only perception within individuals" (p. 332).

At this time, when the social structure is changing rapidly, and in accord with our GLS Model of Family Functioning with its emphasis on the individual – family -- community systems, we consider Benson and colleagues' finding that some family factors "represented family mesosystem characteristics or the interface between family and other systems" to be especially important. Furthermore, Benson and colleagues found that the family's social and cultural orientation was the strongest predictor of satisfaction for the adolescents. Thus, in view of the current rate of social change and community turmoil, such research as that of Benson and his colleagues is meaningful.

Despite advances in the study of family functions and functioning in recent decades, many problems remain. Some are grievous. Family function and mental and/or substance abuse disorders in one or more family members are confounded as, for example, the view that his or her having such a problem signifies that he/she has come from, has been, or is in a dysfunctional family. Although it is difficult even to conceptualize any truly independent variables, the illness equals dysfunction tautology haunts family research. True, since at least Aristotle's time, the traditional family functions have been to meet its two fundamental purposes: to bear and rear children to take their place in society when they are adults and to provide for and regulate the parents' affectional and sexual needs. However, purposes and functions often are indistinguishable, especially when the rearing of children means, implicitly or explicitly, <u>healthy</u> children.

The illness = family dysfunction tautology is illustrated by the defining of a dysfunctional family as being "one in which one or more members experience symptoms that interfere with age -- and role -- appropriate functioning". This results from the system's difficulty in responding to change in the extrafamilial (loss of breadwinner's job) or in the intrafamilial (first child goes to school, grandparent dies, sudden illness) environments...Dysfunction may appear at a point when coping capacity is exceeded, because the previously effective patterns of responding are no long effective.... Challenging ineffective coping behaviors and uncovering unrecognized and submerged strengths are the tasks of therapy" (Siever and Liebeman, 1990).

In the first edition of her comprehensive multi-edited *Normal Family Processes,* Walsh (1982) emphasized the need to "develop models for family coping and competence." She stated that the clinical emphasis "has been primarily on dysfunctional family patterns" (p. xiii). Also, she pointed out that "concepts of 'normality' and 'health' are often confounded, and myths of 'the normal family' abound" (p. xiii), it was difficult to "define a normal family ...(or) to impose criteria of normality that lacked empirical validation" (p. xv). Therefore, she chose, "as most other investigators had, to limit selection criteria to a negative, or conservative, definition of normality: absence of severe psychiatric symptoms of any nuclear family member" (p. xv). However, as she "became increasingly aware of the diversity of patterns in nonsymptomatic families...any singular concept of a homogeneous normal control group (of families) had to be called into question...(and she) became interested in delineating the typical processes, positive strengths, and diversity that characterized normal families".

Walsh concluded that " "Functional" refers to " a judgment about the utility of structural or behavioral patterns in achieving objectives" (p. 6). In contrast, "norms" refer to "ranges of conduct deemed permissible." Family norms are influenced by "normative expectations" and societal value judgments" (p. 6).

Family systems orientation, Walsh stated, "is based on the perspective of normality as a process." However, in her summary of major models of family normality or dysfunction based on various clinical models, she stated that the "structural, strategic, and behavioral models view normality in functional terms (in that) it does not maintain or reinforce symptoms in any members" (p. 25). Walsh described the many models that have been developed from clinical work with families and pointed out that there is considerable overlap.

She noted that a number of investigators have attempted to develop integrative models. We have been impressed by the conceptualization and applicability of Fleck's integrative model of family functioning and family pathology that is based on his many years of clinical experience and research with concepts of GST. His five essential system parameters are:

1. Leadership which is depended on the parental personalities, the marital coalitions, parental role complementarities, and use of power;
2. Boundaries which involve the children's ego development, generational boundaries, and family-community permeability;
3. Affectivity which includes interpersonal intimacy, equivalence of family trials, tolerance for feelings, and unit emotionality;
4. Communication: responsiveness, verbal/nonverbal consistency, expressivity, clarity in form and syntax, and abstract and metaphysical thinking; and
5. Task/goal performance involving both nurturing and meaning, separation mastery and family triangles, behavior control and guidance, peer relationship management, family unit leisure, coping with crisis, emancipation, and postnuclear family adjustments.

* *

We think that studies of family function in the modern/postmodern era need to be aimed primarily toward improving family functioning in the hope that it can enhance family stability and well-being. Also, we hope that enhanced stability will contribute toward the prevention and amelioration of illness and augment the treatment of family members' mental and substance abuse disorders when necessary. Thus, family function/functioning needs to be focused on how well the family is functioning and on how well it is meeting its essential purposes. When possible, family research needs to identify specific areas of functioning that might benefit from interventions.

Our GLS model of family function is tightly based on general living systems theory and its conceptualization of the 19 subsystems whose functioning is essential for all levels of biosocial organization from the cell to the supranational. Accordingly, we define family function strictly in terms of functioning, from the specific biological matter-energy processes needed for life to the transmittal of information, from the biochemical at the cellular level to the electronic at the individual or group level. The emphasis is on functioning, on carrying out the concrete and the abstract tasks of daily life that enable families to fulfill their two basic functions.

Therefore, we are reporting on the development and use of our GLS Family Functioning Model and its assessment instrument. James G. Miller, who developed General Living Systems Theory, and Jesse Miller (1980), described the GLS approach to family studies as neutral. We have attempted to distinguish between family functioning and illness/substance abuse disorders and think that such an approach and method are needed in our increasingly pluralistic multi-ethnic, society that will require a remarkable degree of adaptability to meet the challenges of the new postmodern era.

References

Angell, R. C., (1941). *Foundations for a Science of Personality.* New York: Charles Scribner & Son.

Bane, M. J. & Ellwood, D.T., (1989). One fifth of the nation's children: Why are they poor? *Science,* 245, 1047-1053.

Beavers, W. R., Hampson, R. B., & Hulgus, Y. F., (1985). Commentary: Systems approach to family assessment. *Family Process 24, 398-405.*

Beavers, W. R. & Hampson, R. B., (1990). *Successful families: Assessment and intervention.* New York: W. W. Norton.

Beavers, W. R., Hampson, R. B., (1993). Measuring family competence: The Beavers systems model. In: Walsh, F. (Ed.) *Normal family processes,* (2nd. ed.). The Guilford Press, pp. 73-103.

Belsky, J., (1985). Experimenting with the family of the newborn. *Child Development, 56, p. 409.*

Belsky, J., Rovine, M. & Fish, M., (1989). The developing family system. In: M. Gunnar (Ed.) *Systems and Development, Minnesota symposium on child psychology, Vol. 22.* Hillsdale, NJ: Earlbaum.

Belsky, J., Spanier, G. B. & Rovine, M., (1983). Stability and change in marriage across the transition to parenthood. *J of Marriage and Family,* 45(3), 567-577.

Benedict, R., (1934). *Patterns of culture.* Boston: Houghton Mifflin.

Benson, M. J., Curtner-Smith, M. E. Collins, W. A., et al., (1995). The structure of family perceptions among adolescents and their parents: Individual satisfaction factors and family system factors. *Fam Process, 34(3):323-336.*

Bishop, D. S., Epstein, N. B., Baldwin, L. M., & Miller, I. W., (1988). Older couples: The effect of health, retirement, and family functioning. *Family Systems Medicine,* 6, 238-247.

Bleuler, E., (1909). *Dementia praecox or the group of schizophrenics.* (Trans. 1950, J. Zinkin). New York: International Universities Press.

Bloom, B. L., (1985). A factor analysis of self-report of family functioning. *Fam Process, Vol 24(2):225-239.*

Boake, C. & Salmon, P. G. (1981). Demographic correlates and factor structure of the Family Environment Scale. *J of Clin psychology, 39(1):95-100.*

Boas, F. Cited inn Hatch, E. (1973), *Theories of Man and Culture.* NY: Columbia Univ. Press, pp. 48-53.

Booth, C., (1892). *Life and labour of the people in London* (Vol. 1). London: Macmillan.

Bruére, Martha, (1913). *The utilization of family income.*

Buck, cited in Epstein, N. B., Bishop, D., Ryan, C., et al., (1993). The McMaster model view of healthy family functioning. In F. Walsh (Ed.): *Normal family processes* (2nd ed.). New York, The Guilford Press.

Burgess, E. W. & Locke, H. J., (1945). *The family: From institution to companionship.* New York: American.

Burgess, E. W. & Locke, H. J., (1960). *The family: From institution to companionship* (2nd ed.). New York: American.

Bussell, D. & Reiss, D., (1993). Genetic influences on family process: The emergence of a new framework for family research. In: Walsh, F. (Ed.) *Normal family processes,* (2nd ed.). New York: The Guilford Press, pp. 161.184.

Byington, M. F., (1910). *Homestead: The households of a mill town.* Philidelphia: Russell Sage Foundation.

Caplow, T., Bahr, H. M., Chadwick, B. A., et al., (1982). *Middletown families: Fifty years of change and continuity.* University of Minnesota Press, Minneapolis.

Cooper, J., Sartorius, V. S., (1977). Cultural and temporal variations in schizophrenia: A speculation on the importance of industrialization. *Br. J Psychiat., 130, 50-55.*

Darwin, C., (1909). *Origin of species.* New York: P. F. Collier & Son.

Deal, J. E., Wample, K. S., Halverson, C. F., (1992). The importance of similarity in the family relationship. *Family Process, 31(4): 369-381.*

Dickens, C. (1958). *Hard Times.* NY: Harper & Row.

Dunne, J. Stocker, C., Plomin, R., (1990). Assessing the sibling relationship. *J of Child Psychol and Psychiat, 31, 983-991.*

Dugdale, R. L., (1910). *The Jukes: A study in crime, pauperism, disease, and heredity.* New York: Putman.

Egeland, J. A. & Hostetter, A., (1983). Amish study I: Affective disorders among the Amish, 1976-1980. *American Journal of Psychiatry, 104, 56-61.*

Elder, G. H., Jr. & Rockwell, R. C., (1979). Economic depression and postwar opportunity in men's life: A study of life patterns and health. In R.G. Simmons (Ed.): *Research in community and mental health: An annual compilation of research, vol. I (pp. 249-302).* Greenwich, CT: Jai Press.

Elder, G. H., Jr., (1974). *Children of the Great Depression: Social change in life experience.* Chicago: University of Chicago Press.

Engels, F., (1972). *The origin of the family, private property and the state.* New York: Pathfinder.

Epstein, N. B. & Bishop, D. S., (1981). Problem centered systems theory of the family. In A. S. Gurman & D. P. Kniskern (Eds.), *Handbook of family theory.* New York: Brunner/Mazel.

Epstein, N. B., Bishop, D. S. & Baldwin, L. M., (1984). McMaster model of family functioning: A view of the normal family. In: *Family studies review yearbook*, pp. 75-101. Beverly Hills, CA: Sage.

Epstein, N. B., Segal, J. J. & Rakoff, V., (1962). *Family categories schema.* Unpublished manuscript, Jewish General Hospital, Department of Psychiatry, Montreal.

Epstein, N. B., Bishop, D., Ryan, C., et al. (1993). The McMaster view of healthy family functioning. In: Walsh, F. (Ed.) *Normal family processes.* New York: The Guilford Press, pp. 128-160.

Erikson, E. H., (1959). Identity and the life cycle. In: *Selected Papers.* New York: International Universities Press.

Fisher, L., Ransom, D. C., Terry, H. E., (1993). The California family health project VII. Summary and integration of findings. *Fam Process, 32(1):69-86.*

Friedmann, M. S., McDermut, W. H., Solomon, D. A., et al., (1997). Family functioning and mental illness: A comparison of psychiatric and non clinical families. *Family Process,* Vol 36(4), pp. 357-367.

Galsworthy, J., (1922). *The Forsyte Saga.* NY: Scribner.

Goddard, H. H., (1973). *The Kallikak family.* New York: Arno.

Goldsmith, O., (1909). *The deserted village.* New York: Dodd-Mead.

Goodsell, W., (1915). *A history of the family as a social and educational institution, Vol. III.* New York: Macmilllan.

Hampson, R. B., Beavers, W. R. & Hulgus, Y. F., (1988). Commentary: Comparing the Beavers and Circumplex Models of family functioning. *Family Process, Vol. 27(1), 85-92.*

Hampson, R. B., Beavers, W. R. & Hulgus, Y. F., (1990). Cross-ethnic family differences: Interactional assessments of white, black, and Mexican-American families. *Journal of Marital and Family Therapy, 16(3), 307-309.*

Harrington, M., (1963). *The other America: Poverty in the United States.* Baltimore: Penquin.

Harris, M., (1968). *The rise of anthropological theory: A history of theories of cultural.* New York: Crowell.

Henry, J., (1963). *Culture against man.* New York: Random House.

Hill, R., (1949). *Families under stress: Adjustment to the crises of war, separation and reunion.* New York: Harper.

Jost , H., (1896). In: E. Strömgren (Ed.), (1950) *Proceedings of the Congres International de Psychiaterie Paris VI, Psychiatrie Sociale.* Paris:Hermann, pp. 155-188.

Kabacoff, R. I, Miller, I. W., Bishop, E. S., et al., (1990). A psychometric study of the McMaster family assessment device in psychiatric, medical and non-clinical samples. *J of Family Psychology, 3(4), 431-439.*

Keitner, G. I., (Ed.) (1990). *Depression and families: Impact and treatment.* Washington: American Psychiatric Press.

Kendler, K. S., McGuire, M., Gruenberg, A. M., et al., (1993). The Roscommon family study: I. Methods, diagnosis of probands and risk of schizophrenia in relatives. *Archives of General Psychiatry, 50(7), 527-540.*

Kendler, K. S. (1996). Parenting: A Genetic-epidemiologic perspective. *Am J Psychiat, Vol. 153(1):11-20.*

Kendler, K. S., (1996). The identification and validation of distinct depressive syndromes in a population of female twins. *Arch Gen Psychiat, Vol. 53(5):391-399.*

Kerr, M. E. & Bowen, M., (Eds.). *Family evaluation.* New York: W. W. Norton.

Kluckhohn, C., (1949). *Mirror for man: The relation of anthropology to modern life.* New York: McGraw-Hill, pp. 17-44.

Köller, J., (1950). In: E. Strömgren (Ed.), *Proceedings of the Congrés International de Psychiaterie Paris VI, Psychiatrie Sociale.* Paris: Hermann, pp. 155-188.

Koos, E. L., (1946). *Families in trouble.* New York: King's Crown.

Kraepelin, E., Cited in Rose, A. M. (1966) (Ed.): *Mental health and mental disorder: A sociological approach.* New York: Norton, p. 219.

Leighton, A H., Lambo, T. A., Hughes, C. C., et al., (1963). *Psychiatric disorder among the Yoruba.* Ithaca, NY: Cornell Univ. Press.

Leighton, A. H., (1959). *My name is Legion. Vol. I of the Stirling County Study.* New York: Basic Books.

Leighton, A. H., (1965). Poverty and social change. *Scientific Am., 212(5): 21-27.*

Leighton, A. H, (1971). Cosmos in the Gallup City dump. In: Kaplan, B. H. (Ed.): *Psychiatric disorder and the urban environment.* New York: Behavioral Publications, pp. 1-12.

Leighton, D. C., Harding, J. S., Macklin, D. B., Leighton, A. H., et al., (1963). *The character of danger. Vol. III of the Stirling County Study.* New York: Basic Books.

Lerner, M., (1957). *America as a civilization: Life and thought in the United States today.* New York: Simon and Schuster.

Lewis, J. M. & Looney, J. G., (1983). *The long struggle: Well-functioning working-class black families.* New York: Brunner/Mazel.

Lewis J. M., (1988a). The transition to parenthood: 1. The rating of prenatal marital competence. *Family Process* 27, 149-165. pp. 4-12.

Lewis, J. M., Beavers, W. R., Gossett, J. et al., (1976). *No single thread. Psychological Health in Family Systems.* New York: Brunner/Mazel.

Lewis, J. M., Owen, M. T., Cox, M. J., (1988c). The transition to parenthood III, Incorporation of the child into the family. *Fam Process, 27(4):411-421.*

Lewis, J. M., (1989). *The birth of the family: An empirical inquiry.* New York: Brunner/Mazel.

Lewis, O., (1966). *La Vida: A Puerto Rican family in the culture of poverty – San Juan and New York.* New York: Random House, pp. xlii-lii.

Lidz, T., (1980). The family and the development of the individual. In: C. K. Hofling & J. M. Lewis (Eds.), *The family: Evaluation and treatment.* New York, Brunner/Mazel, pp. 45-70.

Loehlin, J. C. & Nichols, R. C., (1976). *Heredity, environment and personality*. Austin, TX: Univ of TX Press.

London, J., (1904). *People of the abyss*. New York: Nelson.

Malinowski, B., (1927). *Sex and repression in savage society*. London: Routledge and Kagin Paul.

Maziade, M., Caron, C. Cote, R., Merette, C., et al. (1990). Psychiatric status of adolescents who had extreme temperaments at age 7. *Am J of Psychiatry. Vol 147(11), 1531-1536*.

Maziade, M. Caron, C., Cote, R. Boutin, P., et al. (1990). Extreme temperament and diagnosis: a study in a psychiatric sample of consecutive children. *Arch of Gen Psychiatry, Vol. 47(5), 477-484*.

Mead, M., (1968). The implications of culture change for personality development. In Freid, M.: *Readings in anthropology, Vol. II, Cultural anthropology*. New York: Thomas Y. Crowell.

Mead, M., (1978). *Culture and commitment. A study of the generation gap*. New York: Doubleday & Co., Inc.

Mendel, G., (1974). In: Ranier, J. D. The genetics of man in health and mental lillness. *Am Handbook of Psychiatry (2nd ed.), S. Arieti (Ed.)*. Basic Books, Inc.: New York, pp. 134-155.

Miller, I. W., Kabacoff, R. I., Epstein, N. B., Bishop, D. S., et al., (1994). The development of a clinical rating scale for the McMaster Model of Family Functioning. *Family Process,* Vol 33(1), pp. 53-69.

Mintz, S. & Kellogg, S., (1988). *Domestic revolutions: A social history of American family life*. New York: The Free Press.

Moos, R. H., Moos, B. S., (1981) *Family environment scale manual*. Palo Alto, CA: Consulting Psychologists Press.

Moos, R. H., (1990). Conceptual and empirical approaches to developing family-based assessment procedures: Resolving the case of the Family Environmnet Scale. *Fam Process, 29(2):199-208*.

More, L. B., (1913). The cost of living for a wage earner's family in New York City. *The Annals of the American Academy of Political and Social Science*, 48, 104-111.

Murphy, J. M., (1972). A cross-cultural comparison of psychiatric disorder: Eskimos of Alaska, Yorubas of Nigeria, and Nova Scotians of Canada. In Lebra, W. P. (Ed.): *Transcultural research in mental health*. Honolulu: The Univ. Press of Hawaii, pp. 213-236.

Novak, A. L. & Van der veen, F., (1969). Differences in the family perceptions of distrubed adolescents, their normal siblings and normal controls. *Proceedings of the Annual Convention of the American psychological Association, 3, 1968, 481-482*.

Novak, A. L. & Van der veen, F., (1970). Perceived parental relationships as a factor in the emotional adjustment of adolescents. *Proceedings of the Annual Convention of the American Psychological Association, 4(Pt. 2), 1969, 563-564*.

Ogburn, W. F., (1922). *Social change with respect to cultural and original nature*. New York: Viking.

Ogburn, W. F. & Tibbitts, C. (1933). The family and its functions. In: W. F. Ogburn (Ed.) *Recent social trends, Vol. I*. New York: McGraw-Hill, pp. 661-708.

Ogburn, W. F., & Nimkoff, M. F., (1955). *Technology and the changing family*. Boston: Houghton Mifflin.

Olson, D. H., (1993). Circumplex model of marital and family systems. In: Walsh, F. (Ed.) *Normal family processes*. New York: The Guilford Press, 104-137.

Olson, D. H., McCubbin, Barnes, H. I., et al., (1983). *Families: What makes them work*. Beverly Hills, CA: Sage.

Parker, G. (1983). Parental "affectionlss control" as an antecedent to adult depression: A risk factor delineated. *Arch Gen Psychiat, 40, 956-960*.

Parsons, T. & Bales, R. F., (1955). *Family socialization and interaction process*. Glencoe, IL: Free Press.

Parsons, T., (1970). *Social structure and personality*. London: Free Press.

Parsons, T. & Shils, E. A., (1951). *Toward a general theory of action.* Cambridge, MA: Harvard Univ. Press.

Pless, I. B. & Satterwhite B., (1973). *Social Science and Medicine,* 7:613-621.

Reiss D., Costell, R., James, C., et al., (1980). The family meets the hospital: A laboratory forecast of the encounter. *Arch Gen Psychiat, 37, 141.154.*

Reiss D. & Oliveri, M. E., (1991). The family's conception of accountability and competence; A new approach to the conceptualization and assessment of family stress. *Fam Process.*

Robins, L. N., (1966). *Deviant children grown up; a sociological and psychiatric study of sociopathic personality.* Baltimore: Williams & Williams.

Rosenthal, D. & Kety, S., (Eds.) (1968). *The transmission of schizophrenia.* London: Pergamon.

Rosa, M., Beals, J., (1990). Measurement issues in family assessment: The case of the Family Environment Scale. *Fam Process, 29(2):191-198.*

Rowntree, B. S., (1903). *Poverty: A study of town life.* London: Macmillan.

Rüdin, E., (1961). In J. Shields & E. Slater (Eds.), *Handbook of abnormal psychology: An experimental approach.* New York: Basic Books.

Rutter, M. & Madge, N., (1976). *Cycles of disadvantage.* Exeter, NY: Heinemann.

Scarr, S. & Weinberg, R. A. 919910. *The nature-nurture problem revisted: The Minnesota adoption studies.* In: I. E. Sigel 7 G. H. Brody (Eds.) *Methods of family research: biographies of research projects, Vol. I: Normal families.* Hillsdale, NJ: Lawrence Earlbaum Associates, pp. 121-152.

Schwab, J. J., Humphrey, L., (1996). Obsessive Complusive Disorder and the family. In G. Neissen, (Ed.) *Zwangserkrankungen Prävention und Therapie.* Verlag Hans Huber, Dallenwill, Switzerland, pp. 155-166.

Schwab, J. J., Bell, R. A., Stephenson, J. J. (1987). Depressive illnes within the family: Some clinical implications. *Am J Soc Psychiat., 9(5), 341-346.*

Schwab, J., Stephenson, J. J., Ice, J. F., (1993). *Evaluating family mental health: History, epidemiology, and treatment issues.* Plenum Press: New York.

Silver, C. B., (Ed. & Trans.) (1982). *Fredric LePlay: On family, work, and social change.* Chicago: University of Chicago Press.

Siever, M., Liebeman, R., (1990). Family-oriented treatment of children and adolescents. In: R. Michels, A. M. Cooper, S. B. Guze, et al., (Eds.). *Psychiatry, Vol. II.* New York: Basic Books, Inc.

Sigafoos, A., Reiss, D., Rich, J., et al., (1985). Pragmatics in the measurement of family functioning: An interpretive framework for methodology. *Fam Process, Vol. 24(20, 189-203.*

Smith , R. W. & Preston, Fred W., (1977). *Sociology: An Introduction.* NY: St. Martin Press.

Spencer, H., (1882). *The study of sociology.* New York: Appleton.

Steinbeck, J., (1939). *The grapes of wrath.* New York: Viking.

Stephenson-Hinde, J., Akister, J., (1995). The McMaster Model of functioning: Observer and parental reading in a non-clinical sample. *Family Process 34(3):337-347.*

Strauss, M. A. (1979). Measuring intrafamily conflict and violence: The Conflict Tactics Scale. *J Marr and the Family, 41, 75-85.*

Swartz, R. S., (1995). Molecular medicine: Jumping genes. *New England J. of Medicine, 332 (14), April 6, 1995, pp. 941-944.*

The World Almanac and Book of Facts, (1998). Mahwah, NJ. Funk & Wagnalls Corp.

Thomas, W. I., (1923). *The unadjusted girl.* Boston: Little Brown.

Vierkandt, A., (1896). *Naturvölker und kultuvölker ("Natural peoples and cultural peoples").* Lipzig: Duncker & Humbolt.

Walsh F. (Ed.) (1993). *Normal Family Processes,* (2nd ed.), New York: Guilford Press.

Walsh, F., (1982). Preface and conceptualizations of normal family functioning. In: Walsh F. (Ed.) *Normal family processes.* New York: The Guilford Press, xiii-xv and pp. 3-44.

Walsh, F. (1993). Conceptualization of normal family process (2nd ed.). In: F. Walsh (Ed.) *Normal Family Proceses.* New York: The Guilford Press, pp. 3-72.

Weber, M., (1958). *The Protestant ethic and the spirit of capitalism.* (Trans. T. Parsons). New York: Scribner's.

Wertheim, E., (1973). Family unit therapy and the silence and typology of family systems. *Fam Process, 12, 361-376.*

Westley, W. A. & Epstein, N., (1969). *The silent majority: Families of emotionally healthy college students.* San Francisco: Jossey-Bass.

Winokur, G. E., Tsuang, M. T. & Crowe, R., (1982). The Iowa 500: Affective disorders in the relatives of manic and depressed patients. *Am J Psychiatry,* 139 (2), 209-212.

Wynne E. C., (1984). The epigenesis of relational systems: A model for understanding family development. *Family process,* 23(3) 297-318.

Zimmerman, C. C. & Frampton, M. E., (1935). *Family and society: A study of the sociology of reconstruction.* Boston: Van Nostrand.

Zimmerman, C. C., (1947). *The family and civilization.* New York: Harper & Bros.

Zimmerman, C. C., (1972a). 1971 Burgess Award Address: The future of the family in America. *J of Marriage and the Family, 323-333.*

Zimmerman, C. C., (1972b). The future of the family in American: II. The rise of the counter revolution. *Internat. J of Sociology of the Family,* 2(2), 1-9.

CHAPTER 3
The Background and Development of General Living Systems Theory
With the assistance of Roger A. Bell, Ed.D. and John Bell, M.S.S.W.

In this chapter, we look, first, at the development of general systems theory (GST) and family systems theory and therapy during the latter half of the 20th century. Then, we discuss the elaboration of GST as general living systems theory (GLST) by James G. Miller (1978) and describe its basic principles upon which we based our family functioning model and clinical assessments. We conclude with a summary of the application of GLST to psychiatry and to the family.

The Development of GST

The development of GST in the 1950s and 1960s was one of the major advances in scientific theory in the 20th century. In discussing the rise of such an interdisciplinary theory, Ludwig von Bertalanffy (1962) and other theoreticians emphasized that classical science had been concerned almost exclusively with linear causality, one cause $\rightarrow$ one effect, and two-variable problems, and was essentially nomothetic in that it attempted to establish general laws that had explanatory and predictive value from single cases or events. Although such a basically Newtonian theory of science and its applications could solve many problems in physics, its inadequacies, even in the "hard" sciences, were revealed by Einstein's (1922) announcement of the theory of relativity in 1908 and its proof in 1919, and by Niels Bohr's ((1922) description of the uncertainty principle in 1927. Concepts of linearity and two-variable approaches were too restrictive to be used satisfactorily in the rapidly developing biological, social, and behavioral sciences; they could not account for "interactions in multi-variable systems, organization, differentiation, self-maintenance, goal-directedness, and the like" (von Bertalanffy 1966, p. 707). There was a need for theoretical constructs and interdisciplinary theory that did not preclude teleologic considerations.

In his review of the development of systems theories, Buckley (1967) pointed out that, in the 19th century, social and behavioral science research usually was based on 17th and 18th century mechanical models that were seen as "social physics". Its processes were "social mechanics", or based on organic models which postulated that society and its institutions were analogous to organic entities and had a life cycle. Some of those mechanistic and organic concepts included principles fundamental to GST. Buckley noted that de la Mettrie's (1742) "Man a Machine," which has long been held in disrepute as being purely mechanistic, emphasized the systems principle, organization; the major difference between the organic and inorganic or between the living and non-living was the way in which their materials were organized. In the 1860's, Claude Bernard introduced concepts of the regulation of "the animal machine" on principles which have been fully exploited only in 20th century machines--the principles underlying thermostats, electronic controls, and servomechanisms (p. 37). Bernard, who laid the foundation for modern physiology on concepts of systems and equilibria, emphasized the vital importance of regulation of the "milieu interieur", the organism's internal systems.

In the 1870's, in the USA, Josiah Willard Gibbs, the co-founder of "statistical mechanics", conceptualized physicochemical systems. His influence led to L.J. Henderson's formulation of the famous Henderson-Hesselbach equation (1915) for the acid-base equilibrium in the body. The emphasis on systems and the processes needed to maintain them in equilibrium, evidenced by Walter B. Cannon's (1932) homeostasis, stimulated Henderson's interest in social systems. Henderson, a biochemist, a physician, and, later, a sociologist, considered health to be a state of harmony within the organism that was maintained by systems in equilibrium. Likewise, in social systems "every relation is therefore in a state of mutual dependence with everything else, ordinary cause-and effect analysis of events is rarely possible."

Henderson analogized between the regulation of physicochemical systems and social systems. He maintained that the concepts of systems and equilibria, especially those propounded in 1916 by Pareto, the Italian economist-sociologist, in "Mind and Society," were in many respects similar to those of Gibbs' physicochemical system (Henderson, 1935). Pareto presented a conceptualization of the social system that was analogous to the concepts of systems in the natural sciences. Individuals are the components of the social systems, and sentiments, or their manifestations in words and deeds, are the social system's equivalent of, for example, temperature or pressure and their influence on physical and chemical systems. The parts and forces of the social systems are in a state of mutual dependence. Inasmuch as many phenomena cannot be explained in cause and effect terms, it is necessary to analyze mutually dependent variables, especially, "the interactions of individuals in their manifold relations, with their sentiments and interests, with their sayings and doings" (Martindale, 1960, p.185).

Henderson (1935) emphasized: "This system of Pareto's ... makes possible, in some measure, the consideration of all interactions between persons. Like Gibbs' system, it is clear and simple.... Pareto's generalization of the social system is 'The most convenient conceptual scheme now available.... For many purposes a family may be considered as a social system" (Martindale, 1960).

Although the increasing complexity of the modern world, along with the rise of the biological and social sciences, made an expansion of scientific concepts necessary, concepts of social systems were relatively unknown until, according to Russett (1966), in the 1930's, Henderson, "a man of science" fixed the "idea of the social system in the vocabulary of social thought". In 1937, Ludwig von Bertalanffy (1960) presented the principles of GST at a University of Chicago seminar but did not publish until shortly after World War II when "a change in the intellectual climate had taken place, making model building and abstract generalizations fashionable" (von Bertalanffy, 1962, p. 3). He emphasized that the root of GST is the organismic conception in biology, especially the "concept of the organism as an open system which he advanced in the 1920's" (von Bertalanffy, 1962, p. 709). Claude Bernard's concept of the internal milieu and Walter Cannon's principles of homeostasis were fundamental to the development of GST. Some parallel advances in the behavioral sciences that influenced the development of GST were Köhler's (1929) Gestalt theory, and, later, Kurt Lewin's (1951) organismic concepts and basic concepts of field theory.

After World War II, GST incorporated elements of: a) information theory with its emphasis on information as a measurable quantity; b) cybernetics with its principles of feedback; c) game theory with "rational competition between two or more antagonists for more maximum gain and minimum loss" (von Bertalanffy, 1961, p. 3); and, d) decision theory with its analysis of rational choices based on outcome.

Systems concepts have become essentials of a great deal of scientific research. Von Bertalanffy (1962) stated that "The concept of 'systems' is to become a fulcrum in modern scientific thought" (p. 1) inasmuch as such concepts as wholeness or organization that previously were regarded as unscientific or metaphysical, were now amenable to scientific analysis. In discussing systems theory, Ackoff (1959) declared, "We are participating in what is probably the most comprehensive effort to attain a synthesis of scientific knowledge yet made" (p. 1). His optimism was warranted. Systems science has become a major field of study and research, and in the 1990s, systems theory has been seen as having extensive applicability, as evidenced by the development of systems engineering, operations research, and human engineering.

In 1966, von Bertalanffy noted that "the concept of 'systems' has gained increasing influence in psychology and psychopathology." Gordon Allport (1960) referred to it in his revised edition of "Personality as System;" Karl Menninger (1963) used principles of GST in his mental health classic "The Vital Balance;" and Rapaport (1956) noted its "epidemic-like popularity in psychology of open systems" (p. 144).

In accord with the principles of GST, mental disorders are seen as disturbances of "system functions of the psychophysical organism" (von Bertalaffny, 1966, p. 713). For example, cognitive disturbances are products of the mentally ill person's brain, mood disturbances involve deceleration or acceleration of bodily as well as mental processes, and disorders involving lack of motivation are characterized by a reduction of autonomous activity and a loss of spontaneity" (von Bertalanffy, 1966 p. 715).

Von Bertalanffy (1966), concluded that, in the behavioral sciences, systems theory has significance for scientific reasons: a) "the system concept provides a theoretical framework which is *psychophysically neutral*" (p. 716); and b) *Cartesian* dualism and the resulting mind-body problem is incorrect and is obsolete inasmuch as systems concepts provide a common scientific language for physical and mental processes. He emphasized that the theoretical constructs of GST are interdisciplinary and thus transcend the traditional compartments of science and are applicable to many scientific fields.

Buckley (1967) cited von Bertalanffy's (1966) assertion that organism and mechanism have fused in cybernetics and in GST and concluded that GST: a) provided a common vocabulary for behavioral and social disciplines; b) was a technique for evaluating complex organizations; c) could be seen as a synthetic approach to interrelationships of parts; d) was a viewpoint that saw sociocultural systems in terms of information and communication; e) studied relations rather than entities and emphasized process and transition; and f) was operationally definable.

The development of GST in the 1950's gave an impetus to family research. In their review of Family Research 1930-1990, Steggell and Harper (1991) stated that by the 1960's, one-half of family researchers worked with systems theory.

System Theory and the Family

Although the term, system, began to be used in the 19th century as Western Nations became industrialized, it was used only occasionally in reference to the family; neither Edward Shorter's (1975) "The Making of the Modern Family" nor Lawrence Stone's (1977) "The Family, Sex and Marriage in England 1500-1800" mention the family as a system nor refer to a family system. Two examples of the early use of the term are the <u>family</u>

system of employment which Marx (1952) described as the hiring of all the family members (even 4-year-old children) in the sweatshops of England in the 1860s and 1870s, and, in the USA, Dugdale's (1910) description of the use of the family system of discipline or segregation in prisons which he advocated in order to distance the prisoners with good behavior from the incorrigibles and to potentiate constructive peer influences.

Probably, the first use of the term as we now think of it was in Burgess' 1925 description of "The Family as a Unity of Interacting Personalities" in which he enunciated the concept of the family system. Also, during the 1920s, such family scholars as W. F. Ogburn, (1922) began to focus on family functions which they saw as changing rapidly; the compassionate family was becoming prominent and the institutional family was declining.

In the 1950's, the foundation for a "systems approach" to family study and therapy was established by von Bertalanffy's (1956) introduction of GST and Alfred Adler's (1964) support. J.C. Flügel's great, neglected 1921 study and Nathan Ackermann's (1937) pioneering promulgation of "family psychiatry" stimulated increased interest in the family's influence on the development and course of mental disorder. Even the concept of the "schizophrenogenic mother" surfaced. Early studies emphasized Sullivan's (1953) theory of interpersonal relations and object relations theory. Bateson (1956, 1972), Bowen (1988), Fleck (1980), Jackson (1957), Lidz & Lidz (1949), Minuchin (1967), Ruesch (1951), Spiegel and Bell (1989), Wynne (1958), Haley (1963), and their colleagues developed methods for family studies of mental health and illness based on systems concepts and strategies. Jackson and Satir (1961) emphasized an interactionist-oriented approach to family therapy based on the concepts of "human nature" and of the social order being products of communication. The distinctive behavior patterns that characterized a given individual were regarded as developing and being reaffirmed by day to day interactions with associates. An individual's defenses and symptoms, thus, were products of interactions, many of which had been developed within the family system over the early years. Consequently, the primary emphasis in study and treatment needed to be the interactionist-oriented approach to the family inasmuch as any members' reactions were responses that occur in an interpersonal contest.

A second major contributor to family systems study was T. Lidz, who, with R. Lidz, (1949) insisted that the family is a true small group that is unique. The Lidz's differed from Jackson and his colleagues in that they considered the interactionist emphasis to be somewhat limited and, instead, stressed the family's generational and gender differences, especially, members' roles and functions as essentials of study and treatment. As described by Goldenberg and Goldenberg (1990), the systems orientation viewed the family as a group of interrelated parts that could be understood only when seen in their totality, not as individual units. Interactions within the family were considered to be the determinants of behavior and, usually, a family member's mental disorder was seen as evidence of a malfunctioning family system.

In "Foundations of Family Therapy: A Conceptual Framework for Systems Change", Hoffman (1981) described the development of family systems therapy, beginning with the work of Bateson's (1956) group in California in the early 1950's. In her *Comment*, Hare-Mustin (1981) noted that Hoffman pointed out that family therapy was one of the few areas of behavioral science research that was influenced by the epistemological shift away from linear cause and effect systems concepts and circular thinking. Also, Hoffman (1981) offered a synthesis "that weaves together the diverse theories and concepts around which family theory and therapy evolved".

Family theorists and therapists declared strenuously that their concepts and techniques stood in sharp contrast to psychoanalysis with its therapeutic focus on the individual and its seemingly limited concepts. The use of the term, "family systems," spread in epidemic fashion; those who did not subscribe to it enthusiastically were disdained.

Steinglass (1984) emphasized that family systems theory was a conceptual model built around 3 concepts: 1) The family as a system -- "The behavior of the family system is best understood as a product of its organizational characteristics". A member's behavior is a product of various interactive relationships, and "Marital dysfunction is a product of malfunctioning communication channels within the family system" (pg. 583). 2). "Families behave in patterned, predictable fashion because, as systems, they operate according to morphostatic (regulatory) principles.... Families tend to establish a sense of balance or stability and to resist any change" and thus maintain the family equilibrium or family homeostasis described by Jackson (1957). 3) Systemic growth (morphogenesis) holds that families are open systems that "move toward greater organizational complexity over time as a function of the information available to the system" because information reduces uncertainty. Steinglass (1984) stated that the critical feature of "family systems therapy is the therapist's reliance on pattern-recognition vs. deductive reasoning as the basic vehicle for analyzing family behavior and psychopathology" (584). He classified the major schools of family systems in three groups:

1). Structural family therapy (Minuchin, et al., 1967), which places the focus on the family's behavior during the interview. "Pathology is defined in terms in what are thought to be dysfunctional family structures, e.g., problems that arise from maladaptive coalitions, dysfunctional boundary permeability, and inappropriate emotional distance of family members, one to another".

2). Strategic family therapy, which focuses mainly on symptom behavior by analyses of intra-session behaviors. Therapeutic techniques include the assignment of tasks and correctives and the use of paradoxical interventions (Erikson, 1978) Selvini-Palozzoli and Associates (1978).

3). Intergenerational approaches by Bowen and associates (1961) that used family genograms to identify patterns of relationships and behaviors. Their focus has been on triangulated interaction patterns and relationships and on relationships characterized by fusion not differentiation.

In the 1960-1990 era, numerous studies were based on systems concepts. In some ways, the newly developed family systems therapies of the 1950's and 1960's broadened the then relatively narrow focus of many individual psychotherapies; however, frequently, "systems" was neither defined nor described. Bowen (1988) declared that the term, systems, being was used so indiscriminately that it had become almost meaningless.

Family systems theory and therapy were attacked on two fronts. First, in the 1970's, the causes and treatment of mental disorder began to be seen as resulting not from just a defective family system, but from genetic and other biological factors, as evidenced by early findings from twin and other studies and the effectiveness of psychotropic medications. The second was the reaction to strict allegiance to popular "systems" theories that developed in the 1980's and the increasing acceptance of the tenets of postmodernism as evidenced, for example, by the use of family narratives and the tardy recognition of differential gender issues and of families being subjected to socioeconomic and other external stressors.

Systems theorists and therapists responded. They proclaimed that the increasing problems of alcoholism, drug dependence, and mental disorders, along with both the extensive character and social pathologies and the prevailing family stress and instability, were all attributable to dysfunctional family systems (Bradshaw, 1998). During the late 1970's and 1980's, when the "culture of complaint" and the "blame mentality" pervaded American society, enthusiastic systems theorists and therapists even insisted that 90% of American families were "dysfunctional". Nevertheless, the reaction to the strict systems concepts and strategies has been accelerated by Lynn Hoffman (1990) and others' renunciation of the established principles and practices of systems theory and therapy in favor of the new postmodernist theories and approaches.

Rosenblatt (1994) maintains that the literature of family therapy over the past 30 years has been filled with descriptions of the therapeutic use of metaphor to facilitate family change. In his analysis of the theoretical metaphors that "are the bases for thinking about family systems" he stated that in the "transfer of meanings and entailments from one domain to another", the metaphors were "precious tools" but, like all metaphors, they can be limiting. For example, the family systems metaphor can obscure individual responsibility. Also, the metaphor of the family system, fundamental to systemic family therapy, may make it difficult to detect random events and easy to overlook the importance of precedents in family life. Systemic metaphors "may blur different situations in which it might be more useful or ethical to see linear cause and effect instead of system circularity". Specifically, the metaphor of the family boundary can obscure the artificiality of the concept and its neglecting, for example, what happens at the margins. Also, the systems metaphors of both generational structure and gender structure, as well as such concepts as triangulation and family coalitions, can be constraining.

Rosenblatt maintained that new metaphors need to be constructed. He suggested the metaphor of the family as a container, and also that thinking of "the family as a tapestry in process" enables one to see families as still emerging in patterns and textures that unfold out of recurrences ("grocery shopping, opening the mail, paying bills, etc.) and weaving additional family material. The tapestry metaphor avoids the metaphor of family structure along with those such as family differentiation, gender structure, and coalitions that obscure the ever changing nature of family relationships and make it difficult to gain perspectives and see how family structures are never complete. For example, certain families function well at the seemingly pathological extremes of differentiation or of cohesion.

Feminists and social scientists also loudly criticized the concept of the family system because it was considered an entity in itself that ignored issues of gender, class, and race, and was basically cybernetic and mechanistic. Criticism mounted as critics maintained that such principles of family systems theory as power differentials were "myths" and that some systems concepts, such as seeing family violence as evidence of a dysfunctional sadomasochistic relationship, were rationalizations for the status quo that blamed the abuser and the abused equally. The so-called objectivity and neutrality of the therapist were declared fictional. Also, the family systems' views of patients' symptoms as often functional (necessary in order to stabilize the family system) were dismissed as simplistic, if not fallacious. Finally, family systems theory was indicted for not having a cultural or historical context as well as for embracing ontological descriptions of the world and of the structure of reality. Thus, systems theory and therapy are being deemed outmoded and inadequate.

In "Constructing Realities: An Art of Lenses", Hoffman (1990) described her "move away from a cybernetic-biological analogy of family-systems therapy to family therapy that has many of its roots in social construction theory.... In therapy, we now listen to a story and then we collaborate with the persons we are seeing to invent other stories or other meanings for the stories that are told." This development of a family narrative accepts the multiple influences of race, class, gender, family and language, and leads to meaningful explanations of and compromise, but useful, solutions to marital and family problems.

General Living Systems Theory (GLST)

James G. Miller (1978), who developed (GLST) from GST during the past 50 years, emphasized that its aims are to eliminate disciplinary boundaries and to provide an integration of biological and social approaches to "the nature of man, and a new approach to psychopathology, diagnosis, and therapy" (p. 75). He defined a system as "a set of units with relationships among them. The state of each unit is constrained by the state of other units.... A concrete system...is composed of multiple constituent units that are themselves systems at a lower level... (and) are studied by physical and biological scientists... (whereas) abstracted systems are topics of study by personologists and social scientists. Examples of units of concrete systems are parts of an automobile or human organs, while the units of abstract systems are abstracted or selected (e.g. roles or relationships) by researchers for study" (pp. 75-76). Information is "a signal, symbol, message, or pattern of a message as it is used in its technical meaning in communications theory". Markers carry information from a sender to a receiver; examples are writing paper, radio waves, and DNA. "Money is a special sort of information that flows in social systems" (p 76).

Living systems are open systems that maintain negative entropy (negentropy) by taking in more complex units of matter-energy or higher levels than they output. Miller emphasized the uniformities of living systems at various levels because they are composed of molecules containing carbon and certain amino acids that constitute protein, and live in a water-oxygen world. "Moreover, they all have arisen from the same primordial genes or DNA template (and have been) diversified by evolutionary change" (p. 76). Consequently, survival of both complex and simple organisms is dependent upon their carrying out similar subsystem processes resulting in "formal identities across levels of systems". Life is conceptualized as an emergent, a characteristic of complex organisms that emerged at the level of the cell. "At the organism level, with the evolution of man, the capacity to use symbolic language emerged" (p. 77).

One of Miller's major emphases is on the conceptualization of all living systems as being hierarchically organized according to levels, e.g. atoms, cells, organs, organisms, group, etc. The functioning of each is dependent on the functioning of the same 19 essential matter-energy and/or information subsystems.

Structure and process are essentials of all living systems and their subsystems. Structure refers "to the arrangement of a system's subsystems and components in three-dimensional space at a given moment of time"; an example is the proximity of the sense organs to the brain. Subsystem processes (actions) are not "limited to a single component but may be dispersed into a number of components" which can cover a range of components; for example, the pancreas has both a digestive and an endocrine function. Prostheses (e.g. dentures, pacemakers) carry out many functions; for the family, grandparents may be thought of as prostheses when they assist with parenting tasks. Subsystem structures and/or processes may have or may develop pathologies which produce impairments.

Subsystems

All living systems must carry out the 19 critical subsystem processes needed to survive and to perpetuate themselves. The 19 consist of 3 sets: the 8 that process matter-energy, the 9 that process information, and the 2 that process both. As shown in Table 1, for the family as a system the analogous matter-energy and information subsystems, along with some examples of the structure, process, and pathologies of each are paired across the left and right columns (Miller and Miller, 1980).

The subsystem processes in the family system are illustrated by the following examples adapted from Miller and Miller (1980).

The 8 matter-energy processing subsystems are:

1. The ingestor that brings matter-energy across the boundary from the environment.

   Structure -- Components are members who bring matter-energy into the family

   Process -- Traditionally, a division of labor with the women responsible for shopping for groceries and clothing, and the men for tools, automobiles, etc., but there is now increased sharing of these tasks.

   Pathologies-- Bringing in inadequate or inappropriate food or clothing, excessive time shopping, conflicts about selection of food or clothing.

2. The distributor that carries inputs to and/or outputs from the subsystems around the system to various components -- blood and blood vessels are distributors;

   Structure -- Components are family members who distribute matter-energy to each other. Artifacts are cars, delivery services, etc.

Process --   Adults usually do most of the distributing except for special occasions when, for example, a child "passes out the gifts."

Pathologies --   Unequal distribution of food, toys, clothing among the children or the giving of unsuitable drink to family members.

3. The <u>converter</u> changes inputs for use; for example, conversion is carried out by cooking and in organs and cells by such physical and chemical processes as the chewing, and the enzymatic digestion of food;

Structure --   Components are all family members except the small children. When neighbors and relatives help with cooking, the subsystem function thus is dispersed. Food processors are artifacts.

Process --   Traditionally, a division of labor with women doing the cooking but, increasingly, men are sharing this task.

Pathologies --   Improper cooking with lack of cleanliness and infectious diseases resulting.

4. The <u>producer</u> synthesizes materials for growth or repair of damage (e.g. wound healing) to the system, or provides "energy for moving... the system's outputs of products, wastes, or information markers to its suprasystem (next higher system -- e.g. the family is the individual's suprasystem)" (p. 78). This subsystem often is downward dispersed: cells carry out many of the chemical processes for organisms, and workers are the producers in factories;

Structure --   Components are the adults and children who maintain the home and/or take care of family members' health. Artifacts are the instruments and tools.

Process --   Activities/duties are taken over or allocated on the basis of sex and age roles, but often there is sharing, and in busy, urban/suburban families, much of the producing is dispersed to outside services.

Pathologies --   Inadequate upkeep of the home to the extent that it is depressing or dangerous.

5. The <u>storage</u> subsystem retains deposits of matter/energy in the organism and home and thus stores supplies for future use;

Structure --   Members are responsible for storing and maintaining food, clothing, etc.

Process --   Groceries, clothing, tools, etc. are stored for future use. Also, usually the process is upwardly dispersed to supermarkets and department stores that maintain stores of goods.

Pathologies -- Cannot find needed things, spoilage or damage, accidents from clutter of unstored tools.

6. The extruder carries matter-energy out of the system; e.g., extrusion of bodily wastes via the excretory organs and, in societies, trash removal systems for a community;

Structure -- Components are family members. Artifacts consist of garbage cans.

Process -- All members and family pets put out wastes.

Pathologies -- Accumulation of waste and home is unaesthetic.

7. The motor subsystem moves the system or its parts around the environment. The automobile is the motor for the family; the transportation industry moves persons in the community.

Structure - Components are family members who drive the automobile, ride bicycles, etc. Use of buses is an example of upward dispersal. Artifacts are cars, boats, baby carriages.

Process -- Families travel on vacations, go to work or school together, etc.

Pathologies -- Inadequate transportation facilities, failure to coordinate schedules, conflicting choices.

8. The supporter "maintains the spatial relationships among components" (p. 78); e.g. bones form the supporter for organisms, a house for a family.

Structure -- Houses, furniture, automobiles.

Process -- Provides rigid support and shelter for the family

Pathologies -- Insufficient space with crowding.

The 9 information processing subsystems are:

1. The input transducer that brings information on markers into the system-- cells' input transducers are their receptors, the families' can be their television sets.

Structure -- Components are family members who receive information from work or school and report/discuss it. The process is upwardly dispersed when messages are delivered by a service worker. Artifacts are the radio, telephone, and the internet.

Process -- The members' memory and coding capabilities allow for omissions, distortions, and errors.

Pathologies -- Deliberate falsification, distortion or withholding of information.

2. The internal transducer subsystem receives markers from other subsystems and carries information about need for alterations of activity. Persons who report to groups are the internal transducer components for organizations;

Structure --   Components are all family members although the mother usually knows most about how other subsystems are functioning.

Process --   Members discuss what is happening and express feelings about events, family members, and the self.

Pathologies --   Common in families and can be serious. Members who cannot/will not express feelings contribute to pathology by reducing the function of this important subsystem.

3. The channel and net comprise the routes whereby information is transmitted throughout the system. Examples in organisms are neural pathways, in families' person-to-person communication;

Structure --   Components are family members who transmit information from the input transducer and internal transducer subsystems to other members. Members may communicate via computers. Artifacts are telephones; often, process is upwardly dispersed to the media.

Process --   All family members are in the net but all channels may not be open; information may not go equally over all channels or be largely one-way, e.g. from parent to oppositional child.

Pathologies --   Are common; members' coalitions exclude others or emotional distress may interrupt the flow.

4. The decoder changes information from the input transducer or internal transducer into "a private code that can be used internally by the system." In organisms, sensory information is decoded in its passage through the central nervous system. In groups, the decoder translates information from the outside;

Structure --   Components are members who explain the meaning of an input to the family.

Process --   Parents explain messages/events to the children in accord with the family language.

Pathologies --   Failure to decode restricts learning, or distorted explanations lead to paranoid views.

5. The associator subsystem "carries out the first stage of the learning process (by) forming enduring associations among items of information in the system" (p. 79). As Miller and Miller (1980) explain, groups are dependent on the members' associative capacities to carry out this subsystem process;

Structure --   Components are family members who make critical associations (first stage of learning) to increase others' understanding of information.

Process --   Family members interact e.g., by discussions at dinner or helping children with homework.

Pathology --   Is mainly the inability or failure of family members to associate information in ways that increase understanding and learning.

6. The memory subsystem stores information and carries out the second stage of learning inasmuch as the process includes both storage and retrieval of information. For individuals, the brain is the organ of memory as are the minutes of meetings for groups;

Structure --   Components are family members who store information in their own nervous systems, and/or who keep family records or photograph albums. Financial records and birth certificates are artifacts.

Process --   Information storage has 4 functions: a) reading into storage; b) maintaining it in storage; c) loss and alteration in storage; and d) retrieval.   Monetary "information" is stored in banks.

Pathologies --   Include losing records or not being able to store enough money for family needs/emergencies.

7.   The decider is an executive subsystem; the 4 stages of its process are: identification of purposes, and their analysis, synthesis, and implementation.   In humans, the brain makes decisions; in organizations, executives do so.

Structure --   Components are family member(s), who make decisions for the family.   In patriarchal families, the father controls decision-making. In modern families, parents share or divide decision-making with the wife/mother making decisions about the children and the husband/father making financial decisions, but increasingly, there is more equality in decision making.

Process --   The decision process has 4 stages: a) setting goals; b) analyzing their desirability and feasibility of alternatives; c) synthesizing, or determining strategy for problem solving; and d) implementing.

Pathologies --   Appear with failure to decide about cost-effectiveness or one person's making arbitrary decisions; decision-making often is irrational and power struggles may determine outcomes (Miller and Miller, 1980).

8. The encoder subsystem processes information brought by other subsystems so that it can be interpreted. It makes the "private" code public. In families, encoding explains or alters "personal" messages so that they are acceptable.   Organizations' speech writers or public information offices function as encoders;

Structure --	Components are family members who transact family "business" for example, by writing about the mortgage or dealing with school formalities.
Process --	Involves a change from family language to that suitable outside the home and often involves dealing with the suprasystem. Encoding is upwardly dispersed when accountants prepare tax forms.
Pathologies --	Arise when messages are distorted during encoding or do not convey critical information; resulting losses impair functioning of other family subsystems.

9. The <u>output transducer</u> puts out information/markers to others in the environment. Telephone messages, letters, and even hand signals are output transductions, as is blushing. Spokespersons are output transducers for groups.

Structure --	Components are family member(s) who pay bills or handle family affairs by transducing information from family to environment.
Process --	Examples are contacting schools, handling family business, voting.
Pathology --	Results from failure to comply with financial/other demands.

The <u>2 subsystems that process both matter-energy and information</u> are:

1. The <u>reproducer</u> that gives rise to other similar systems. The reproducing process "involves transmission of information -- the blueprint, template, or charter of the new system -- and the organization of matter-energy to compose the new systems" (Miller, 1978, p. 77). The mating dyad is the family reproducer, and information that provides for a charter is the reproducer of a corporation. The reproducer is the only subsystem not necessary for survival of the individual but is necessary for perpetuation of the species.

Structure --	Components are the man and woman; wedding rings are artifacs;
Process --	The mating dyad reproduces individuals (not families) who become members of new families and the process in the family involves transmitting values and establishing rules.
Pathologies --	Infertility, incestuous matings, or bigamy with legal problems, failing to foster healthful development.

2. The <u>boundary</u> at the perimeter of the system holds the components together, protects from exterior forces, and allows for passage of matter-energy/information to and from the environment. Examples are, for the

organism, the skin that prevents excessive input or output, and for a group, a doorkeeper.

Structure --	Components are the members of the family except infants. Their boundary is the dwelling. But the information boundary "is continuous in space-time" by virtue of the use of telephones (artifacts), etc. (p. 151).
Process --	Boundaries function as barriers, filters, or selectors of the flow of matter-energy and information that cross the boundary and thus "maintain a steady-state differential between the interior of the system and its environment."
Pathologies --	Failing to exclude intruders with loss of privacy, poor protection of children in the yard, or impact of media on adolescents.

Subsystem processes are limited by: a) the rate at which matter-energy information is processed; b) the amount that can be processed per unit of time; c) the number of omissions and errors made in the processing; d) the meaning of the information processed; and e) costs to the systems of carrying out the process.

Inasmuch as living systems are open systems, they have dynamic relationships with their environments with which they exchange matter-energy and information. Systems and subsystems maintain steady states with their suprasystems as well as with their internal environments. Either deficient or excessive input or output can be stressors that strain the system or subsystems which then require adjustment processes to maintain health and ensure survival. The term, adjustment process(es), is applicable to both matter-energy and information because of their parallel actions

Adjustment processes maintain a steady state by altering the rate of inputs or outputs by both positive and negative feedback. At five levels -- cell, organ, organism, group, and organization -- information input overload is handled by similar adjustment processes although they obviously vary in complexity according to the level and the subsystem involved. As the rate of information input increases, the system attempts to increase its processing but, when overloaded, shows evidence of strain as it adjusts, "at first, by randomly omitting some of the signals in the input (of) information" (Miller, 1978, p. 81). Later omissions are compounded by processing errors.

Adjustment processes are classified as matter-energy input, internal transmission, or output, and as information input, internal transmission, or output. Adjustment processes entail some "cost" to the system that, in organisms, may involve expenditures of money (a type of information) or loss of time. Also, adjustment costs may become pathological (e.g. compulsive checking to ensure safety), or are fundamentally pathological (e.g. use of alcohol). With increasing stress, a greater number of subsystems become involved until "no further components with new adjustment processes are available (and) the functioning of the system collapses" (Miller, 1978, p. 82). We are seeing many families in which there is stress and strain from information input overload: adolescents are acting out and parents are complaining of stress, anxiety, depression, and/or alcohol dependence.

The Application of GLST to Psychiatry

GLST has both conceptual and clinical applicability to psychiatry. Conceptually, it offers a resolution of the mind-body dilemma by viewing the mind as being for information processing and the body for matter-energy processing, and by acknowledging their interactions. Other issues concern decoding and encoding that involve, for example, the interpretation of messages from the environment as being either benign or threatening, the evaluation of interpersonal communication, or the expression of thoughts and emotions.

Karl Menninger (1963) outlined a GLST theory of personality that has four major schemes: a) adjustment, or individual-environmental interactions; b) the organization of living systems; c) psychological regulation and control (ego psychology); and d) motivation, especially to avoid or lessen anxiety. The ego is the decider subsystem. The id's drives toward love and aggression "are concerned with the governance of the organism's subsystems" (p. 82) (decoding information, output transducing, reproducing). The introjected superego "is concerned with the governance of the organism's suprasystem" (e.g. staying within speed limits in the community, or reporting all income to the government for tax purposes).

Pathologies result from either insufficient or excess matter-energy and/or information inputs, from inputs of inappropriate or maladaptive matter-energy or information, or from abnormalities in the internal matter-energy and/or internal information processes. Examples at five levels of stressors altering steady states and producing strains because adjustment processes do not cope with them adequately are:

1. Cell level -- addictive drugs affect enzymes and thus alter decoder processes and the interpretation of information;
2. Organ level -- thromboses occlude arteries and thus alter the brain function by reducing matter-energy;
3. Organism level -- Menninger identified pathological adjustment processes at 5 degrees of internal-processing pathology: a) nervousness or mild adaptive discontent; b) neurotic disorders; c) aggression and violence; d) psychotic states with denial of the validity of environmental inputs; and e) extreme disorganization or suicide. Pathologies at the level of the organism include failure of adjustment processes because of lack of

information input (e.g. psychosis with sensory deprivation), or exhaustion of adjustment processes by excessive information inputs (e.g. crowding);

4. Group level -- lack of matter-energy leads to conflict and excess to strain; centralization of the channel-net with only one person carrying out the information processing for the group is conducive to group psychopathology (e.g. gang warfare); and excess matter-energy and/or information inputs from chronically ill person(s) or in-laws in the home produce pathology;

5. Organization level -- either lack of or excess matter-energy and/or information produces problems/inadequate performance.

GLST is applicable to diagnosis and therapy. Miller and Miller (1980) emphasized 3 diagnostic principles: a) every process should be accurately identified with the structure that carries it out; b) it is necessary to trace routes of matter-energy and information flow; and c) "The existence of the 19 critical subsystems in all living systems can serve as a basis for agreement among diagnosticians" inasmuch as the functioning of each subsystem can be tested to ascertain if it is in a steady state. Identification of the type/location of subsystem malfunction often is a prerequisite for treatment. Inadequate matter-energy or information inputs can be remedied, for example, by treating deficiency states with vitamins or, in delirium, correcting perceptual conditions by spectacles or hearing aids.

Diagnostic strategies include: a) identification of each of the 19 subsystems; b) specification of the variables to be measured; c) formulating and using indicators that make quantitative readings of the variables; d) systematic examination of each subsystem; and e) examination of abnormal variables in order to identify pathological syndromes. Our GLST Family Functioning Assessment provides for a comprehensive clinical evaluation of each of those 5 strategies.

In family therapy based on principles of GLST, the goals are to change structures and processes in the family and/or the environment to relieve strains and allow subsystems to return to their normal range of function. In the therapeutic process, the family is seen "not simply as a set of individuals but as a system in itself made up of interacting human beings" (Miller and Miller, 1980, pp. 175-76). Also, it is possible to look at each member as a system at the organism level and to determine whether pathology lies at the member (organism) level, the family (group) level, at the community/suprasystem (organization) level, or at all of those levels when the family is in the midst of such social pathologies as drugs, crime, and poverty.

Thus, GLST does more than provide a conceptual or descriptive approach to the family. It offers "a means for explaining and predicting interpersonal and family processes... by testing relationships among various subsystem variables in one or more subsystems" (p. 176). Methodical research at various levels of living systems and an analysis of their complexity have the potential to increase our understanding of families and social groups.

GLST and the Family

In "The Family as a System," James and Jessie Miller (1980) pointed out that principles of GLST relate the family, as a system, to the other environmental, social, and biological systems with which it interacts. They defined the family as a group level system with "a set of organisms, commonly called <u>members</u>, who, over a period of time or multiple interrupted periods, relate to one another face-to-face" (p. 145).

Table 1 – The Critical Subsystem

A. Both matter-Energy and Information
1. The Reproducer -- Gives rise to similar subsystems -- (tested by asking family about transmission of values, rules, and discipline of children).
2. The Boundary -- holds components of system together and protects them -- (tested by asking about visitors to the home and regulating use of telephone and regulating television).

B. Systems paired

Process Matter-Energy	Process Information
3. Ingestor -- Brings matter-energy across into organism (tested by asking about who brings in groceries).	11. Input transducer -- Brings markers-information)--into the organism (tested by asking about who brings "news" into the family").
	12. Internal transducer -- Receives and processes information from other subsystems (tested by asking about handling information within the family and dealing with feelings).
4. Distributor -- Carries goods and news around the system (tested by asking about handing out goods or by giving attention to others).	13. Channel and Net -- The network for transmitting information within the system (evaluated by observation of videotape).
5. Converter -- Changes material for use (tested by asking about cooking).	14. Decoder -- Alters information for family use (tested by who explains to family members).

6. Producer -- Forms associations, repairing (tested by asking about care of home, cleaning, care of yard, etc.).

7. Storage -- Retains various forms of matter-energy (tested by asking about who stores goods and adequacy of available space for storage).

15. Associator -- Forms associations among items of information in the system (not tested).

16. Memory -- Stores various sets of information (tested by asking about keeping diaries, photographs, etc.).

17. Decider -- Executive receiving and transmitting information within the system (tested by asking about how/who makes the decisions for the family, handling money, etc.).

18. Encoder -- Alters family information for transmittal to others outside the family (tested by asking who tells others about family news/activities.

8. Extruder -- Transmits matter-energy out of the system (tested by asking about who removes garbage/wastes).

9. Motor -- Moves the system around the environment (tested by asking about family transportation, driving).

10. Supporter -- Maintains spatial relationships within the family (tested by asking about number of rooms/bedrooms, space).

19. Output transducer -- Puts out information into the environment (tested by asking who pays the bills, attends PTA meetings).

Adapted from the "The Family as a System: by (Miller and Miller, 1980) and simplified for use in this research.

A family group is distinguished from an organization by not having echelons. Kinship systems are not considered families because they are abstract or conceptual systems of related persons who, for example, can regulate marriage and prescribe behaviors. In contrast, families are concrete systems "whose organism components interact in carrying out matter-energy and subsystem processes" (p. 147). The 19 subsystems processes are carried out by the members who are components of many, if not all, of the family's subsystems. The family's suprasystem is a kinship or a community group.

A systems analysis of the family, therefore, includes a review of its normal structure and process and an evaluation of each subsystem and of the system as a whole for pathology. It is necessary to ascertain which members constitute the various subsystems, which subsystems are dispersed to other living systems (e.g. relatives), whether artifacts or prostheses are used, and the costs in matter-energy, information, money, or the time needed for functioning/adapting.

Family Adjustment Processes

As Miller and Miller (1980) explain, such adjustment processes as both negative and positive feedback guide the components' use of information to change future outputs. Negative feedback decreases the number of inputs or slows them and reduces strain in the system. Positive feedback uses information about past inputs and increases outputs. Thus, negative feedback, if not excessive, maintains a steady state in the system, but positive feedback does not do so inasmuch as it tends both to diminish control of the system and to increase activity so that a subsystem malfunctions or even fails. In families, internal feedback mechanisms among components (family members) enhance adjustments, as does external feedback that flows into the system. Family members can modify each other's behaviors when cues are accurately perceived and sensitively received. The resulting interpersonal sensitivity can produce harmony and increase the mental hygiene functions of the family as members make adjustments to reduce interpersonal strain (p. 171).

Members' communications with and reactions to each other are adjustments that modify behaviors and maintain a steady state. Likewise, in the family's interactions with the community and neighbors it receives feedback. A common example of negative feedback is the school counselor's requesting a meeting with family members to discuss an adolescent's behavior problems. When the result is a reduction in disturbed behavior, one can see that the negative feedback from the school led to salutary adjustments in the family system. Miller and Miller (1980) point out that, unfortunately, poverty-stricken, crime-ridden, demoralized communities flood the family system with positive feedback that increases conflict, delinquency, and family violence. The changes in and fragmentation of the family that occur often call for profound adjustments by each member and the group. Essential services, especially for the children, need to be carried out in families of divorce by the remaining members who often are overburdened to the point that the family is considered dysfunctional. An example of pathological adjustment described by Wallerstein (1989) is that of a young child's becoming overburdened when he or she has to become the mother's emotional support following divorce. Or, a widow may become overly dependent on her adult children following her husband's death.

The "empty nest" syndrome with its emotional distress can develop when parents have lost the information inputs and other stimuli supplied by daughters or sons who left home. Conversely, the addition of a family member with the birth of a baby or the return of an adult child to the home after he or she had been "launched," increases inputs and adjustments are required to maintain a steady state. Thus, either the loss or gain of a member can change the rate and quality of family interactions and affect the functioning of subsystem processes and the family system.

According to Miller and Miller (1980), families are integrated "when their multiple, simultaneous, separate processes are under the control of centralized decision-making and work toward common purposes and goals" (p. 173). Over the course of the family life cycle, the degree of integration or family cohesion and marital and sexual satisfaction change as members are added, reach adolescence, seek their own identities, leave the family, become ill, and die. Generally, cohesion and satisfaction tend to be high during the first few years of the family life cycle, and drop to their nadir during the adolescent stage when the teenagers are experimenting with independence, but slowly increase after the children leave home, again to reach a high level as the end of the cycle approaches (Schwab, et.al. 1993).

In concluding their excellent discussion of GLST and the family, Miller and Miller (1980) pointed out that GLST uses terms that are somewhat unfamiliar and may be thought of as jargon. Although they are technical, the terms are neutral and allow for the use of similar concepts and language in various disciplines. Miller and Miller (1980) emphasize that the 19 subsystems critical to the function of the family system have been identified and described and that GLST applies to families in health and disease and during development, and to members' interactions, as well as to diagnosis, treatment, and prevention.

In summary, the application of GST to family study and treatment has had about four decades of acceptance, at times even uncritical acceptance. GLST is a significant development of GST that has been used in research and in work with groups and organizations. Miller (1978) defined the principles and described the concepts of GLST precisely and Miller and Miller (1980) discussed its specific use with families. Our research with the application of GLST to family study thus differs from that of other systems theorists in the past and their work with GST in that it is defined, explicated, and firmly rooted in theory. As described in Chapter IV and presented in the Appendix, we have developed a GLS Assessment Instrument that uses conventional, descriptive language and is pragmatic. We present specific examples of each subsystem's activities to assess whether and how well family members carry out its specific functions, their problems with each subsystem, the severity of the problems, methods of resolution, and satisfaction with them and the results. To the best of our knowledge, we have been the first to apply GLST systematically to family research, as we describe in the next four chapters.

References:

Ackerman, N., (1937). The family as a social and emotional unit. *The Bulletin of the Kansas Mental Hygiene Society.*

Ackoff, R. L., (1959). Games, decisions, and organizations. In *General systems IV, 1959,* pp. 145-150.

Adler, A., (1964). *Problems of neurosis.* New York: Harper and Row.

Allport, G., W., (1960). The open system in personality theory. *J Abnormal and Social Psychiatry,* 61.

Bahr, S. J., (Ed.), (1991). *Family research: A sixty year review, 1930-1990.* Vol. I, New York, Lexington Books, Macmillan Books.

Bateson, G., Jackson, D., Haley, J., et al., (1956). Toward a theory of schizophrenia. *Behavioral Science, 1(4), 231-264.*

Bateson, G., (1972). *Steps to on ecology of mind.* Chandler, Scranton.

Bernard, C., (1865). *Introduction to the study of experimental medicine.* New York: Macmllan (1927).

Bohr, N., (1924). Cited in W. C. Dampier: (1966) *A history of science and its relations with philosophy and religion.* Cambridge, MA: University Press Cambridge, pp. 389-399.

Bowen, M., (1961). Family psychotherapy. *Am. J. Orthopsychiatry,* 31(1): 40-60.

Bowen, M., (1988). Epilogue: An odyssey toward science. In M. E. Kerr and M. Bowen (Eds.): *Family evaluation.* New York: W. W. Norton.

Bradshaw, J., (1998). *Bradshaw and the family.* New York: Bantam Books.

Buckley, W., (1967). *Sociology and modern systems theory.* Prentice Hall, Inc., Englewood Cliffs, NJ.

Burgess, E. W. The family as a social system. In: *The urban community: Selected papers from the proceedings of the American Sociological Society 1925.* Chicago: University of Chicago Press.

Cannon, W., (1932). *The Wisdom of the Body.* New York: W. W. Morton.

Dugdale, R. L., (1910). *The Jukes: A study in crime, pauperism, disease and heredity.* New York: Putnam.

Einstein, A., (1922). The meaning of relativity. Cited in W. C. Dampier (1966): *A history of science and its relations with philosophy and religion.* University Press Cambridge, pp. 398-412.

Erickson, E. H., (1959). Identity and the life cycle. In: *Selected papers.* New York Internat. Univ. Press.

Erikson, K.T., (1978). *Everything in its path.* New York: Harper & Row.

Fleck, S., (1980). The family and psychiatry. In A. M. Freedman and H. I. Kaplan (Eds.),

The comprehensive textbook of psychiatry (3rd ed.). Baltimore: Williams and Wilkins, pp. 13-530

Fleck, S., (1983). A holistic approach to family typology and the axis of DSM-III. *Arch. Gen. Psych.*, 40, 901-906.

Flügel, J. C., (1921). *The psycho-analytic study of the family*. London: Internat. Psychoanalytical Press.

Gibbs, W., (1942). Cited in M. Rukeyer: *Willard Gibbs*. Garden City, NJ: Doubleday, Doran, & Co., Inc.

Goldenberg, I. & Goldenberg, H., (1990). *Family theory: An overview*. Montrey, CA: Wadsworth.

Haley, J., (1963). *Strategies of psychotherapy*. New York, Greene and Stratton.

Hare-Mustin, R. T., (1983). Focusing on relationships in the family. *Harvard Educ. Rev.* 53(2), 203-210.

Henderson, L. J., (1915). *The fitness of the environment*. New York: Macmllan Co.

Henderson, L. J., (1935). *Pareto's General Sociology*. Cambridge, MA: Russell & Russell.

Hoffman, L., (1981). *Foundations of family therapy: A conceptual framework for systems change*. New York: Basic Books, Inc.

Hoffman, L., (1990). Constructing realities: An art of lenses. *Family Process*, Vol. 29, pp. 1-12.

Hofling, C. K. & Lewis, J. M., (Eds.) (1980). *The family: Evaluation and treatment*. New York: Brunner/Mazel.

Jackson, D., (1957). The question of family homeostasis. *Psychiatry Quarterly Supplement*, 31, 75-90.

Jackson, D., Satir, V., (1961). A review of psychiatric developments in family diagnosis and family therapy. In: N. W. Ackerman, F. L. Bentman, S. N. Sherman (Eds.) *Exploring the base for family therapy*. New York: Family Service Association of America.

Köhler, W., (1929). *Gestalt psychology*. New York: Liveright.

La Metterie, J. O. L'Homme machine (1747). Discussed in Durant W. and Durant A. (1965): *The age of Voltaire, The story of civilization IX*. New York: Simon and Schuster, pp. 617-622.

Lewin, K., (1951). Field theory in social science. In D. Cartwright (Ed.), *Social science: selected theoretical papers*. New York: Harper and Row.

Lidz, R. & Lidz, T., (1949). The family environment of the schizophrenic. *Am. J. of Psychiat.*, 106, 332-345.

Martindale, D. (1960). *The nature and types of sociological theory*. Boston: Houghton Mifflin Co.

Marx, K., (1952). *Das kapital*. In R. M. Hutchins (Ed.): *Great books of the western world*. Chicago, IL, Encyclopedia Britannica.

Menninger, K. A., (1963). *The vital balance*. Viking, New York.

Miller, J. G., (1975). General systems theory. In *Comprehensive textbook of psychiatry II, Vol. I*. A. M. Freedman, H. I. Kaplan, B. J. Sadock (Eds.). Williams & Wilkson Co., Baltimore.

Miller, J. G., (1978). *Living systems*. New York, McGraw-Hill, Inc.

Miller, J. G. & Miller, J. L., (1980). The family as a system. In C. K. Hofling & J. Lewis (Eds.): *The family: Evaluation and treatment*, pp. 141-184. New York: Brunner/Mazel.

Minuchin, S., Montalo, B, Guerney, B.G., Jr., et al., (1967). *Families of the slums: An exploration of their structure and treatment*. New York: Basic Books.

Ogburn, W. F., (1922). *Social change with respect to culture and original nature*. New York: Viking.

Paré, D. A., (1996). Culture and meaning: Expanding the metaphorical repertoire of family therapy. *Family Process*, Vol. 35(1), 21-42.

Rapaport, A., (1956). The promise and pitfalls of information theory. In *Behavioral Science I*, 303-315.

Rosenblatt, P.C., (1994). *Metaphors of family systems theory.* New York: Guilford Press.

Ruesch, J., Bateson, G., (1951). *Communication. The social matrix of psychiatry.* New York: W. W. Norton.

Rukeyser, M., (1942). *Williard Gibbs.* Garden City, NY: Doubleday, Doran & Co., Inc.

Russett, C. E., (1968). *The concept of equilibrium in American social thought.* Yale University Press: New Haven.

Schwab, J. J., Stephenson, J. J., Ice, J. F., (1993). *Evaluating family mental health, History, epidemiology, and treatment issues.* New York: Plenum Publishing Co.

Selvini Palozzoli, M., et al., (1978) *Paradox and counterparadox.* New York: Jacob Aronson.

Shorter, E. E., (1975). *The making of the modern family.* New York: Basic Books.

Speigel, J. & Bell, N., (1959). The family of the psychiatric patient. In Silvano Arieti (Ed.), *American Handbook of Psychiatry*, vol. I, pp. 114-149. New York: Basic Books.

Steggell, G. L., Harper, J. M., (1991). Family interactions patterns and communication processes. In *Family Research. A Sixty-Year, 1930-1990 Vol. I,* Stephen J. Bahr (Ed.). Lexington Books: Toronto, p 117.

Steinglass, P., (1984). Family systems theory and therapy: A clinic application of general systems theory. *Psychiatric Annuals*, 14:8. 582-586.

Steinglass, P., (1985). Family systems approach to alcoholism. *Journal of Substance Abuse Treatment*, 2, 161-167.

Stone, L., (1977). *The family, sex and marriage in England 1500-1800.* Weidenfeld and Nicolson: London.

Sullivan, H. S., (1953). *The interpersonal theory of psychiatry.* New York: W. W. Norton.

von Bertalanffy, L., (1950). General system theory, Main currents in modern thought. *General Systems* 1, 1-10.

von Bertalanffy, L., (1952). *Problems of life.* New York, John Wiley & Sons.

von Bertalanffy, L., (1966).. General system theory and psychiatry. In S. Arieti: (Ed.) *American handbook of psychiatry.* Vol. III. New York, Basic Books, pp. 705-720.

von Bertalanffy, L., (1962). General system theory – A critical review. *Yearbook of society general living systems theory,* 7, 1-21.

Wallerstein, J., (1989, Jan. 22). Children after divorce: Wounds that don't heal. *New York Times Magazine*, pp. 18-26.

Wynne, L. C., et al., (1958). Pseudomutality in the family relationships of schizophrenics. *Psychiatry*, 21, 205-220.

CHAPTER 4
Background, Research Methods, and the Epidemiologic Study

Introduction

In the early 1980s, we began to direct our research efforts toward family studies because we were seeing many patients with family problems and we had mounting concern about the well-being of the family. The senior author's work on the epidemiology of the mental disorders during the preceding 20 years supplied a basis for a family research program (Schwab, et al. 1977, 1978). We developed plans to test methods for epidemiologic studies of family well-being, particularly family mental health. As described in the first volume in this series, three other influences coalesced to stimulate our interest in family research (Schwab, Stephenson, Ice, 1993). One was the publication in 1978 of James G. Miller's definitive volume, General Living Systems. Inasmuch as he was the President of the University of Louisville and a Professor in our Department, we were in a favorable position to learn first-hand about systems theory. Another was the development of such instruments for field studies as the Diagnostic Interview Schedule (DIS) that was being used effectively in the Epidemiologic Catchment Area (ECA) studies (Robins, et al., 1979, 1984). The third was the realization that although the ECA studies were both definitive and comprehensive, the results of additional research modeled on them would probably be limited. There was need for the entire field of psychiatric epidemiology to make both a conceptual and a methodologic leap forward. The well-designed ECA studies were supplying new data about the frequency, distribution, and correlates of mental disorder in the general population, but they had not evaluated dynamic group factors. Therefore, in our pilot feasibility study we attempted to raise the level of the epidemiologic unit, conceptually and methodologically, from that of the individual to that of the small group, the family.

In view of the instability of the family at this time and the rapid change in family structure in the USA at the end of the 20th century, it is not possible to present a generally agreed-upon definition of the family. Therefore, for the purposes of our studies, we define the family in GLS terms as a set of individuals living in a household who interact and are bound together by common, shared properties (legal, affectional, or other) (Schwab, et al., 1993, p. 231).

We used three major approaches to study family mental health and well-being comprehensively. First, we conducted a fairly exhaustive review of the history of the family in Western Society during the past 5,000 years and of related studies of family mental health and illness. The second was the centerpiece of our program. We designed a community study and carried out four waves of interviews with a random sample of families from the general population in their homes over a four-year period of time. We were especially interested in the sequential relationships between family organization and functioning and the onset and course of mental illness. Specifically, we looked on one hand at the interactions, associations, and influences between the occurrence of stressful life events (SLE) and/or living with chronic stressors and the characteristics of the family environment, and, on the other, the absence, presence, or development of mental illness symptomatology and/or substance abuse/dependence. Also, we gathered information on what was happening socioeconomically in the community during the years we conducted the study. One of our convictions is that the family is not an isolated social unit but that it influences and is influenced by other individuals and institutions, the community, and the broad sociocultural processes in our society. Therefore, we collected census tract and other social indicator data to obtain information about the families' neighborhoods and communities. General living systems theory (GLST) was especially valuable because it provided a paradigm we could use to evaluate associations between the mental health of family members at one level, family well-being at another, and the influences of the community and society at still another level.

Our third approach was to carry out a retrospective case study of child psychiatry patients and their families from 1923 to 1988 (Schwab, et al., 1993). It was designed to augment our efforts by providing a longitudinal perspective for the community study and also to help tie together our historical, epidemiologic, and clinical efforts. Many of the results of the study of the history of the family in Western Society are presented in the first volume (Schwab et al, 1993). Also, it contains a description of the methods for and the results of the epidemiologic study along with a summary of the historical 1923-1988 case study. However, we have not reported the results of our work with the Bell and Schwab general living systems family functioning assessment instrument that we designed. We used it in the second follow-up (the third wave of our home interviews) and repeated it with a case-control study of 2 groups of families, 8 with a child in treatment at our Bingham Child Guidance Clinic and 8 neighborhood control families. In addition, we have used it with a number of married couples who have consulted us for assessment of problems and therapy. We consider the development and preliminary results of the use of the general living systems (GLS) family functioning model and assessment instrument to be the most important part of our work.

Description of Louisville and Historical Notes

We conducted our research in Louisville, Kentucky, a city in middle America with a metropolitan-area population of almost one million persons. It has a traditional city structure with a center, suburbs, and exurbs and is an appropriate site for a prospective study of families inasmuch as the community is relatively stable. Except for a moderate increase in population, there have been no major demographic changes since World War II. Also, we believed that the study would be acceptable to the community for several reasons. One was that for many years there had been excellent rapport between the University, with its urban mission, and the community . Another was that our research base, the medical school (the eleventh oldest in the United States), is the pride of the city. Third, there had been a marked increase in adolescent suicides in the late 1970s that alarmed the community about mental disorder and relationships between depression and suicide (Shafi and Shafi, 1992). Fourth, previous studies in Louisville (Roper, 1950; Bell & Sundel, 1975; Matheny & Dolan, 1980) had good response rates.

Louisville was one of the first cities to be established west of the Appalachian Mountains. In early 1778, 11 married couples, 26 children, four bachelors, and one Negro slave traveled in rafts down the Ohio River from Redstone, Pennsylvania and established a settlement on the site of present-day Louisville. Thus, the story of Louisville began with families, not explorers or merchants, but men and women and their children who were looking for a place to live and work, and love and grow together. Immigrant groups from France and also from the southern German states, who were fleeing from the turmoil of the French Revolution and the Napoleonic Wars, came to Louisville (named for Louis XVI of France) and Jefferson County (named to honor Thomas Jefferson).

The University of Louisville, the first municipal university in the USA, was chartered in 1798. A number of medical schools were started in the early 1800s but they generally lasted only a few years. In 1837, the Louisville Medical Institute, which was supported by the city, merged with the Louisville Collegiate Institute to become the University of Louisville School of Medicine. In the 1890s, about one-half of all physicians practicing west of the Mississippi River had had some training in Louisville.

From its early years, Louisville was a center for Roman Catholic and major Protestant Churches. The first Archdiocese of the Roman Catholic Church west of the Appalachian Mountains was in nearby Bardstown, Kentucky; in 1841, it was moved to Louisville. In 1845, the Southern Baptist Convention was constituted, and in 1877 the Southern Baptist Theological Seminary moved to Louisville. The Presbyterian Theological Seminary of Louisville was founded in 1893, and since 1989, Louisville has been the national headquarters of the Presbyterian Church. During the 19th century, many monasteries, nunneries, retreats, and shrines were built throughout the area. During the Civil War, Kentucky remained in the Union but sentiments were ambivalent. It was a border state; sometimes family members fought on opposing sides. There were some major battles in the southern part of the state and some guerrilla skirmishing near Louisville. After the War, Louisville became an Ohio River town and, by the 1890s, a railroad hub.

During World War I, "Louisville changed overnight from a big little city to a little big city" (Riebel, 1956, p. 149). It suffered during the Great Depression because it was the home of a number of diverse industries, but it expanded rapidly during World War II and continued to attract industries afterwards. It had a stable economy until the sharp recession of the early 1980s.

During the years in which we did most of our fieldwork, 1981 to 1986, Louisville underwent extensive economic changes. (Coomes, P. personal communication, 1991) It lost its relatively heavy concentration of industries, and unemployment was high during the 1980s. Recovery from the recession did not begin until about 1985; however, even though much heavy industry had moved away, most people did not leave Louisville for jobs elsewhere as they did in many parts of the Midwest. The population was stable because it tended to be relatively old and many continued to have jobs because of their seniority. Also, many people felt "settled," owned their homes, and had relatively low mortgage payments. But, job loss was the major economic theme during the years of our study. We were interviewing families at a time when there was little construction and when the recession in this region was at about its worst. That unfortunate fact supports the reliability of our use of the city and county directories as sources for our sample inasmuch as they probably reflected the actual households in the area to a truer extent than they would during a period of rapid urban and suburban building. In the late 1980s, the city came out of the recession as employment increased fairly steadily.

In 1980, the population of Jefferson County was 685,004--urban 654,938 and rural 30,066. There were slightly more females, 359,392, than males, 325,612. The median age was 30.1 years, for males, 28.8 years, and for females, 31.7. About 85% of the population were whites; almost all of the remaining, 109,702 were blacks. The total number of families was 182,954; the mean number of persons per family was 3.22.

As explained in our earlier volume (Schwab, et al., 1993) we obtained background data on Louisville and on the sociodemographic and major health characteristics of the census tracts in which our families lived from the Needs Assessment Study conducted by Warheit and Bell (1983). Also, Bell, Warheit, Holzer and their colleagues had conducted social indicator analyses of the greater Louisville area in the late 1970s that included an analysis of 52 social indicators, a rank-ordering of all census tracts in the County, an evaluation of socioenvironmental risk factors for mental disorders, and the development of profiles of areas of greatest need for mental health services. (Bell, Warheit, Buhl, et al., 1978).

The Epidemiologic Study

Approaches and aims

For the epidemiologic study, one of our first tasks was to develop methods. To the best of our knowledge, such a study had not been carried out previously although there had been studies of clinic families and of volunteer families. We needed to adapt instruments and procedures, such as those that we had used in our earlier epidemiologic studies of individuals, for use with families, and we also needed to develop new approaches and methods so that we could obtain data at the level of the family as well as the individual. We were funded by the National Institute of Mental Health (NIMH) Grant No. MH 36140, 1983-1985) for three years in order to test methods for epidemiologic studies of families and to evaluate the feasibility of such studies by carrying out research with a random sample of 50 families over time.

The specific aims were to: a) gather, manage, and analyze individual and family-level data over time; b) evaluate conceptual, methodologic, and analytic issues in family research; c) assess both ongoing (step-by-step procedural) and overall feasibility; and d) use the findings to establish a basis for longitudinal family studies. We hoped that our conceptualizations and methods would be tested by other researchers and that the findings could be used to formulate hypotheses for future family studies.

Issues

The main conceptual issues included defining the family unit for study, designing a family functioning model, and developing family-level measures of symptomatology, health, and stress that, for example, went beyond just averaging all members' scores to arrive at a family mean score inasmuch as such methods contain obvious distortions and there is a loss of information involved in averaging. When possible, we used raters' discussions and consensus to arrive at whole family scores and ratings and found they provided a pragmatic, clinically-based feasible way to move from individual-level data to family-level data. Also, that approach allowed us to apply our extensive clinical experience to evaluations of symptoms, persons, and families.

The procedural issues included the following steps: 1) the recruiting and training of field interviewers; 2) using the table of random numbers to select a random sample of households from the Louisville and Jefferson County Directories; 3) designing and developing a comprehensive interview schedule that would include essential personal and family history data, symptoms as assessed by the Diagnostic Interview Schedule (DIS), physical and mental health status, an SLE inventory, attitudes toward marriage and the family, and characteristics of the family as measured by the Family Environment Scale (FES) (Moos and Moos, 1981). We modified the adult schedule for use with the children and adolescents, and with children used the Diagnostic Interview Schedule for Children (DISC) (Costello, Edelbrock, Dulcan et al., 1984). Other diagnostic instruments we used were: a) the Center for Epidemiologic Studies Depression Scale (CES-D) (Radloff, 1977); b) the Short Michigan Alcohol Screening Test (SMAST) (Selzer, Vinokur & Van Roijen, 1975); c) the Child Behavior Checklist (CBCL) (Achenbach & Edelbrock, 1983); and d) the Denver Development Screening Test (DDST) (Frankenburg, Dodds, Fandal, et al., 1975). 4) Sending a letter and supporting documents to eligible families to inform them briefly that they had been selected for a family health study that was supported by prominent city and University officials as well as by the NIMH. 5) Having two interviewers visit the household one week after the letter had been mailed in order to explain the project, obtain written informed consent, and make an appointment for the first interview. Also, the interviewers obtained preliminary information about the composition of the household, relationships, etc. 6) At all 3 times (T-1, T-2, and T-3), 2 or 3 interviewers went to the families' homes and interviewed each adult and child individually (separated from each other) for about 1½ hours. We gathered information on major sociodemographic factors, including occupation and income, health histories and current health status, marital and sexual satisfaction/dissatisfaction levels, and symptoms and indicators of illness by using the various scales and inventories mentioned.

Criteria for Symptomatic Status

A person was considered to be symptomatic if he/she met any of the following criteria:
1) A CES-D score of 17 plus;
2) On the DIS -- a) 4 or more depression symptoms; b) 3 or more panic symptoms; and c) 3 or more symptoms of phobias;
3) A SMAST score of 3 or above;
4) Positive responses to the alcohol and drug items on the DIS;
5) A child psychiatrist's rating of moderate or severe symptomatology on the DISC (children ages 7 through 15 years);
6) The presence of 30 or more positive items on the CBCL; and/or
7) The child psychiatrist's rating of the DDST's as showing a developmental lag.

The presence of 1 or more symptomatic persons in the family gave the family symptom status.

The Family Functioning Interviews

After family members had individually completed the various interviews, we used portable video equipment (with a wide-angle lens and recorder) to videotape the family members, as a group, in their homes while we and they proceeded with the GLS Family Functioning Assessment Interview. Later the videotapes were rated 3 or 4 times by experienced clinicians to give us a graphic picture of family life "in action" in the home.

As will be discussed, at T-1, the videotaped family functioning task involved setting individual and family goals for the forthcoming year. At T-2, we gave the list of SLE to the family members, as a group, and asked about their occurrence and effects on family members. At T-3, we gave the newly developed GLS Family Functioning Assessment (see Appendix).

The videotaping approaches were acceptable to the families. The interviewers reported that the families liked the T-3 Family Functioning Assessment Interview the best, but we had learned a great deal from the earlier interviews, particularly the T-1 interviews that focused on the members' individual and family goals.

For the T-1, baseline study, 26 of the 43 families (60%) agreed to be videotaped. At T-2, of the 34 families continuing in the study, 26 (74%) were videotaped, and at T-3, 25 (71%) of the 34 families were videotaped. A small, hard-core group of about 25% of the families refused to be videotaped. Families likely to decline to be videotaped were couples in their sixties or couples or single parents over age 50 with adult children in the home. Only three younger families refused; one did so because of religious reasons and two because of the public nature of their employment (in one, a member was a judge and in the other, a member was a public school teacher). A few families that had declined at T-1, agreed to be videotaped at T-3, but two families that had been videotaped previously declined to be videotaped at T-3--one was in the process of moving and the other "had had enough of the study." We learned that presenting the videotaped questions and tasks to the family "up front" lowered anxiety about and resistance to being videotaped.

The trained personnel interviewed each child and adult individually in their homes for about one and one-half hours at each of the three times: a) at baseline with the Time-1 interview; b) six months later with the first follow-up, the T-2 interview; and c) nine months after that for the second follow-up, the T-3 interview. In addition, the families were videotaped in their homes while they completed the "family interview." The videotapes were rated to obtain observer-based as well as self-report data. At T-4, one year after the T-3 interview, we conducted the follow-up interview described in Chapter 5.

The 19 families in the current family functioning study are a core group on which we had interview data at all 4 times and videotapes at the first 3 times. The data on the core group and in the videotapes have not been reported.

Data Management and Analyses

We used the commercial software package, SIR, for the management and organization of the data on the 75 adults and 54 children in the core epidemiologic study. For the data analyses, we used the statistical procedures in SPSS, including chi-square, analysis of variance, cluster analyses, discriminant function analyses, and logistic regressions. We found that discriminant function analyses and logistic regressions could predict symptom status, even though the results were limited by the relatively small size of the sample.

Results

Some of the results of the baseline, T-1 epidemiologic study were surprising (Schwab, et al., 1993). We did not know what to anticipate inasmuch as we had not been able to find comparable data from an epidemiologic study of a random sample of families from the general population that had been carried out in the USA.

Prevalence of Symptomatology at Time-1

At Time-1, 15 (18% of the total sample) members and 12 (28% of the total) families had a DSM-III lifetime diagnosis of one or more mental disorders. The most common were major depression, panic disorder, or alcohol abuse/dependency.

No family member met full DIS criteria for the diagnosis of a mental disorder at T-1; however, during the course of the study, three members in different families did so. As described (Schwab, et al., 1993) at T-1, 25 (58%) of the 43 families met the criteria we established for being symptomatic--those 25 families contained 44 symptomatic members. Thus, we had evidence of significant symptomatic distress among the families in the community. In 13 (52%) of those 25 families, one member was symptomatic, but the other 12 (48%) families were multisymptomatic in that in 6 (24%) of them, 2 members were symptomatic, and in the other 6 (24%) families, 3 or more members were symptomatic. At T-1, members living at home who were most likely to be symptomatic were the adult daughters (100%), followed by the adult sons (90%), young daughters (60%), and mothers (50%). Those less likely to be symptomatic were the fathers (38%) and young sons (29%).

The adult daughters tended to be symptomatic predominantly on the CES-D that assessed current emotional distress, the adult sons on the alcohol and/or drug problem checklists, the mothers on the CES-D and symptoms on the depression and panic lists in the DIS, and the fathers for depression symptoms. The CES-D was the measure that most often revealed the family members' distress--13% of family members were in the high risk range; others were the depression symptom list in the DIS--11% of family members, drug problems--10%, alcohol problems--6%, panic symptoms--6%, and phobic symptoms--4% of the family members.

Many of the symptomatic family members were subclinical or subsyndromal cases. Their being uncovered by a study such as ours is one of the "uses of epidemiology" (Morris, 1957). Unfortunately, very few symptomatic family members were receiving care; only 4 families had members who received mental health care during the preceding year.

Attrition

Between the Time-1 and T-2 interviews (first follow-up), 2 (5%) of the 43 families moved away and 7 (16%) dropped out of the study. A disproportionately high number, 8 (89%) of those 9 families were symptomatic. They tended to be single-parent, poor, and often black families that had multiple problems and a great deal of symptomatology. Almost all of them had young and/or adult children at home. Most of the adult children were symptomatic--the sons with alcohol/drug problems and the daughters with depressive symptoms, panic, and/or phobias. Those families pleaded that the study took too much time; however, it appeared that the interviews were surfacing disturbing problems that had been avoided because there were no solutions in sight. Special efforts are needed to retain such families in research programs; also, therapists need to make additional efforts to understand these families' burdens and to provide concrete help with crises along with "working through" the resistance to therapy.

Change and Variability in Symptomatology and Family Composition Over Time

The second most important result was that there was substantial variability in family symptomatology and composition from one time to the next over the 15 month period in which we conducted our baseline and two follow-up family interviews. Inasmuch as the research was designed to test feasibility, we used the T-2 interviews mainly to test innovative and alternative approaches and procedures. Thus, the interview procedures as well as the data differed from those obtained at both T-1 or T-3 when the procedures were generally similar.

The 34 families that completed the second and third follow-up, the T-2 and T-3 interviews, constituted a panel for Time-1 -- Time-3 comparisons. At Time-1, in 17 (50%) of those 34 families, 26 (25%) of the 129 family members were symptomatic; 1 member was symptomatic in 11 (65%) of those 17 families, but 2 or more members were symptomatic in the other 6 (35%) families. The adult sons and daughters were the members most often symptomatic, the sons with alcohol and drug problems and the daughters with affective distress and phobias. Compared to the 17 asymptomatic families, the 17 symptomatic families were somewhat larger, more of them contained adult children (few of whom were employed), and the heads of the families were older and had less education and lower incomes.

Prevalence of Symptomatology at Time-3

At T-3, we found somewhat less symptomatology than at T-1. Of the 34 families at T-3, in 15 (44%) families, 19 (56%) members were symptomatic; 1 member was symptomatic in 12 (80% of those 15 families), but 2 or more members were symptomatic in the remaining 3 (20%). At T-3, as at T-1, the adult sons and daughters were the family members' most often symptomatic and the fathers least often. Also, as at T-1, the symptomatic males tended to report alcohol and drug abuse problems and the females' depression symptoms. Finding less symptomatology at reinterviews (the regression toward the mean) has been reported often in epidemiologic studies, especially when interviews are only months or a year or so apart.

Time-1 – Time-3 Comparisons

Symptom patterns that tended not to change from T-1 to T-3 were the depression symptoms on the CES-D and/or the DIS. Also, the symptoms of dysphoria were the ones that "developed" over the 15-month period between T-1 and T-3, whereas panic and phobic symptoms and some of the alcohol and drug problems tended to clear up.

We divided the 34 families into 4 subgroups according to their symptom status at both times. The first contained the 14 (41%) of the 34 families that were asymptomatic at both T-1 and T-3. Of the 8 (24%) that changed in symptom status from T-1 to T-3, 3 families (the second subgroup) changed from asymptomatic to symptomatic (family 15-18 month incidence rate 9%) and in the third subgroup, 5 families changed from symptomatic at T-1 to asymptomatic at T-3 (family 15-18 month remission rate 15%). The 12 (35%) families in the fourth group, unfortunately, were chronic--symptomatic at both T-1 and T-3. All of the families that were symptomatic at both times had either young children or adult children at home; often the parents tended to be older than most parents in the study, and there was a persistence and also a multiplicity of symptoms in the same family members over time. Thus, over the 15-18 months, the family good mental health rate was 41%, the incidence rate 9%, the remission rate 15%, and the chronicity rate 35%.

In the 34 families, the members most likely to be symptomatic at T-1 and/or T-3 were the adult sons, 60%, and the young daughters, 50%, followed by the adult daughters, 43%, and the mothers, 30%. Fathers and young sons had the lowest percentages with symptomatology, 23% and 19%, respectively.

The composition of some of the families also changed over the 15-month period. In the 34 families, there were 5 (15%) major changes; 3 persons entered families (2 were born and 1 adult returned home) and 2 left to marry. Inasmuch as the family is a dynamic, complex group, we suggest that family researchers and therapists need continually to assess possible changes in composition as well as interactions within the family.

Family Risk Factors

The three major family risk factors were the structural (belonging to a single-parent family or having adult children at home), low socioeconomic status (SES), and stress. Of the 43 T-1 families, 8 (89%) of the 9 single-parent families were symptomatic in contrast to 17 (50%) of the 34 families with two parents. We found that the risks associated with having adult children at home were serious; at T-1, 12 (75%) of the 16 families with adult children at home were symptomatic, and 73% of the adult children were symptomatic--usually with alcohol or drug problems. Often, the mothers in those families were suffering from affective distress. The adult children seemed to be distorting the family structure and were contributing to symptomatology within the family.

Low SES--reflecting low educational, occupational, and income levels-- has both direct and mediating effects that are deleterious. The families headed by fathers and/or mothers with less than high school educations and by heads who were unemployed or had only part-time employment, as well as those with annual family incomes of $12,000 (1983 dollars) or less, were significantly more likely to be symptomatic than their better educated, employed, higher-income counterparts. These findings bring to mind that in the first systematic family research, in the 1850s and 1860s, LePlay found that the adequacy of "family budgets" was related strongly to family stability (Silver, 1982). Our results revealed that the symptomatology often associated with low family incomes was an unfortunate aspect of American life in the 1980s when "the bottom 40% of families had actual declines in income" (Caruthers, 1992).

Although we had studied stressful life events (SLE) in patients and random samples of the general population for about 20 years, we were surprised at the extent of differential reporting by various family members at T-1 about whether a particular SLE had occurred during the preceding 6 months (Stephenson J. J., Schwab J. J., Bell R.A., 1990). Consequently, to develop methods and to evaluate feasibility, at T-2, we gave the SLE inventory to the family as a group while they were being videotaped. Fewer SLE were reported than we anticipated; we think that certain events were not reported because of the group setting and lack of confidentiality. (Stephenson, et al. 1990). Therefore at T-3, we returned to the method that we had used at T-1; each member was asked about the occurrence of SLE and their effects during the confidential individual interview.

To evaluate stress at the family level, we took the information from the level of the individual, i.e. each family member's responses to the SLE inventory and questions about who was affected and to what extent, and why the event had occurred, and, then, as a panel, we grouped related events and their effects into family stress themes that we rated for each family to obtain family-level data. For example, a stress theme that involved work might include such SLE as a family member's being laid off from one job, obtaining a new job at a lower wage, having less family income, another member's starting work, and reduced expenditures for the children's education.

We placed the themes in three major categories: a) the <u>intrafamilial</u> that involved only the members of the household; b) the other <u>relatives'</u> themes that involved family members not living in the household; and c) <u>friends'</u> themes. As a panel, we rated the stress themes in each category as either positive or negative, included ratings of the theme's impact on the family, and gave them overall family stress scores that ranged from plus 4 (positive, e.g. achievements) to minus 4 (negative--severe stress) to compare the family-level stress and its type to the presence or absence of symptomatology.

As to be anticipated, work/finances was by far the most common intrafamilial stress theme inasmuch as the interviews took place during the recession of the early to mid 1980s. The symptomatic group's mean intrafamilial stress theme rating was negative (-1.8 ± 3.5), significantly different than the asymptomatic group's positive rating (0.6 ± 1.7). Also, the symptomatic group's mean other-relatives' stress rating (-0.8 ± 2.2) was more negative than the asymptomatic group's mean rating (-0.1 ± 1.7). The friends' mean stress-theme ratings (-1.0 and -1.2) were about the same and negative because the themes concerned mainly such events as friends dying or moving away. The most common intrafamilial negative stress themes were work/finances, minor law violations, and hospitalizations; the main positive theme was a personal achievement. The most common negative other-relatives' stress themes were work/finances and hospitalization; the most common positive ones were engagement/marriage and a personal achievement.

The second major finding about family stress involved the associations between the family life cycle stages and stress. Our five-stage classification of the family life cycle consisted of 1) the beginning family—just the couple; 2) young children at home (oldest child 12 years); 3) adolescents at home (oldest child 18 years); 4) adult children at home; and 5) aging couple alone. Mean intrafamilial stress theme scores were positive for the families in the first or second stage of the family life cycle, but negative for those in the third-, fourth-, and fifth stages. Our finding a high level of stress and symptomatology, not just in the third or adolescent stage (the usual finding) but also at the next stage when many parents were in their fifties and had adult children at home turned out to be indicative of problems stemming from the continued presence or return of adult children to the parental home.

The third major finding from the study of the effects of SLE on the families was that there was little agreement among the family members about their occurrence. All the family members reported only 35 to 40% of the total SLEs that had occurred. The wife/mother reported an additional 30%, the husband/father another 20%, and the children's reports added still another 15-20%. We were surprised at the lack of agreement about even the occurrence of SLE and consider it to have clinical importance.

The fourth major family stress finding was that the Time-1 intrafamilial stress theme rating was a significant predictor of the Time-3 intrafamilial stress ratings. Such a finding has grave implications for families that are battered by SLE; unfortunately, their stressors continue to occur and to exert deleterious influences.

After conducting the baseline and first follow-up (T-2) interviews with the families, we realized that in order to obtain a more complete understanding of the effect of stress upon the family, it would be necessary to supplement the SLE Inventory for adults and adolescents with evaluations of chronic stressors. We were particularly interested in the "hassle" of everyday life, especially stressors related to marriage, work/school, finances, parent-child relationships, and the neighborhood. We developed a comprehensive chronic stressor rating form that each interviewer rated after the second follow-up, the T-3 interview, on a seven-point (no stress to high stress) continuum for the families for which she had been the primary interviewer at all three times. Our work with chronic stressors was built on Ilfeld and his colleagues' (1977) research in Chicago. They reported, for example, that chronic stressors explained a much greater degree of the variance in 2,500 respondents' depression scores than the conventional sociodemographic variables. At T-3, we also gathered data about the families' chronic social stressors which Ilfeld (1977) had found were significantly associated with depression symptoms in his study of inner city adults in Chicago. The most significant were financial difficulties and job stressors for the men and for the women, chronic marital difficulties and parenting.

In 1989, Gary's study of 1,018 African-American adults in Norfolk, Virginia also found that chronic stressors, "the hassles of everyday life", especially financial, relationship, and alcohol were strongly associated with high CES-D scores.

The Family Environment

We found that the Moos and Moos (1981) Family Environment Scale (FES) we used to evaluate the characteristics of each family's environment yielded more information about the family than we had anticipated. Earlier, Boake and Salmon (1981) had reported that the norms for Louisville were different from those reported for the Bay Area populations on which the FES had been standardized. We used the Louisville norms, which were somewhat higher on cohesion and on moral-religious emphasis and lower on conflict and on intellectual-cultural and active-recreational orientations, than those reported for the Bay Area Sample.

The FES subscale scores revealed significant differences between the symptomatic and asymptomatic families. The symptomatic had significantly lower mean cohesion and expressiveness subscale scores, slightly higher conflict scores, and a tendency toward lower independence, intellectual-cultural orientation, and active recreational-orientation subscale scores than the asymptomatic. Also, the symptomatic had higher family incongruence scores than the asymptomatic. The scores on the various subscales differed somewhat according to the type of problem. For example, families that had high scores on the CES-D, which assesses emotional distress during the preceding week, had significantly lower cohesion, expressiveness, and moral-religious emphasis subscale scores and a higher family incongruence score than those with low CES-D scores, and those with drug problems had significantly lower mean cohesion and intellectual-cultural orientation scores and a significantly higher mean conflict score than their counterparts.

Predictors of Symptomatic Status

We used the T-1 FES subscale and family incongruence scores in discriminant function analyses and logistical regressions to determine how well they predicted both the T-1 and T-3 symptom status. As described more fully in our first volume (Schwab, et al., 1993), the discriminant function analyses correctly classified 76.8% of the 43 T-1 families' symptom status. Also, the 17 of those 43 families with young children were classified into symptomatic and asymptomatic groups with 100% accuracy. Depression symptom status was correctly classified in 86.1% of the families. Low cohesion subscale scores generally were the most powerful predictors of overall symptomatology; high conflict subscale scores were predictors of drug problems; and, low independence scores were the best predictors of child psychopathology. The logistical regressions correctly classified from 63% to 84% of the families on overall symptom status. Again, a low mean cohesion score was a powerful predictor of symptom status.

We then used the T-1 FES subscale and family incongruence scores in discriminant function analyses and logistical regressions to see how accurately they predicted family symptom status 15 months later at T-3. For those discriminant analyses, a linear combination of 6 T-1 FES subscale scores correctly classified 82% of the families as being either symptomatic or asymptomatic 15 months later. For the logistical regressions, the T-1 cohesion scale scores alone correctly predicted 62% of the families' T-3 symptomatic status. We regarded these associations between the characteristics of the family environment and family well-being and, sometimes even specific types of symptoms and problems, as having both research and clinical importance. The most striking findings were the associations between low cohesion scores and depressive symptoms, between high conflict scores and depressive symptoms, between high conflict scores and drug problems, and between low independence scores and the children being symptomatic.

The Time-4 study

One year after completing the second follow-up study (third wave), we developed a brief interview schedule that could be used to obtain additional, Time-4 (T-4) follow-up information on the families from a key informant. We trained a female medical student to conduct the T-4 interviews in the home with a family member. The key informant approach had been used in such early epidemiologic studies as Andrew Halliday's (1828) pioneering work in Scotland, the 1832 Connecticut study by Amariah Brigham (1963), and Jarvis' (1855) classic Massachusetts study as well as in many social science studies in this century and by the U.S. Bureau of Census. We used that approach because we had limited financial support and also because we wanted to evaluate the feasibility of the key informant approach for family research. The T-4 interview was shorter than the interviews conducted previously.

The revised schedule included many items about whether changes had occurred in the family composition, health, work, and finances since the T-3 interview about 15 months earlier. We relied for symptom assessment on the CES-D given to the key informant and on a "second family CES-D" that would be completed by the same key informant about the other family members. Also, we included our SLE inventory and the FES used previously, and added Cantril's "Ladder of Life" (Cantril, 1965) to gauge each family's hopes and fears and its optimism-pessimism level. There were no family videotaped interviews at T-4. The results of the T-4 study are reported in Chapter V.

We thought that the basic T-1 and T-2 interviews had yielded important data about the families we were studying, especially their health status, well-being, and factors related to emotional distress and to behavioral or substance abuse disorders. But, we did not yet have either the method or the information from any source that would enable us to assess family functioning objectively in terms of both the family's 2 traditional functions--rearing children to become autonomous members of society, and meeting the partners' emotional and sexual needs--and also its 5 essential functions we described: maintenance of the group; perpetuation of the group; regulation of the adults' sexuality; provision of emotional support for all family members; and learning and enculturation--the inculcation of values, beliefs, and skills. Therefore, to complete this initial series of studies of family functioning, we developed and tested our general living systems theory (GLST) family functioning model at T-3, and then extended the research by carrying out a case-control study of 8 families that had a child receiving mental health care at the Bingham Child Guidance Clinic and 8 matched families in the same neighborhood with no child or adult in mental health treatment. The results of those two efforts to evaluate family functioning and its associations with families' mental health/illness are presented in the next two chapters.

References

Achenbach, J. M. & Edelbrock, C. S., (1983). *Manual for the child behavior checklist and revised child behavior profile*. Burlington, VT: Queen City Printers.

Bell, R. A. & Sundel, M., (1975). *The Louisville Metropolitan health and family life study.* Unpublished manuscript.

Bell, R. A., Goldsmith, H. F., Lin, E., et al., (Eds.) (1980). Social indicators for human service systems. *Louisville, KY: Department of Psychiatry and Behavioral Sciences.*

Bell, R. A., Warheit, G. J., Buhl, J. A., et al., (Eds.), (1978). Social Indicators for human service systems. Louisville, KY: *Univ. of Louisville Dept. of Psychiatry and Behavioral Sciences.*

Boake, C. & Salmon, P. G., (1981, Oct. 22). Demographic correlates and factor structure of the Family Environment Scale. *J of Clinical Psychology,* 39(1), 95-100.

Brigham, A., (1963). Cited in Brigham, A.: Remarks on the influence of mental cultivation upon health (1832). Excerpted in Hunter, R., & McAlpine, I. (Eds.) *Three hundred years of psychiatry, 1535-1800: A history presented in selected English texts.* London: Oxford University Press, pp. 821-825.

Brown, G. W. & Harris, T., (1978). *Social origins of depression: A study of psychiatric disorders in women.* New York: Free Press.

Cantril, H., (1965). *The pattern of human concerns.* New Brunswick, NJ: Rutgers University Press.

Caruthers, C., (July 8, 1992). Surge of children living in poverty. *Wall Street Journal, A2.*

Coomes, P., (1990). *Personal Communication.*

Costello, A. J., Edelbrock, C., Dulcan, M. K., et al., (1984). Development and Testing of the NIMH Diagnostic Interview Schedule for Children in a clinic population. Final Report. Rockville, MD: Center for Epidemiologic Studies, National Institute of Mental Health.

Frankenberg, W. K., Dodds, J. B., Fandal, A. W., et al., (1975). *Devener developmental screening test reference manual (rev. ed.).* Boulder: University of Colorado Medical Center.

Gary, L. R., Brown, D. R., Milburn, N. G., et al., (1989). Depression in black American adults: Findings from the Norfolk Area Health Study. Washington DC: Mental Health Research and Development Center, Howard University.

Halliday, A., (1828): *A general view of the present state of lunatics and lunatic asylums in Great Britain and Ireland, and in some other kingdoms.* London: Thomas & George Underwood.

Ifeld, F. W., (1977). Current social stressors and symptoms of depression. *Am J of Psychiatry,* 134(2), 161-166.

Jarvis, E., (1885). Report on insanity and idiocy in Massachusetts by the Commission on Lunacy, under resolve of the Legislature of 1854. Boston: William White Printer, to the State.

Matheny, A. P., Jr. & Dolan, A. B., (1980). A twin study of personality and temperament during middle childhood. *J of Research in Personality,* 14, 224.

Moos R. H. & Moos B. S., (1981). *Family environment scale manual.* Palo Alto, CA: Consulting Psychologists Press.

Morris, J. N., (1964): *Uses of epidemiology (2nd. ed.).* Baltimore: Williams & Wilkins.

Radloff, L. S., (1977). The CES-D Scale: A self-report depression scale for research in the general population. *Applied Psychological Measurement,* I, 385-401.

Riebel, R. C., (1954). Photographic and narrative history of Louisville.

Robins, L. N., et al., (1979). *The National Institute of Mental Health DiagnosticInterview Schedule (DIS.).* Bethesda, MD: National Institute of Mental.

Robins L. N., Helzer, J. E., Weissman, M. M. et al., (1984). Lifetime prevalence of specific psychiatric disorders in 3 sites. *Arch Gen Psychiat,* 41(10) 942-948.

Robins, L. N., Regier, D. A., (Eds.), (1991) *Psychiatric disorders in America: The epidemiologic Catchment Area Study.* Published by the Free Press, New York.

Roper, E., (1950). *People's attitudes concerning mental health: A study made in the City of Louisville.* Louisville, KY: Elmo Roper.

Schwab, J. J., Bell, R. A., Warheit, G. J., & Schwab, R. B., (1979). *Social order and mental health: The Florida health study.* New York: Brunner/Mazel.

Schwab, J. J., Schwab, M. E., (1978) *The sociocultural roots of mental illness: An epidemiologic survey.* Plenum Medical Book Co., New York.

Schwab, J. J., Stephenson, J. J., Ice, J. F., (1993). *Evaluating family mental health: History, epidemiology, and treatment issues.* New York, Plenum.

Selzer, M. L., Vinokur, A. & van Lorijen, L., (1975). A self-administered Short Michigan Alcoholism Screening Test. *J of Studies on Alcohol,* 36, 117-126.

Shafii, M., Shafii, S. L., (1992). *Clinical guide to depression in children and adolescents.* Washington DC: American Psychiatric Press.

Silver, C. B., (Ed. & Trans.) (1982). *Fredrick Le Play: On family, work and social change.* Chicago: University of Chicago Press.

Stephenson, J. J., Schwab, J. J., Bell, R. A., (1990). Stressful life events and risks for depression in the family. *Stress Medicine,* 6, 145-155.

CHAPTER 5
Pilot Study I - Results - The Assessment of Family Functioning

During the four years devoted to field work, we developed and tested a model of family functioning that: a) would be based on general living systems theory (GLST); b) could be measured at the family (not just at the individual) level; c) would focus more on family system processes -- performance of the tasks and interactions of everyday life -- than on characteristics of the family; d) could be independently rated to provide observer-based data to complement family members' self-report data and interviewers' descriptions; e) would diminish value judgments; and f) was not tautological in that family functioning was not equated with health or illness. Thus, our major aim was to develop and test an assessment instrument that could be used to study family functioning as an independent variable in research in which the dependent variable would be members' mental and/or physical distress, although we recognize that such variables are inevitably linked.

To develop the model, we looked at the evolution of theory for family research and used modifications of other researchers' models of family functioning to evaluate their appropriateness and feasibility for our study. We found that we wanted to design our own model because, generally, others were usually assessing characteristics of the family or family competence, ostensibly to meet its basic purposes, not family functioning. Also, except for a few notable ongoing studies, most tended to equate competent functioning with health and well-being and thus were circular when used in studies of health and illness.

There have been two major approaches to the study of family functioning. The simplest, least expensive, and most common has been family members' self-reports on scales measuring such variables considered to be indicators of family function as cohesion, decision-making, adaptability, family style, power, and /or affective involvement. The other approach consists of observers' ratings of the family and/or videotapes of it for many of those same variables while the family was engaged in solving a problem. Whether and how the family members resolved the problem were usually considered less important than the observers' ratings of such variables as the quality of communication, other interactions, power, decision-making, or boundaries. A combined self-report -- observer-rated approach obviously is the most comprehensive but is bound to be both expensive and laborious. Inasmuch as we were developing a research instrument that later could be used in clinical work, our study included both family members' subjective reports and objective observer-based ratings of the families' videotaped interviews.

THE ASSESSMENT OF FAMILY FUNCTIONING

We studied the families at 4 times, 3 times with interviews in their homes at 6-9 months intervals and then for the fourth time with a 1 year follow-up interview. The assessment instrument based on the GLS model of family functioning that we developed and used at Time-3 (T-3) became the centerpiece of our study. At Time-1 (T-1) and Time-2 (T-2), to evaluate the families, we used mainly their Family Environment Scale (FES) subscale and the members' difference scores, along with observers' ratings of videotapes of the families for such indicators of family functioning as clarity of communication, quality of emotional tone, and degree of adaptability while they were carrying out an assigned task. The results of our use of the T-1 and T-2 approaches will be presented and compared to the findings from the use of our GLS instrument at T-3 that assessed the processes of everyday family life directly.

SECTION A - TIME-3 (T-3)

CHARACTERISTICS OF THE FAMILIES STUDIED

Of the 34 families in the sample, we did not have complete data on 15 of them for a number of reasons; 9 families declined to be videotaped at T-3, and some tapes were imperfect. Also, 8 of those 15 families did not participate in the T-4 follow-up. As shown in Table 5.1, those 15, as a group, differed somewhat from the study group of 19. They included more elderly and fewer young families and had more adult children in their homes than the families that completed the study. Our assessments of family functioning are based on the core group of 19 families that participated in all 4 phases of the research (except for 2 families that missed T-4). Thus, we would have a 3 to 4 year longitudinal perspective on the families' lives.

At T-1, 5 (12%) of the original 43 families were African-American, but after the lengthy, probing T-1 interview, 4 of them dropped out for a number of reasons. Therefore, the group of 19 contained the only African-American family (5%) that continued with the research.

The group of 19 families that completed the study had annual family incomes and economic levels that were about the same as those of the 15 non-completers, but their physical health ratings were not as good as those of the non-completers even though the 15 consisted of disproportionately more elderly families. Also, the group of 19 had poorer mental health ratings, 8 (42%) of the 19 completing families were symptomatic in contrast to only 3 (20%) of the non-completer families.

The 19 T-3 families were in many ways representative of families in middle America in the 1980's. There were 18 couples and 1 single parent; 10 of the families had children under the age of 18 in the home and 2 others each had 2 adult children in their homes -- a total of 37 adults, 18 children, and 4 adult children. The parents' age distribution was 4 elderly (65-84yr.), 5 middle-aged (40-64yr.), and 10 young (24-39yr.) families. Family incomes crossed the socioeconomic spectrum, ranging from 5 having excellent incomes, quite a bit higher than the median for the census tracts in which they lived to 3 families at the poverty level. Sixteen (84%) of the families were in good or excellent physical health; 1 family was in fair health, and only 2 were in poor physical health.

Table 5.1. Comparative Data - Drop-outs and Completers

	Drop-out Fam - n-15	Completers - n-19
No. of Children	24 (1.6 per fam)	22 (1.16 per fam)
No. of Adult Children	13 (54%)	4 (19%)
No. Fam-Elderly Par.	5 (33%)	4 (20%)
No. Fam-Young Par.	4 (26%)	11 (55%)
Annual Fam. Income		
Excellent	4 (26.6%)	5 (22.7%)
Poverty Level	2 (13.3%)	3 (13.6%)
Physical Health		
Excellent	0.46	0.42
Poor	0.08	0.16
Mental Health		
Symptomatic	3 (20.5%)	8 (42.1%)
Asymptomatic	12 (80%)	11 (57.9%)
No.-Number Par.- Parent Fam -Family		

FAMILIES' SYMPTOMATIC STATUS

At Time-3, 8 (42%) of the 19 families met the criteria for being symptomatic, i.e., at least 1 member was having definite symptoms of a mental disorder or a drug or alcohol problem, as discussed in Chapter IV. That 42% is about the same as the percentage of symptomatic families in the original group of 43 studied about 2 years earlier at Time-1 (Schwab, Stephenson, and Ice, 1993).

In the 8 symptomatic families, 1 person was symptomatic in 4 (50%) of them, and 2 persons were symptomatic in each of the other 4 (50%.). Thus, of the 59 members in the 19 families, 12 (20%) were symptomatic: 4 (35%) of them were wives/mothers, 3 (25%) were young daughters, 2 (17%) were husbands/fathers, 2 (17%) were young sons, and 1 (8%) was an adult son living at home. On the various symptom measures, 6 adults were positive on the CES-D and 3 on depression symptoms; 3 young children were positive on the CBCL and the other 2 on the Child Psychiatrist's independent ratings of their videotapes.

THE GENERAL LIVING SYSTEMS (GLS) MODEL

As described in Chapter 3 (pp. 5-25), the GLS Family Functioning Model that we developed specified Miller's (1978) 19 essential subsystems or processes that are carried out at all levels of biosocial organization, including the family. We analyzed the data in a number of different ways and decided that presenting the data according to levels of family functioning appeared to be the most meaningful approach.

Classification of Functioning Groups - The GLS Approach

The 3 investigators -- a psychiatrist, a child psychiatrist, and a psychologist -- rated each of the 17 subsystems on the family videotapes for level of functioning on a 0-100 point scale according to the specific criteria that we developed (note 1). For example; Was the subsystem active? If so, were there disruptions in the system functioning? How long did they last? To what extent did the subsystem fulfill its purpose? What was the degree of disruption of other subsystems? (See Appendix for the Subsystems Functioning Criteria Scale). High scores indicated a high level of functioning and lower scores lesser levels of functioning. We ranked the families from the highest to the lowest level of functioning according to the number of subsystems each family carried out at varying levels of effectiveness, 100%, 95-99%, 80-94%, etc., and then used the frequency distributions, not arbitrary cut-off points, to classify the 19 families into the following 3 groups: 8 high-functioning (HF) families, 6 mid-functioning (MF) families, and 5 low functioning (LF) families.

THE HIGH FUNCTIONING (HF) GROUP --T-3

The 8 HF families consisted of 2 elderly couples, 4 middle-aged families (2 couples, 1 single parent with 2 adult daughters, and, 1 couple with a 16 yr. old daughter), and 2 young families (1 childless couple and another with an 8 yr. old daughter). Of the 8 families, 4 had ratings of excellent on our

5-point income scale (excellent, good, fair, poor, poverty) based on census norms; 2 were rated as having good, and the remaining 2 as having fair annual family incomes. Thus, none was at either the poor or the poverty level. On their physical health ratings, 3 were excellent, and 5 were good. Of the 8 HF families, 2 (25%) were symptomatic. The following case vignette is illustrative of an HF family.

Family A was an impressive, very well functioning young family. The father was an educational officer in the military and the mother was a 5th grade school teacher. The 9 year old daughter was a skilled ice skater who also played the piano; she helped around the house and was both responsible and compliant, but not overly so. She appeared to be a "super kid" and both parents obviously were proud of her. They lavished attention and affection on her. She responded positively and returned their affection. The father did a great deal around the house; he helped with cleaning, and even put on a new roof. His wife described him as a perfectionist, but he showed no indicators of having obsessive-compulsive disorder (OCD) or of an obsessive-compulsive personality. The mother was outgoing and, like her husband, was spontaneous, open, and giving. She kept a daily journal of family activities and maintained an orderly household. The family performed many subsystem functions jointly, including decision-making. Communication was excellent, especially when it was factual. The family emphasized hard work, achievement balanced with pleasure, helping others, altruism, and shared "Christian values".

THE MID-FUNCTIONING (MF) GROUP

The 6 MF families consisted of 1 elderly couple with 2 adult sons at home, 1 middle-aged couple with a 16 year old daughter and 2 sons ages 15 and 12, and 4 young families (1 childless couple, another couple with a 13 year old son, a third with 2 sons ages 8 and 1, and a fourth with a 9 year old son). Of the 6, 1 family had an annual income rating of excellent, 4 had income ratings of fair, and 1 had a poverty level rating. On their T-3 physical health ratings, 3 were good and 3 were fair. Two (33.3%) of the 6 MF families were symptomatic. The following case vignette is illustrative of an MF family.

Family B, was a young couple in their mid to late twenties with 2 sons, ages 8 and 1. The father, who had a salaried job, took pride in having personally remodeled their home extensively. Their income level, which was rated as fair, had improved significantly in the past one and one-half years.

Although they were functioning fairly well at the T-3 interview, the mother had had a post-partum depression earlier in the year that they described as "a horrible thing" with a "great deal of crying" which lasted almost 2 months. Her mother and aunt had come to live with them in order to help keep the household running. She had been advised by her physician to see a psychiatrist, but refused to do so, and "began to snap out of it". They had no physical health problems at the time of the T-3 interview.

On their subsystems ratings, the family, generally, was seen as functioning well, but their ratings on 2 subsystems, the *Encoder* (processing "information" for the family from other subsystems) and, especially, the *Output Transducer* (transmits information to the outside) were less than optimal. Also, they had some problems of mild severity with the *Storage* (storing supplies, etc.), *Distributor* (of goods), and *Decider (*executive decision-making) subsystems.

The parents carried out conventional family roles. They shared decision-making and many other family functions. Also, they shared conventional values that they transmitted to their 8-year-old son, who was a compliant boy. The marriage seemed sound; they were invested in themselves, the children, and their home. Communication was very good. They were self-contained and had little involvement with friends, neighbors or community, as evidenced by their having some problems handling business affairs and outside matters.

THE LOW FUNCTIONING (LF) GROUP

The 5 families in the LF group included 1 elderly couple and 4 young families: 1 was a couple with a 9 year old daughter; another was a mother with her live-in boyfriend and her 2 daughters ages 15 and 8; the third was a couple with 3 sons ages 12, 7, and 5 (the only African-American family in the study); and the fourth young family was a mother with her live-in boyfriend and her sons ages 7, 5, and 2. Four (80%) of the 5 families had income levels rated as poor; the fifth was at poverty level. On their physical health ratings, there were 1 excellent, 2 fair, and 2 poor ratings. Four (80%) of the 5 LF families were symptomatic. The following case vignette is illustrative of an LF family

Family C consisted of a husband and wife in their early 30's and their 8 year old daughter. He worked as an independent contractor remodeling houses and she worked at seasonal jobs. Both wanted full-time jobs with regular paychecks. They were struggling financially and had an income rating of poor. Also, their general health rating was low. The wife had had many symptoms of anxiety and depression, and she talked about losing her temper, getting into bad moods, and then yelling or going to bed. The husband, who appeared generally restrained, had had an "alcohol problem". Also, there was serious illness in the extended family.

There were some difficulties with family role functions. The mother did not like either grocery shopping or cooking, which she did as quickly as possible. She found it necessary to handle all the money and balance the checkbook inasmuch as he spent carelessly. Both were involved in decision-making but she worried after decisions were made.

The marriage seemed solid although they reported sexual dissatisfaction. They were close to her mother and father whom they saw frequently and telephoned often. Both were devoted to their daughter who said little during the interview, but she listened intently and was listened to when she spoke. She was an almost straight A student, shared their values, and enjoyed swimming. She had no behavioral problems.

In summary, the HF group contained fewer young parent families and fewer children than either the MF or, especially, the LF group. Also, the economic level of the HF group was higher than the MF and much higher than the LF groups' levels. The symptomatic status of the HF group was better (only 25% symptomatic) than the MF group (38% symptomatic) and, especially, the LF group (80% symptomatic).

PROBLEMS, THEIR SEVERITY, AND SUBSYSTEM FUNCTIONING

One of our aims was to evaluate the associations between subsystem functioning, the number of problems with each subsystem, and their severity. Therefore, for each family we gathered data about the number of problems per subsystem, and whether they had been resolved? and How? Then we rated the severity of each family's problems according to specific criteria (See Appendix). Table 5.2 presents the families' rank positions in each of the three functioning groups, symptom status, age of parents, number in the family, economic level, total number and severity of each family's subsystem problems, and the problem/severity rank.

Number and Severity of Subsystem Problems

The 8 families in the HF group averaged 4.25 subsystem problems per family, and in the MF group, the 6 families averaged 5.5 problems per family; however, the 5 families in the LF group had many more problems, an average of 11 per family. Also, the average severity of the problems reported by the three functioning groups varied greatly, from a low of 1.1 per family in the HF group and 1.5 in the MF group to the high of 5.7 in the LF group.

Rankings of Families for Subsystem Problems/Severity

We then ranked the families (1-19, from few to many) according to the number of subsystems with problems weighted for severity. The families' rankings generally (at a 79% level) matched their positions in the 3 functioning groups; however, for 4 (21%) of the 19 families, there were inconsistencies. First, 2 HF families (0094 and 0111) that ranked at 7th and 8th positions in functioning (at the lower end of the HF group) had P/S rankings similar to MF families' of 10.5 and 14.0 on number of problems weighted for severity. The second inconsistency was that 2 MF families (0081 and (113) had few problems of little severity and P/S rankings similar to the HF families, at positions 7 and 2 respectively. In contrast to those inconsistencies in the HF and MF groups, the ranking of the LF group families for number and severity of problems closely matched their relatively low family functioning level.

The 2 HF families that were functioning at higher levels than indicated by their moderately large number of problems of borderline severity apparently were able to cope with or otherwise surmount their problems and continue to function at a reasonably high level. They were:

1. Family 0094 was an elderly, asymptomatic couple in excellent health with an income level rating of good and a low stress level. Independent observers described them as having a good sense of humor that they used effectively, and they were rated as having a very high coping potential and a high level of resources. He was a retired mechanic and she a retired nurse. They had reared 5 children successfully and were a close knit family with strong family ties.

2. Family 0111 was a young symptomatic couple; both were professionals with advanced degrees and both were ambitious. Their health was excellent, their economic level was fair (he was in graduate school), and they were rated as being at a mid-stress level, but they had no chronic stressors. On the FES, they were high on *Cohesion* and low on *Intellectual/Cultural Orientation* and on *Control*. Independent observers rated their resources as high, but their coping potential was considered only

fair inasmuch as they were having family conflict about when they would have a child. She had been in therapy because she and her sister had interpersonal difficulties with their mother.

Table 5.2. Comparative Data of Functioning Groups at Time-3

STUDY I Family I.D.	T-3 Symp. Status	Age of Par.	No.in Fam.	Econ Level	Total Prob	Severity Weight	P/S Rank	Func Rank
HF Group								
177	As	E	2	Fair	0	0	0.5	1
151	S	M	3	Ex	3	1	4.5	2
85	As	Y	3	Ex	4	1	4.5	3
129	As	M	3	Ex	4	0.7	4	4
127	As	M	2	Good	5	0.3	3	5
82	As	M	2	Ex	4	1.3	8	6
94	As	E	2	Good	6	2	10.5	7
111	S	Y	2	Fair	8	2.7	14	8
MF Group								
81	S	Y	2	Fair	3	1	4.5	9
141	As	Y	4	Fair	6	2	10.5	10
157	S	E	4	Pov.	6	1.7	9	11
121	As	Y	3	Fair	10	2	12	12
113	As	M	5	Fair	1	0	0.5	13
160	As	Y	3	Ex	7	2.3	13	14
LF Group								
162	As	Y	5	Poor	11	3.7	16	15
108	S	Y	5	Poor	8	2.7	15	16
128	S	Y	4	Poor	11	6.7	18	17
11	S	Y	3	Poor	11	5	17	18
8	S	E	2	Pov.	14	9.3	19	19

Par.-Parent   Fam.-Family   Econ-Economic
S-Symptomatic   E-Elderly   Ex-Excellent
As- Asymptomatic   M- Mid-age   Pov.-Poverty
Symp.-symptom   Y- Young   P/S.-Problem/Severity
    No.-Number   Func.-Functioning

The other inconsistencies were that 2 MF families with relatively low mid- range functioning ratings had disproportionately low rankings on number and severity of problems. Apparently, they just were not functioning optimally.

3. Family 0113 was a mid-age couple with 2 teen-agers and a school-age child. The family was asymptomatic, had fair health, and was at a fair economic level, but upwardly mobile. They were rated as having low stress and had no chronic stressors. The father, a first generation immigrant from Germany, was authoritative, had high expectations for his children, and expected them to follow his work ethic. He had trouble with the nuances of the English language, and was working as a skilled laborer. The father declared: "Nothing is a problem in this family". Thus, he displayed rigidity and an attitude of denial. His American wife was obese and was described as a "couch potato". They had minor problems with *Storage* (storing supplies etc.), *Memory* (storing of information in photo albums), *Encoder* (processing of information from other subsystems), *and Reproducer* (dealing with values, rules and discipline) subsystems.

4. Family 0081 was a young, childless couple that expressed disappointment about not having children and was having controversy about when they should. They were symptomatic, had a good health rating, and were rated at mid-level stress. Although the marriage appeared to be strong, each tended to have his or her own individual activities. They alluded to a major illness in the past year. Difficulties were evident on only one subsystem, the *Internal Transducer* (dealing with family information and feelings).

These inconsistencies, as shown in Table 5.2, indicate that the actual number of problems and their severity alone, without consideration of a family's coping potential and resources, were not always reliable indicators of family functioning.

Table 5.3 shows the ranking of the 17 subsystems according to the total number of families that had problems with each and also the number of families in each of the three functioning groups reporting problems with the subsystems. Of the 17 subsystems, the *Storage* (storage of goods and supplies) and *Producer* (care of the house and yard) were reported most often as being troublesome -- by 14 (82%) and 12 (70%) of families respectively. In contrast, 4 subsystems -- the *Distributor* (of goods), *Input Transducer* (brings information into the family), *Decoder* (explains information), and *Motor* (moving about, transportation), each posed problems to only 2-3 (15%) families. As shown in Table 5.3, examination of the number of families in each of the 3 functioning groups reporting problems with each subsystem revealed that for the 8 HF families, 3 (18%) subsystems gave no problems to any of them, and 8 (47%) subsystems each gave problems to only 1 family. Also, there were no subsystems with which all of the families reported having problems, and only 3 (18%) subsystems were reported as giving problems to as many as 4 (50%) of the 8 HF families.

Table 5.3. Rankings of Subsystems for Number of Families with Problems

STUDY I T-3			
Rank Order of Subsystems High to Low	No. of Fam with Problems		
	HF	MF	LF
	n-8	n-6	n-5
1.0 Storage	5	4	5
2.0 Producer	5	3	4
3.5 Decider	1	3	5
3.5 Boundary	4	3	5
5.0 Internal Trans.	2	2	4
6.0 Converter	1	2	4
7.25 Reproducer	1	0	5
7.25 Extruder	2	1	3
7.25 Ingestor	2	1	3
7.25 Output Trans.	1	2	3
11.5 Supporter	0	1	4
11.5 Encoder	1	2	2
13.0 Memory	1	2	2
14.5 Motor	0	1	2
14.5 Decoder	1	1	1
16.5 Input Trans.	1	0	1
16.5 Distributor	0	0	2

In the 6 MF families, 3 (18%) subsystems did not give problems to any of them, and each of 5 (29%) gave problems to only 1 family. Only 3 (18%) subsystems -- *Storage* (of goods and supplies*)*, *Producer* (care of house and yard*)*, *and Decider* (executive decision making*)*, gave problems to as many as 3 (50%) of the families, and no subsystem gave problems to all 6 families. We noted that the percentages of families having problems with subsystems was the same as in the HF group.

In contrast, for the 5 LF families, all of the subsystems (100%) gave problems to at least one family; 5 (29%) subsystems each gave problems to 4 (80%) of the families; and 4 (24%) subsystems posed problems for all 5 (100%) families. Only 2 subsystems gave problems to just one of the 5 families.

In summary, we can see that 13 (76%) of the 17 subsystems gave problems to the 8 HF families, and 14 (82%) gave problems to the 6 MF families; but, all 17 (100%) subsystems gave problems to at least one of the 5 LF families. Thus, a comparison of group levels of functioning with the number of subsystems giving problems revealed few differences between the HF and MF groups; however, both of them differed greatly from the LF group for which all of the subsystems gave problems to 2 or more of the 5 families.

The Subsystems that Most Often Gave Problems to the GLS Functioning Groups

In each of the 3 functioning groups, of the 17 subsystems, the *Storage* (of goods and supplies*)* and *Producer* (care of house and yard) were reported by most of the families as giving trouble. Inasmuch as these two pertain to adequate storage space and to both house cleaning and upkeep of the yard, we can see that how well they are carried out are indicators of how well a family is handling the chores of everyday life. In the HF group, the subsystems posing problems to most families were the *Storage, Producer,*and *Boundary* (regulation of visitors, telephone and television). In the MF group, they were *Storage, Producer* and *Decider*; and, in the LF group, all 5 families had problems with the *Storage, Decider,* and *Reproducer* (values, rules and discipline) subsystems, and 4 of those 5 families also had problems with an additional 5 subsystems -- the *Converter* (preparation of food), *Producer, Boundary, Supporter* (space in the house), and *Internal Transducer* (dealing with information and feelings).

Subsystems that Differentiated the 3 GLS Functioning Groups

The number of problems with the following 6 subsystems reported by the families varied greatly and also differentiated the 3 functioning groups.

1. The *Decider* subsystem gave problems to only 1 (12.5%) of the HF families, but to 3 (50%) of the MF families, and to all 5 (100%) of the LF families. The tasks associated with this subsystem are both general -- How are decisions made and by whom? -- and also specific -- How are decisions about money made and by whom? How is it determined whether money is spent or saved? Thus, the functioning of the *Decider* subsystem is integral to family life and is known to be a source of conflict as well as a sensitive barometer of family pressures and stress. We speculated that the functioning group differential with the *Decider* subsystem might be attributable, in part, to the families' very different economic levels. Those in the LF group had relatively low incomes.

2. Somewhat surprisingly, the *Boundary* subsystem (regulation of visitors entering the house, and the use of the telephone, and television) was associated with more problems for the HF group (50%) and, especially, for the LF group (80%), than the MF group (17%). It is difficult to explain these group differences inasmuch as the 2 groups with higher percentages of families with *Boundary* problems were the relatively affluent HF group and the LF group composed of poor families. The MF group, composed mainly of middle-income families, had only one family with *Boundary* problems. Also, the composition of the families gave no clues about the distribution of problems with the *Boundary* subsystem.

3. The *Internal Transducer* subsystem that deals with keeping track of and dealing with information about family activities and feelings within the family was associated with more problems for the LF group (80%) than for either the HF (25%) or MF (33%) groups. These differences probably reflect the LF group's large percentage (80%) of symptomatic families, low socioeconomic levels, and large family size. Thus, we think that how well the *Internal Transducer* subsystem functions can be a sensitive indicator of family well-being.

4. The problems with the *Reproducer* subsystem, pertaining to transmission of family values, discipline, and rules, were closely associated with functioning levels. Only 1 of the 14 HF and MF families had problems with this subsystem, whereas all 5 (100%) of the LF families had problems with it. This extreme difference between the groups raises questions about factors that influence the transmission of values. They include, for example, the influence on children and other family members of television and schools, the generation gap, secularism, and socioeconomic status. In one family, a mother stated that "in this day and age it is difficult to transmit values".

5. Another subsystem with which there were marked group differences was the *Supporter* that deals with the use of space and sleeping arrangements in the home. None of the HF and only 1(17%) of the MF families had problems with it, in contrast to 4 (80%) of the LF families. The differences in socioeconomic levels and adequate living space probably accounted for the absence or presence of problems with the *Supporter* subsystem inasmuch as LF families were at the poor or poverty level.

6. The *Converter* subsystem that refers mainly to preparation of food, cooking, and the number of meals the family eats together each week also was differentially associated with level of functioning. Of the 8 HF families, only 1 (12.5%) had *Converter* subsystem problems as did only 2 (33%) of the MF families, in contrast to 4 (80%) of the LF families. We think that problems with the *Converter* subsystem reflect some of the difficulties common to many of the families in the USA at this time. Family

life styles have changed greatly, with both parents often having to work outside the home and to follow different, often arduous schedules that leave little time for "family life". Consequently, family members tend often to get by with fast foods, TV dinners, and the latch-key children preparing their own food.

In summary, in the HF group, 1 of the 6 subsystems, *the Boundary (that deals with regulating visitors, telephone and television.)* that differentiated the 3 groups, posed problems for (50%) of families, and another, *the Internal Transducer (that deals with information and feelings),* posed problems for 25%; 3 subsystems, *the Decider (executive decision-making), Converter (preparation of food),* and the, *Reproducer (deals with values, rules and discipline)* gave problems to 12.5%, and 1 subsystem the *Supporter (that deals with space and sleeping arrangements)* posed no problems for any HF families. In the MF group, the percentages of families reporting problems ranged from 50% (*Decider*) to 33% (*Internal Transducer, Converter*) to 17% (*Boundary, Supporter*). In contrast, for the LF group, the percentage of families reporting problems ranged from 80% (*Boundary, Internal Transducer, Converter, Supporter*) to 100% of the families (*Decider, Reproducer*).

Thus, of the 17 subsystems, the 6 presented above -- the *Decider, Boundary, Internal Transducer, Reproducer, Supporter, and Converter*) -- were critically associated with family functioning. We think they can be used in a shortened version of the interview schedule inasmuch as the number of problems with them sharply differentiated the three GLS functioning groups.

GLS FUNCTIONING LEVELS, ECONOMIC LEVELS, SYMPTOM STATUS AND STRESS

The stress ratings, as shown in Table 4, were based on both the number and severity of Stressful Life Events (SLE) that had occurred and also the number and types of chronic stressors affecting the families. Of the 19 families, 11 (58%) had low stress ratings, 4 (21%) had mid-stress, and 4 (21%) had high stress ratings. Of the 11 low stress families, 6 (56%) were in the HF group and 4 (36%) were in the MF group; but only 1 (9%) was in the LF group. Two (50%) of the 4 mid-stress families were in the HF group and the other 2 (50%) were in the MF group. All 4 (100%) of the families with high stress ratings were in the LF group. Thus, overall, there were definite associations between higher functioning levels and lower stress ratings and also between lower functioning level and higher stress ratings.

We also found a strong association between overall stress ratings and symptomatic/asymptomatic status. Only 2 (18%) of the 11 low stress families were symptomatic; in contrast, 2 (50%) of the mid-stress families were symptomatic as were 4 (80%) of the 5 high stress families.

Our analysis of the GLS functioning group levels, stress levels, and symptom status showed that in all 3 GLS groups there were associations between lower stress levels and being asymptomatic. An exception was that in the LF group, 1 high stress family (0162) was asymptomatic probably because of its high coping potential. We also looked at the families' socioeconomic levels and symptom status and found the anticipated definite association between lower economic levels and being symptomatic.

Chronic Stressors

We were especially concerned about the negative, probably deleterious, association between chronic stressors and family well-being. There were striking differences according to functioning group levels in both the number and type of chronic stressors reported by the families.

For example, as shown in Table 5.4, only 3 (38%) of the 8 HF families and 1 (17%) of the 6 MF families reported chronic stressors in contrast to 4 (80%) of the 5 LF families. Moreover, in the HF and MF groups, the chronic stressors were health, family environment, and parenting problems. Whereas, in the LF group, the chronic stressors were varied -- financial, crowding in the home, health, and discipline of the children.

Of the 8 families with chronic stressors, 4 (50%) were symptomatic; 3 of them had 2 or more stressors each. The other 4 (50%) families reporting chronic stressors were asymptomatic; of them, 3 reported only 1 chronic stressor each but, surprisingly, the other asymptomatic family, which was in the LF group, had 4 chronic stressors. When we examined the chronic stressors, we also assessed the families' Coping Potential and Family Resources to ascertain whether they might enable the families to mitigate the effects of stress.

Table 5.5 summarizes the families' Stress levels, Coping Potential, Family Resources and their Symptom Status. In some families, their relatively high Coping Potential and Resources were associated with asymptomatic status and may have buffered or otherwise mediated the effects of SLE.

Table 5.4. Stress Levels and Descending Order of Functioning Levels

STUDY I T-3						
Family I.D.	Age of Parent	No. in Fam.	Econ. Level	Stress Level	No. of Chr. Stressors	Symp Status
HF Group						
177	E	2	Fair	Low	No data	As
151	M	3	Ex	Mid	0	S
85	Y	3	Ex	Low	0	As
129	M	3	Ex	Low	0	As
127	M	2	Good	Low	1	As
82	M	2	Ex	Low	1	As
94	E	2	Good	Low	1	As
111	Y	2	Fair	Mid	0	S
MF Group						
81	Y	2	Fair	Mid	0	S
141	Y	4	Fair	Low	0	As
157	E	4	Poverty	Mid	3	S
121	Y	3	Fair	Low	0	As
113	M	5	Fair	Low	0	As
160	Y	3	Ex	Low	0	As
LF Group						
162	Y	5	Poor	High	4	As
108	Y	5	Poor	No data	0	S
128	Y	4	Poor	High	14	S
11	Y	3	Poor	High	2	S
8	E	2	Pov.	High	5	S

Fam-Family   Econ.-Economic   Chr.-Chronic
E-Elderly   Ex-Excellent   S- Symptomatic
M-Mid-age   Pov.-Poverty   As-Asymptomatic
Y-Young

Table 5.5. Stress, Coping Potential, Family Resources and Symptom Status

STUDY I	T-3 Data				
Stress Levels	GLS Functioning Group	Coping Potential Rating	Family Resources Rating	Symp. Status	No. Chr. Str.
Family I.D.					
High Stress					
162	LF	high	mid	As	4
128	LF	mid	high	S	14
11	LF	mid	mid	S	2
8	LF	mid	mid	S	5
Mid- Stress					
151	HF	high	high	S	0
111	HF	mid	high	S	0
81	MF	mid	mid	S	0
157	MF	mid	mid	S	3
Low Stress					
177	HF	mid	high	As	nd
85	HF	high	high	As	0
129	HF	high	high	As	0
127	HF	high	high	As	1
82	HF	high	high	As	1
94	HF	high	high	As	1
141	MF	high	high	As	0
121	MF	mid	mid	As	0
113	MF	mid	mid	As	0
160	MF	high	no data	As	0

No. Chr. Str. - Number of Chronic Stressors
Symp. - Symptom
nd - no data

For example, Family 0127 had 1 stressor ("Strict" home life), but high ratings on Coping Potential, and Family Resources. Family 0082 also had 1 stressor (problems with the environment), but high ratings on Coping Potential, Family Resources, and both mother's and father's availability. Family 0094 had 2 chronic stressors (chronic health problems and "strict" home life), but had high ratings on Coping Potential, Family Resources, and both mother's and father's availability. Thus, those families' Coping Potential and Resources may have prevented the chronic stressors from having serious effects on the family members' well-being.

We found a tendency for Coping Potential to be positively associated with GLS functioning level. We recognize that our conclusions are only suggestive and now think that a more comprehensive evaluation of SLE, coping ability, and family resources should be an explicit part of the family assessment.

COMPARISONS OF THE FAMILY ENVIRONMENT SCALE (FES) SCORES AND GLS FUNCTIONING GROUP LEVELS

Inasmuch as the FES has been widely used in family studies since the mid- 1970s, we carried out extensive analyses of its results in relation to our GLS family functioning data. At T-3, the 19 families had 190 FES subscale scores; 28 (15%) were high, 132 (69%) were in the normal range, and 30 (16%) were low scores. In the HF group, 23 (29%) were high scores, 48 (60%) were in the normal range, and only 11% were low scores. In the MF group, 5 (8%) were high, 49 (82%) were in the normal range, and 6 (10%) were low. But, in the LF group, 7 (14%) were high, 28 (56%) were in the normal range and 15 (30%) were low. (All scores had been given the same direction so that high scores were "positive" and low scores "negative".)

As shown in Table 5.6, on the Interpersonal Dimension of the FES -- the *Cohesion*, *Expressiveness*, and *Conflict* subscales--we found some definite GLS functioning level -- subscale score patterns. One was the fairly clear-cut association between high functioning level and high *Cohesion*, normal *Expressiveness*, and normal *Conflict* scores. Another was that almost all of the MF families' Interpersonal subscale scores were in the normal range. But, in contrast to the HF and MF families, the LF families

had disproportionately more low *Cohesion*, low *Expressiveness*, and high *Conflict* scores, indicative of problems in the family environment.

The various GLS functioning levels also were associated differentially with the respondents' scores on the two subscales -- *Organization* and *Control* -- in the System-Maintenance Dimension of the FES. Families in the HF group had scores predominantly in the normal range. However, many in the MF group had low *Control* scores. Those in the LF group tended to have low *Organization* scores and were the only families in the study to have high *Control* scores.

Table 5.6. T-3 FES Scores and Functioning groups - Study I

FES Dimensions	GLS Groups								
	HF N-8			MF N-6			LF N-5		
	Number of Families								
	hi	n	lo	hi	n	lo	hi	n	lo
Interpersonal									
Cohesion	6	1	1	2	4	0	1	1	3
Expressiveness	0	6	2	0	5	1	0	1	4
Conflict	8-n			6 -n			3	2	0
Value/Orientation									
Independence	2	6	0	1	5	0	5-n		
Achievement	2	5	1	6-n			1	4	0
Intellectual/Cultural	3	5	0	1	5	0	0	4	1
Recreational	2	5	1	1	5	0	0	4	1
Moral/Religious	1	7	0	0	5	1	0	3	2
Systems/Maintenance									
Organization	7	0	1	6-n			0	2	3
Control	0	5	3	0	2	4	2	2	1

hi- Above Louisville norm
n - Louisville norm
lo- Below Louisville norm

On the Value/Orientation Dimension with its 5 subscales -- *Independence*, *Achievement*, *Intellectual-Cultural Orientation*, *Active Recreational Orientation*, and *Moral/Religious Emphasis* -- the 19 families had a total of 95 possible scores. The HF group had more high scores, 10 (25%), than the MF group's 3 (10%), or the LF group's 1 (4%). The HF group had only 2 (5%) low scores, and the MF group had only 1 (35), but LF group had 4 (16%) low scores.

Thus, as shown in Table 6.5 there were some associations between the different GLS family functioning levels and the FES subscale scores. The high level of functioning associated with high *Cohesion* scores, supported other investigators' (Keitner,1990) and our previous findings (Schwab, Stephenson, Ice, 1993). Also, high functioning level was associated with normal *Expressiveness, Conflict, Organization,* and *Control* subscale scores. On the Value/Orientation Dimension, high functioning was associated with high FES subscale scores indicative of interests and activities in a variety of spheres, especially the *Intellectual/Cultural*, which is associated with mid- to upper socioeconomic status and the Active Recreational Orientation subscale which is associated with higher levels of physical health.

Mid-level functioning was associated with many normal FES subscale scores. One exception was that two thirds of the MF families had low *Control* scores, indicating that those families were on the egalitarian end of the authoritarian/egalitarian continuum.

In fairly marked contrast to the HF and MF groups, the LF group had relatively low *Cohesion*, low *Expressiveness*, and high *Conflict* scores, indicative of many family problems and difficulties. In addition, their low *Organization* scores reflected a relatively low level of family functioning. We and others (Koos, 1946), have found that a low level of *Organization* is common in families having difficulties in many areas, including coping with stress and health problems. Also, the 2 LF families' high *Control* scores, reflecting strong regulation of family members' behaviors, are often indicative of family problems and psychopathology as, for example, have been reported in borderline personality disorder (BPD) families (Weaver and Clum, 1993). The LF families' lack of any high scores on the Value/Orientation subscales probably was indicative of their .lack of resources and relatively low level of functioning. In particular, 2 (40%) of the 5 LF families had low *Moral/Religious Emphasis* subscale scores whereas only 1 (17%) MF and no HF families had a low *Moral/Religious Emphasis* score; 1 HF family had a high score on the subscale.

In summary, on our small heterogeneous random sample of families, the subscale scores on the independent self-report measure, the FES, were generally in accord with the ratings of the observer-based GLS Family Functioning Assessment and thus complement each other. We suggest that an in-depth evaluation of family life requires assessment of both domains, the families' functioning and its characteristics.

FES DIMENSIONS AND SPECIFIC SUBSYSTEMS

Comparisons of the 3 FES Dimensions (Interpersonal, Value-Orientation, Systems Maintenance) and GLS subsystems on the basis of their face validity showed that particular FES dimensions could be represented by the functioning of specific subsystems. The FES Interpersonal Dimension was represented by the GLS *Input Transducer, Boundary,* and *Internal Transducer* subsystems, the Systems Maintenance Dimension by the *Decider, Output Transducer,* and *Reproducer* subsystems, and the Value/Orientation Dimension mainly by the *Reproducer* subsystem. Comparisons of the families' FES subscale scores with their subsystem ratings revealed that low FES Interpersonal Dimension scores tended to be associated with low ratings on the representative subsystems we identified. Also, we noted that high *Cohesion* subscale scores were strongly associated with high functioning ratings on the *Boundary* subsystem for all but 1 family (0094).

The low FES Systems Maintenance Dimension scores on *Organization* and *Control* were associated with low ratings on the GLS *Decider* subsystem, Also, there was a tendency for low *Organization and Control* scores in the Systems/Maintenance Dimension to be associated with low GLS *Output Transducer* and *Reproducer* subsystem ratings.

We were surprised to find almost no definite associations between the *Moral/Religious Emphasis* scores and the *Reproducer* subsystem ratings. In this respect, we noted that about 75% of the families had FES *Moral/Religious Emphasis* scores in the normal range.

In summary, we found a reasonable level of concordance between certain self-report FES subscale scores and specific GLS subsystem functioning ratings. In particular, the important FES Interpersonal Dimension subscale scores were associated with high ratings on the GLS *Producer, Boundary,* and *Internal Transducer* subsystems that pertain respectively to the upkeep and cleaning of the house *(Producer)*, regulation of visitors, television and telephone *(Boundary)*, and keeping track of family members' activities and dealing with their feelings *(Internal Transducer)*. Also, there were similar associations between the scores on the two Systems-Maintenance subscales -- *Organization* and *Control* -- and the ratings of the *Decider (*how decisions are made and by whom), *Output Transducer* (how family business is handled and by whom), and *Reproducer* (values, discipline, rules*)* subsystems. But, we found few associations between the FES Value-Orientation Dimension subscale scores and specific subsystem functioning. In particular, there were almost no definite associations between *the FES Moral/Religious Emphasis* scores and ratings on the GLS *Reproducer* subsystem that concerns the transmission of values, rules, and discipline.

COMPARISONS OF FUNCTIONING LEVELS AND RATINGS OF CONSTRUCTS

To assess aspects of family functioning as comprehensively as possible and to include fairly conventional approaches to that complex topic, we categorized relevant items on the independent observers' rating forms (Form B) into 8 emotional and interactional Constructs that have been used by others to evaluate family functioning and well-being. We formulated the 8 Constructs from 48 Form B items on the basis of their face validity (See Appendix.). For example, the item "How often was the discussion understood by family members"? was included in the Construct, Verbal Communication. The 48 items were categorized into the following 8 Constructs:

(1) Verbal Communication;
(2) Nonverbal Communication;
(3) Family Behavior during the interview;
(4) Emotional Tone during the interview;
(5) Boundaries (intergenerational and extra-familial);
(6) Bonding;
(7) Adaptability;
(8) Individualism-Familism Orientation;

The items in each Construct were rated on a 5-point scale ranging from low to high by 3 independent observers: a child psychiatrist, a psychiatric social worker, and a college level housewife/secretary. For the 19 families, we averaged the 3 observers' ratings of each item, and then, calculated the mean score and standard deviation for the items in each Construct. Families that scored more than 1 standard deviation above or below the mean were considered "high" or "low" respectively on that particular construct.

On the 8 constructs, the 8 HF families had 64 ratings; 10 (16%) were high, 4 (75%) were in the normal range, and 6 (9%) were low. Of their 48 possible ratings, the 6 MF families had 6 (13%) high scores, 39 (81%) normal, and 3 (6%) low ratings. In contrast, of the 5 LF families' 40 possible ratings, none was high, 28 (70%) were normal, and 12 (30%) were low ratings. Thus, overall, on the Constructs, the 3 functioning groups had somewhat different ratings. The HF and MF families had more high ratings and fewer low ratings than the LF families. However, there were only slight differences between the HF and MF groups' ratings.

The HF group tended to have high ratings on the Individualism-Familism Construct, indicative of inclinations toward individualism, and, to our surprise, they had equal numbers of highs and lows on Verbal Communication. The MF group had no strikingly high or low ratings. In contrast, the 5 LF families had no high ratings, but had 3(60%) low ratings on the Individualism-Familism Construct, indicative of a family orientation, and 2 (40%) low ratings on each of the Verbal Communication, Emotional Tone, and Bonding Constructs.

Thus, the major differences between the 3 functioning groups on the Constructs, rated by independent observers, were between the HF and MF groups on the one hand and the LF group on the other. That difference was consistent with findings on other measures that showed relatively few differences between the HF and MF families, but major differences in functioning and other characteristics between them and the LF families with their many low ratings or scores.

SECTION B - A LOOK BACK TO TIME-1 AND TIME-2

A) THE FAMILIES' CHARACTERISTICS AND FUNCTIONING AT T-1

To place the families in a temporal perspective and deepen our understanding of the GLS Family Functioning Model, we then looked at how the T-3 GLS functioning groups had performed at Time 1 (T-1, 15-18 mos. previously) and Time 2 (T-2, 6-9 mos. previously) when we were

Table 5.7. T-1 Comparative Data - The Core Group of 19

STUDY I	T-1	T-1	T-1	T-1	T-1
Family I.D.	Stress	H:W Agree	Health	Symp	Cons.
T-3 GLS HF Group					
177	Low	High	Ex	As	Yes
151	Mid	Low	Ex	S	np
85	High	Mid	Good	S	np
129	Low	no data	Ex	As	Yes
127	Low	High	Ex	As	Yes
82	Low	High	Ex	As	Yes
94	Mid	Mid	Poor	As	No
111	Mid	High	Ex	As	np
T-3 GLS MF Group					
81	Mid	Low	Fair	S	Yes
141	Mid	High	Ex	S	np
157	High	Low	Fair	S	Yes
121	Low	High	Fair	As	Yes
113	Mid	Low	Fair	S	Yes
160	Low	Low	Fair	As	No
T-3 GLS LF Group					
162	High	Mid	Fair	As	No
108	Mid	Low	Fair	S	np
128	High	Low	Good	S	Yes
11	High	Mid	Ex	S	np
8	Low	Low	Poor	S	np

Cons.-Consensus on goals
np- non-participant
H:W- Husband:Wife Agreement
Ex.-Excellent

S-Symptomatic
As- Asymptomatic
Symp. -Symptom Status
Econ.- Economic

using other methods (e.g. goal assessment and husband:wife agreement about the number of SLE that had occurred) to assess aspects of family functioning. There were no differences in the composition of the families in the months between T-1, T-2, and T-3.

The major functioning group differences at T-1 were that most of the families in the HF and MF groups had good or better economic levels than the families in the LF group, almost all of which were at the poor or poverty level. A second difference was that only 1 (13%) HF family and 1 (17%) MF family was at high stress, and 4 (50%) HF and 2 (33%) MF families were at low stress. In contrast, 3 (60%) of the LF families were at high stress and only 1 (20%) was at a low stress level. Also, the physical health status of the families in the groups differed; in the HF group 6 (75%) were in excellent health and only 1 (13%) was in poor health. But in the MF group only 1 (17%) had an excellent health rating; the remaining 5 (83%) had a health rating of fair. In the LF group, the physical health status of the families varied considerably: 1 (20%) was excellent 1 (20%) was good, but 2 (40%) were fair and 1 (20%) had a rating of poor.

The symptom status at T-1 varied with the GLS Functioning levels defined at T-3: 2 (25%) of the HF families, 4 (66%) families in the MF group, and 4 (80%) of the LF families were symptomatic.

Table 5.7 summarizes the T-1 data according to T-3 GLS Functioning groups, and shows the associations between stress level, the level of husband/wife agreement on the occurrence of SLE Consensus/non-Consensus on family goals and other variables.

Husband/Wife Agreement on Occurrence of Stressful Life Events

We examined the percentages of husband/wife agreement on the reports of the occurrence of SLE at T-1 and classified the 18 couples[*] into 6 (33%) high agreement, 4 (22%) mid-level agreement, and 8 (44%) low level agreement couples.

Of the 6 couples with high H:W agreement, none was at high stress, 2 (35%) were at mid-stress, and 4 (67%) were low stress. In contrast, 3 (75%) of the mid-level agreement couples were at high stress, and 1 (25%) at mid-stress. But, of the 8 low agreement couples, 2 (25%) were at high stress, 4 (50%) were at mid-stress, and the remaining 2 (25%) were at low stress. Thus, there was an association between high level of H:W agreement and mid or low stress ratings, but no definite associations between mid-level H:W agreement and stress ratings.

Families' T-3 GLS functioning levels were strongly associated with their T-1 H:W agreement levels. Of the 7 T-3 HF families, 5 (71%) had been

---

[*] H:W agreement data were unavailable on the 19th (a single parent) HF family.

high agreement couples, 1 (14%) a mid-agreement, and the other 1 (14%) a low agreement couple. Of the 6 T-3 MF families, 2 (33%) had been high agreement couples, 1 (17%) a mid-agreement, and 3 (50%) were low agreement couples. Moreover, of the 5 LF families at T-1, none was a high H:W agreement, 2 (40%) were mid-agreement and 3 (60%) low level agreement couples. Thus, there was a definite positive relationship between T-1 H:W agreement levels and T-3 GLS family functioning group level.

Perhaps the next most striking finding about H:W agreement was that the level was markedly different between the symptomatic and asymptomatic groups. As shown in Table 5.8, of the 8 T-1 asymptomatic families, 5 (63%) were in the high H:W agreement group, 2 (25%) were in the mid-agreement group, and 1 (12.5%) was in the low agreement group. In sharp contrast, only 1 (10%) of the 10 T-1 symptomatic families was in the high H:W agreement group: 2 (20%) were in the mid-agreement group, and 7 (70%) were in the low agreement group.

Table 5.8. T-1 Symptom Status and T-1 Husband:Wife Agreement

T-1 Symptom Status	T-1 Husband:Wife Agreement		
	High	Mid	Low
Symptomatic n=10	1 (10%)	2 (20%)	7 (70%)
Asymptomatic n=9 less 1 single parent	5 (63%)	2 (25%)	1 (12.5%)

A comparison of T-1 H:W agreement and T-3 symptom status 15 to 18 months later revealed that T-1 agreement levels had predictive value. At T-3, of the 8 symptomatic families, only 1 (13%) had been a high H:W agreement couple, 1 (13%) was a mid-H:W agreement couple, and 6 (75%) of them were low agreement.

Family Characteristics and Interactions: T-1 FES Scores

To assess different aspects of family functioning at T-1, we used 2 methods. One was an observer-based approach; independent observers rated videotapes of the families while they were engaged in a task -- attempting to reach consensus about their family goals for the forthcoming year. The other approach was to obtain their scores on the widely used self-report scale, the FES, which we administered to all adults and adolescents. Table 5.9 shows the distribution of the T-1 FES scores according to the T-3 GLS functioning levels.

Table 5.9. T-3 GLS Functioning Level, T-1 FES Scores, Symptom Status, and Goal-setting

T-3 Family I.D.	T-1 Interpersonal Dimension			T-1 Value/Orientation Dimension					T-1 Sys/Main Dimension		T-1 Goalsetting Rating
S at T-1	Coh.	Exp.	Con.	Ind.	Ach.	I/C	Rec	M/R.	Org.	Ctrl.	
HF Group											
177	n	n	n	H	L	n	n	n	n	L	H
S 151	H	n	n	n	H	n	H	n	H	H	M
S 85	H	n	n	n	H	H	n	n	n	n	np
129	n	H	n	n	n	H	n	n	n	n	L
127	H	n	n	H	H	H	n	H	n	n	H
82	n	n	n	H	H	H	n	n	n	L	M
94	n	H	n	H	n	H	n	n	L	L	H
111	n	n	n	n	n	n	n	n	n	L	np
MF Group											
S 81	n	n	n	n	n	n	H	L	n	L	M
S 41	n	n	n	n	n	n	n	L	n	n	np
S 157	n	n	n	H	L	n	n	n	n	L	np
121	n	n	n	n	n	n	n	L	n	n	M
S 113	n	n	n	n	n	n	n	n	L	n	L
160	n	n	n	n	n	n	n	n	n	n	L
LF Group											
162	n	n	H	n	n	n	n	n	n	H	M
S 108	n	n	n	n	H	H	n	n	H	n	np
S 128	L	n	n	n	n	n	n	L	L	n	L
S 11	n	n	n	n	n	n	n	n	L	L	np
S 8	L	L	n	H	L	L	L	L	L	L	np

S-Symptomatic   Sys/Main - System Maintenance   M/R - Moral Religious
Coh. - Cohesion   Ind. - Independence   H - High Performance
Exp. - Expressiveness   Ach. - Achievement   M - Mid-Performance
Con. - Conflict   I/C - Intellectual/Cultural   L - Low Performance
Org. - Organization   Rec. - Recreation   np - Non-participant
Ctrl. - Control
n - Louisville norm   L - below Louisville norm
H -above Louisville norm

At T-1, the 19 families had 190 FES subscale scores; 30 (14.5%) were high;134 (70.5%) were in the normal range; and 26 (14%) were low scores.

At T-1, of their 80 FES scores, the GLS HF group had 21 (27.5%) high scores, 52 (65%) in the normal range, and only 6 (7.5%) low scores. In contrast, of their 60 scores, the MF group had only 2 (3.3%) high scores and 7 (12%) low scores; but 51 (85%) were in the normal range, consistent with their mid-level functioning. Of their 50 total scores, the LF group had 6 (12%) high scores and 31 (62%) in the normal range, but 13 (26%) low scores. Thus, we can see that at T-1 the HF group had many more high scores and fewer low scores than either the MF or LF group.

T-1 Stress Levels and T-1 Symptomatic Status - the Core Group of 19 Families

At T-1, 9 (47%) of the 19 families were asymptomatic and 10 (42%) were symptomatic. Both groups contained about equal numbers of persons in the various age and health groupings, but the symptomatic group had more poverty level families (40%) than the asymptomatic (11%).

Table 5.10. T-1 Stress and Symptom Status

Symptomatic Status	Stress Level		
	High	Mid	Low
Symptomatic-n=10	5 (50%)	4 (40%)	1 (10%)
Asymptomatic-n=9	1 (11%)	2 (22%)	6 (67%)
Total Number of families	6	6	7

As shown in Table 5.10, analysis of the T-1 stress levels and symptomatic status revealed that only 1 (14%) of the 7 families in the low stress group was symptomatic and 6 (84%) were asymptomatic. In contrast, 4 (67%) of the 6 families in the mid-stress group were symptomatic and only 2 (33%) were asymptomatic, and 5 (83%) of the families in the high stress group were symptomatic and only 1 (17%) was asymptomatic. Thus, as to be anticipated, there was a strong positive association between higher stress levels and symptomatic status.

Analysis of the families' FES scores and symptomatic status showed relatively few group differences. The 10 symptomatic families had a total of 14 (14%) high scores, 67 (67%) normal, and 19 (19%) low subscale scores, compared to the 9 asymptomatic families' 15 (17%) high, 69 (76%) normal and 7 (8%) low subscale scores (See Table 5.9).

The HF group contained 2 symptomatic families and 6 asymptomatic families. On the Interpersonal Dimension at T-1, the symptomatic families had 2 (33%) high scores, 4 (67%) normal, and no low scores; the asymptomatic families had 3 (17%) high, 15 (83%) normal, and no low subscale scores.

On the Value/Orientation Dimension, the Symptomatic HF families had 4 (27%) high scores, 6 (60%) in the normal range, and no low subscale scores; the asymptomatic had 10 (33%) high, 19 (64%) normal, and 1 (3%) low subscale score.

On the Systems Maintenance Dimension, the symptomatic HF families had 2 (50%) high, and 2 (50%) normal scores; the 6 asymptomatic families had no high, 7 (57%) normal, and 5 (43%)) low subscale scores.

The MF group contained 4 symptomatic and 2 asymptomatic families. On the Interpersonal Dimension, both the symptomatic families' and the asymptomatic families' scores were mainly in the normal range.

On the Value/Orientation Dimension, the symptomatic had 2 (10%) high, 15 (75%) normal, and 3 (15%) low subscale scores; the asymptomatic had no high, 9 (90%) normal and 1 (10%) low subscale score.

On the Systems/Maintenance Dimension, the symptomatic had no high, 5 (63%) normal and 3 (37%) low subscale scores; the asymptomatic had no high, 4 (100%) normal and no low subscale scores.

The LF group contained 4 (80%) symptomatic families and 1 (20%) asymptomatic family. On the Interpersonal Dimension, the symptomatic had no high, 9 (81%) normal, and 2 (19%) low subscale scores; the asymptomatic had 1 (33%) high, 2 (67%) normal and no low subscale scores.

On the Value/Orientation scale, the symptomatic had 3 (15%) high, 12 (60%) normal, and 5 (25%) low subscale scores; the asymptomatic had 5 (100%) normal subscale scores.

On the Systems/Maintenance Dimension, the symptomatic had 1 (12%) high, 2 (25%) normal, and 5 (63%) low subscale scores; the asymptomatic had 1 (10%) high and 1 (50%) normal subscale score.

T-1 Form B Construct Ratings compared to T-3 GLS Levels of Functioning

As described on page 19, we formulated 8 Constructs from the 152 relevant items on the independent observers' videotape rating form B. These were: Verbal Communication, Non-verbal Communication, Family Behavior, Emotional Tone (high rating -- excessive; low rating -- being quiet and detached), Intergenerational and extrafamilial Boundaries, Bonding, Adaptability, and Individualism/Familism ratio (high rating indicative of Individualism).

At T-1, of the 8 T-3 GLS HF families' 64 construct ratings, 9 (14%) were high, 51 (79%) were in the normal range, and only 4 (8%) were low ratings. Of the 6 MF families' 48 ratings, 6 (12.5%) were high ratings, 35 (73%) were in the normal range, and 7 (15%) were low ratings. But, of the 5 GLS LF families' 40 ratings, only 1 (2.5%) was a high rating, 31 (78%) were in the normal range, and 8 (20%) were low ratings. Thus, the HF and

MF families had larger percentages of high T-1 construct ratings than those in the LF group. Also, the HF group had a lower percentage of low ratings than either the MF or LF families. However, the percentages of ratings in the normal range in the 3 groups were about the same--79%, 73%, and 78%--for the HF, MF, and LF groups respectively, very little different than they were at T-3--75%, 81%, and 70%.

Symptom Status and Construct Ratings at T-1

Analyses of the T-1 construct ratings and symptomatic status revealed that of the 10 T-1 symptomatic families' 80 construct ratings, only 8 (10%) were high ratings, 61 (77%) were in the normal range, and 11 (14%) were low ratings. Of the 9 asymptomatic families' 72 ratings, 8 (11%) were high ratings, 58 (81%) were in the normal range, and 6 (8%) were low ratings. Thus, there were surprisingly few differences in the two groups' ratings.

A few of the families, however, had many more high or low ratings than the others. In particular, asymptomatic HF families, 0177 and 0127, each had 4 high construct ratings, and symptomatic MF family 0081 had 3 high ratings. Two families each had a large number of low construct ratings; of the 8 constructs, symptomatic MF family 0157 had 6 (75%) low ratings and symptomatic LF family 0128 also had 6 (75%) low ratings.

On the whole, we did not find that the construct ratings provided significant data on the families. The ratings generally did not differentiate either families' functioning levels or the symptomatic from the asymptomatic families. It should be noted that these construct ratings were made by 3 independent raters.

T-1 Goal Setting: Videotaping Assessments

As described in Chap IV, to evaluate family functioning at T-1, we videotaped family members as they engaged in a goal setting task. Of the 19 families, at T-1, 4 (21%) declined to be videotaped, a member of another family was too ill to finish the taping, and 2 other families did not complete the paperwork. Consequently, we had complete T-1 videotape ratings on only 12 (64%) of the 19 families. We rated those 12 on (a) their estimates of the probability that they would achieve their first goal (note 2). We then gave each family a combined goal-setting rating based on their estimates of the 3 following factors: 1) the percentage probability they would achieve their goal--low to high rating; (2) the amount of responsibility assigned to the family for attainment (high responsibility--high rating); and (3) the amount of responsibility for attainment attributable to luck/circumstance (low attribution--high rating).

T-1 Goal Setting Ratings and T-3 GLS Functioning Levels (determined 15-18 months later) - The Group of 12

Table 5.11 presents the 12 T-1 families' goal-setting ratings and related variables. On their combined T-1 goal setting ratings, of the 6 T-3 HF families, 3 (50%) had the only high T-1 goal-setting ratings, 2 (33%) had mid-level, and 1 (17%) had a low T-1 goal-setting rating. Of the 4 T-3 MF families, none had a high goal-setting rating, 2 (50%) had mid-level ratings, and the other 2 (50%) had low goal-setting ratings. The 2 T-3 LF families had mid-level T-1 goal setting ratings.

Table 5.11. T-1 Group of 12 - Comparative Data

T-1 Family I.D.	T-3 GLS Levels	T-1 Stress Level	T-1 Symp Status	T-1 Fam Cons	T-1 H:W Agree
High Goal Setting Ratings					
94	HF	M	As	c	Mid
127	HF	Lo	As	c	H
177	HF	Lo	As	c	H
Mid Goal Setting Ratings					
81	MF	H	S	c	Lo
82	HF	Lo	As	c	H
121	MF	Lo	As	c	H
128	LF	H	S	c	Lo
162	LF	H	As	nc	Mid
151	HF	M	S	nc	Lo
Low Goal Setting Ratings					
113	MF	M	S	c	Lo
129	HF	Lo	As	c	no data
160	MF	Lo	As	nc	Lo

Fam -Family   H-High   As-Asymptomatic
Con.-Consensus   M-Mid   S-Symptomatic
c-concensus   Lo-Low
nc-non-consensus
H:W- Husband:Wife Agreement

Comparisons of the 12 families' T-1 goal-setting ratings and their T-3 GLS functioning levels revealed that functioning assessed by the goal-setting ratings tended to be somewhat lower than the GLS functioning levels 18 months later. Also, on looking back we can see that there was agreement between only 5 families' (3 HF and 2 MF) T-1 ratings on the goal-setting task and their T-3 GLS functioning levels -- a 42% level of T-1 -- T-3 agreement.

Consensus Groups

At T-1, 9 (75%) (the consensus group) of the 12 families reached consensus about their family goals after they discussed them as a group while being videotaped; but, 3 (25%) (the non-consensus group) did not. Comparisons of possible associations between the T-1 consensus and non-consensus groups and their T-3 GLS functioning group levels showed a tendency for the consensus group families to be in the higher GLS functioning groups: 5 (55%) were in the HF group, 3 (33%) were in the MF group, and only 1 (11%) was in the LF group. In contrast, of the 3 non-consensus families, 1 (33%) was a T-3 HF family, another (33%) was an MF family, and the 3rd (33%) was an LF family. Also, there was a tendency for the consensus families to have lower (better) T-3 problem/severity rankings than the non-consensus families, 2 of which had high rankings indicative of many problems, some of which were severe. Thus, in these small groups, there were some weak associations between reaching consensus about family goals at T-1 and the families' T-3 GLS functioning levels.

Symptom Status and Consensus at T-1

We then examined possible associations between symptomatic/asymptomatic status, consensual agreement about family goals, and the families' combined goal-setting ratings. In both the consensus and non-consensus groups, 33% of the families were symptomatic. Only 1 (25%), of the 4 symptomatic families believed at a high level of probability that it would reach its goal. However, the 8 asymptomatic families were more optimistic, 5 (63%) believed at a 90-100% level of probability that they would attain their first goal.

T-1 Family Goal-setting Ratings and Stress Ratings

The stress ratings of the 12 T-1 families were classified into three groups: 6 (50%) low stress families, 4 (33%) mid-stress and 2 (17%) high stress families. On the T-1 stress ratings, there were no differences between the high goal-setting group of 3 families and the low goal-setting group of 3; both groups had 2 low level and 1 mid level stress ratings. Neither group had a high stress family. However, of the 6 families with mid-level goal-setting ratings, 2 (33%) had high stress ratings; 2 (33%) others had mid-level stress ratings, and the remaining 2 (33%) had low level stress ratings.

We found somewhat greater differences between the Consensus and Non-consensus groups' stress ratings. Of the 9 consensus families, 5 (56%) were at low stress, 4 (44%) were at mid-level stress, and none was at a high stress level. However, of the 3 non-consensus families, 1 (33%) had a low stress rating, another 1 (33%) a mid-stress, and the third 1 (33%) a high stress rating. Thus, there was a tendency for the consensus families to be at lower stress levels than the non-consensus.

Stress Levels and Symptomatic Status

As shown in Table 5.11, analysis of the T-1 stress levels and symptomatic status revealed that of the 3 (25%) high stress families, 2 were symptomatic and the other 1 was not. Also, of the 3 (25%) mid-stress families, 2 were symptomatic and the other 1 was not. All of the 6 (50%) low level stress families were asymptomatic. But, of the 4 symptomatic families, 3 (75%) were at mid-stress and 1 (25%) at high stress, and. of the 8 asymptomatic families, 2 (50%) were at low stress, 2 (50%) at mid stress, and 1 (13%) was at high stress. Thus there was a fairly clear-cut association between low stress and asymptomatic status, even in this small sample.

Stress Groups, Consensus, and H:W Agreement at T-1

Analysis of Husband:Wife agreement about the number of SLE that had occurred showed that of the 9 goal consensus families, 4 (44%) had a high level of H:W agreement about the occurrence of SLE; 1 (11%) had a mid-level of agreement, and 3 (33%) had a low level of agreement; SLE data were not available on one family. In contrast, 2 of the 3 non-consensus families (0160,0151) had low levels of H:W agreement on the number of SLE that had occurred at T-1, and the third family (0162) had mid-level H:W agreement.

Thus, in this small sample, there was a weak association between the family's reaching consensus on the topic, goal setting for the forthcoming year, and the level of H:W agreement on the occurrence of SLE. Non-consensus was associated with a low level of H:W agreement, but consensus was not associated with a high level of agreement.

T-1 Goal Setting Ratings, Consensus Groups, T-1 FES Scores, and Symptom Status

One of the 3 families (25%) that had high goal-setting ratings had high FES scores, and the other 2 had mid-level scores. Of the 6 (50%) families rated as mid performance on the goal setting task, 1 had high FES scores; 3 had mid- level FES scores, and 2 had low FES scores. Of the remaining 3 (25%) families that had been rated low on the goal setting task, 2 had high FES scores and the other 2 had mid-level FES scores. Of the 12 families' FES scores, there were 5 (42%) with high scores, another 5 (42%) with mid-level scores, and the remaining 2 (17%) with low scores.

The Consensus and the Non-consensus groups' FES scores differed only slightly; the Consensus group had 18% high scores and the Non-consensus group, 20%. Generally, there were few low scores; the Consensus group had 13% low scores whereas the Non-consensus group had none.

Of the 4 symptomatic families in this group of 12, 1 (25%) had high FES scores, 1 (25%) had mid-level FES scores, and the last 2 (50%) had low FES scores. Of the 8 asymptomatic families, 5 (63%) had high FES scores, 2 (25%) had mid-level scores, and only 1 (12%) had low FES scores. Thus, there was a tendency for the asymptomatic families to have higher FES scores than the symptomatic.

Summary

In summary, to assess aspects of family functioning at T-1, we used 3 measures: Family members ability to attain consensus about family goals for the forthcoming year, their goal-setting ratings, and their FES scores. We hypothesized that high levels of family functioning would be associated with the families reaching consensus about their goals and their having both high goal-setting ratings and high FES scores. In addition, we considered a number of mediating variables, especially stress levels, degree of husband-wife agreement about the occurrence of SLE, and symptom status for which there was a definite association between a low level of H:W agreement and being symptomatic.

Our use of the family goal-setting task at T-1 to assess levels of family functioning revealed that 9 (75%) of the 12 families were able to reach consensus about their family goals, but 3 (25%) were not. The T-1 assessment of their functioning on 3 combined ratings about the goals (attainment, responsibility, and attribution), placed them in 3 groups: 3 (25% families in the high level of functioning group, 6 (50%) families in the mid-level, and 3 (25%) families in the low level of functioning group. On the T-3 GLS assessment, there was a tendency for the HF families to have high goal-setting ratings, but the MF and LF families' goal-setting ratings were all at either mid or low levels.

When we completed the Time-1 assessment, we realized that we had learned a great deal about various aspects of family life from our comprehensive interviews of individual members and of the family as a whole. However, the differing approaches that we used yielded only partial, somewhat restricted views of the families and their functioning. For example, there were no major differences between the Consensus and Non-consensus groups' demographic characteristics and percentages that were symptomatic. Also, there was a low level of concordance (33%) between Consensus/Non-consensus group status and FES levels. Consequently, we deemed it necessary to approach the complex topic of family functioning in new and different ways.

To accomplish that goal, we decided to interview all the families in the study, 6-8 months later (T-2). But, first, inasmuch as we had found fairly strong associations between stress levels and various aspects of family life, especially symptom status, to enlarge our view of family functioning we focused mainly on the problem of stress, families' ways of reacting to and coping with it, and its effects on their interactions and functioning.

B) T-2 ASSESSMENT OF THE FAMILIES - 6 MONTHS LATER

Before we started the formal Time 2 interviews, we asked the families about what had happened since T-1. They emphasized that they liked the Time-1 interviews; in particular, the discussion of goals had helped them look at aspects of their family life that they considered valuable.

For the first part of the T-2 assessment, we asked the family members again to complete the FES. In view of our intention to examine various aspects of family functioning and our long-standing interest in studies of SLE, we made the standard SLE interview comprehensive by expanding the number of questions about each life event reported and its effects on families and their well-being. While the family, as a group, was being videotaped, an interviewer read the list of SLE to them, and asked about each event: Had it occurred during the preceding 6 months? If so, When? What caused it? What were its effects? Who had been affected? In what ways?

The 19 families reported a total of 56 SLE (range 0-10), average 2.95 events, per family. We were surprised at the relatively low number of events reported at that time. It seemed that the family members were holding back, not reporting as many SLE as probably had occurred, and definitely fewer than the number reported by members during the individual interviews at T-1 when a total of 79 events (range 0-9), average 4.16 per family had been reported, or at T-3, when a total of 107 events (range 1-16), average 5.63 per family had been reported. We thought that the absence of confidentiality in the T-2 family group SLE interview was at least partially responsible for fewer SLE being reported, as was the limited 6-8 month interval since the previous interview.

Table 5.12. T-2 Stress Groups and Demographic Data

T-2 Family I.D.	T-2 Par Age	T-2 No. of Dependents	T-2 Economic Level	T-2 Health Rating	T-2 Symp Status
High Stress Group					
85	Y	1 f. ch	Fair	G	As
81	Y	0	Ex	Fair	S
141	Y	2 m ch	Poor	Ex	As
8	E	0	Pov	Poor	S
Mid-stress Group					
151	M	1 16 yr	Ex	Ex	S
129	M	2 f Adult ch	Ex	Ex	As
127	M	0	G	Ex	As
94	E	0	G	Poor	As
111	Y	0	Fair	Ex	S
157	E	2m Adult ch	Pov	Fair	S
113	M	1 adol	G	Fair	As
162	Y	2m ch.& 1m Adol	Poor	Fair	As
128 Y		1 ch 1f Adol	Pov	G	S
11 Y		1f ch.	G	Ex	S
Low Stress Group					
177	E	0	Poor	Ex	As
82	M	0	G	Ex	As
121	Y	1 m 13yr	Fair	Fair	As
160	Y	1 m ch	G	Fair	As
108	Y	3 f ch	Pov	Fair	S

E-Elderly	f-female	Ex-Excellent
M-Mid-age	m-male	G=Good
Y-Young	ch-child	Pov-Poverty
Par.-Parent	Adol-adolescent	S-Symptomatic
		As-Asymptomatic

172

T-2 Stress Groups and T-3 GLS Functioning Levels

We classified the families into high, mid, and low stress groups on the basis of: 1) the number of SLE reported; 2) the family members' ratings of the effects of the SLE; and 3) a panel's (1 general psychiatrist, 1 child psychiatrist, and 1 social scientist) rating of the severity of the event and its effects on family life. Of the 19 families, 5 (26%) were rated as low stress, 10 (53%) as mid stress and 4 (25%) as high stress.

Table 5.12 shows the families in the 3 stress groups, their sociodemographic data, and their GLS functioning levels at Time 3. A comparative assessment found no pattern of associations between the stress levels and age, number of dependents, economic level, and physical health status. The families from each of the T-2 stress groups were fairly equally distributed within the T-3 GLS functioning groups.

In the 6-8 months between T-1 and T-2, there were some changes in the families' symptomatic status. Three (30%) of the T-1 symptomatic families became asymptomatic, and only 1 (10%) previously asymptomatic family developed significant symptomatology. Our T-2 focus on stress revealed that 4 families were at higher stress levels at T-2 than at T-1; 2 of the 4 had a much larger number of SLE at T-2 than at T-1; however, 10 (55%) of the 19 families had a decline in their stress ratings. None of the 4 that had increased stress, had become symptomatic; in fact 1 (25%) of them became asymptomatic.

Table 5.13 shows the distribution of the symptomatic/asymptomatic families in the stress groups.

Table 5.13. T-2 Stress and Symptom Status

STUDY I	T-2		
Symptomatic Status	Stress Level		
	High	Mid	Low
Symptomatic- n=8	2 (25%)	5 (62.5%)	1 (12.5%)
Asymptomatic-n=11	2 (18%)	5 (45%)	4 (36%)

These T-1--T-2 changes were paralleled by some changes in the families' FES scores. At T-1, 6 (32%) of the families had high FES scores, but at T-2, more, 9 (47%) families had high scores.

Table 5.14. Stress Groups and FES Scores-T-2

FES Dimensions	T-2 Stress Groups								
	High-N=4			Mid- N=10			Low-N=5		
	Number of families* scores on FES								
Interpersonal	hi	n	lo	hi	n	lo	hi	n	lo
Cohesion	1	2	1	3	5	1	4	1	0
Expressiveness	1	2	1	0	8	1	0	5	0
Conflict	0	4	0	1	7	1	0	5	0
Value/Orientation									
Independence	2	2	0	1	9	0	2	3	0
Achievement	1	2	1	5	5	0	2	3	0
Intellectual/Cultural	0	3	1	4	6	0	1	4	0
Recreational	1	2	1	2	8	0	2	3	0
Moral/Religious	1	1	2	0	8	2	1	4	0
Systems/Maintenance									
Organization	1	1	2	0	8	2	2	3	0
Control	0	3	1	1	5	4	0	3	2

n- Louisville norm
hi-above Louisville norm
lo-below Louisville norm
* Interpersonal Dimension Data missing on 1 Mid-stress
   family

Generally, we found associations between a low stress level and asymptomatic status at T-2 for the families in the T-3 GLS HF and MF groups; the 1 (20%) asymptomatic LF family was in the mid-stress group. The 4 (80%) LF families that were symptomatic were mainly in the high and mid-level stress groups. However, the associations between low stress, symptom status, and FES scores were somewhat inconclusive. It became apparent that we needed a comprehensive method for studying and assessing family functioning that would include evaluations of the families' coping strategies and potential as well as their resources and the interpersonal aspects of family functioning, such as stress, that we discussed for Time-3 at the beginning of this chapter.

C) A LOOK FORWARD TO TIME - 4

To conclude our longitudinal study, about 15 months after completing the comprehensive T-3 GLS family functioning assessments, we carried out a brief T-4 follow-up. Inasmuch as we had limited funding, we shortened the interview schedule for T-4. Also, we interviewed only one person in the family and, thus, used the key informant approach to epidemiologic studies that has been employed fairly successfully in the past, for example, by Halliday (1828) in Scotland and by Jarvis (1854) in his famous Massachusetts study. We recruited a second-year female medical student who was particularly interested in studying families and mental illness and trained her in the use of the questionnaire. She obtained interviews with 17 (89%) of the 19 families in our core group.

One (0113) of the 2 families video-taped at T-3 that did not participate at T-4 was a T-3 asymptomatic MF family consisting of a middle-aged couple and 3 adolescents. Their general economic level had been rated as fair, but better than the median for the relatively economically low census tract in which they lived. Their overall physical health rating was fair but their stress level was low and they had no chronic stressors. On their FES, the rating for Organization was low, but all of the other ratings were within the Louisville norms.

The other (0129) was a single-parent HF family consisting of a middle-aged, divorced Caucasian woman and her two adult daughters. Their general economic level was excellent, above the median for their relatively high-income census tract, and their overall general health rating was good. They were a low stress family, had no chronic stressors, and were asymptomatic at T-3. On the T-3 FES, they had high scores on the Cohesion, Independence, Achievement, and Recreational-Orientation subscales.

At the T-4 follow-up, there was a change in the composition of 1 (6%) of the 17 families; family 0111 had a baby between T-3 and T-4. Seven (41%) of the families considered themselves to be "better off" financially at T-4 than at T-3; 4 of them were symptomatic and 3 were asymptomatic. Six (37%) families reported no change in their financial status; both family 0157 that was at the poverty level at T-4 and family 0094 that was at a good economic level were symptomatic, but the 4 (67%) others were asymptomatic.

Four (24%) families considered themselves "worse off" financially. Two elderly families (0008 was symptomatic and 0177 was asymptomatic) attributed their being "worse off" to increasing costs of medicine and/or inflation. The other 2 were young families; 1 (0141) was an asymptomatic family) that had a lower income and increased expenses, and in the other (0111), which was symptomatic (the wife/mother was in treatment for panic symptoms), the addition of the baby to their family had put a strain on their already thin finances.

Symptom Status at T-4

At T-4, 7 (40%) of the 17 families were symptomatic, and 10 (59%) were asymptomatic. Five (71%) of the 7 that were symptomatic at T-4 had been symptomatic at T-3, they were:

1) LF family 0008 -- the wife had many anxiety and depressive symptoms and was being treated with Librium, and the husband had moderately severe Alzheimer's Disease;

2) LF family 0011 -- the wife was somewhat improved but still had depression and panic symptoms and the young daughter was still having many fears;

3) HF family 0111 -- the wife was still in treatment for panic symptoms;

4) LF family 0128 -- 1 child, who had been in treatment at T-3, was still symptomatic at T-4 because of continuing conduct and school problems and difficulty with friends; and

5) MF family 0157 -- the mother continued to have anxiety and panic symptoms and memory problems, and the son also continued to have problems.

Two families (0094 and 0162) that had been asymptomatic at T-3 were symptomatic at T-4. In 1 family (0094), the husband had increasing memory problems. The eighth symptomatic family (0162), which had been asymptomatic at T-3 (although their son was potentially in trouble), became symptomatic at T-4 because the son's problems had escalated and he had been before the Juvenile Court.

Thus, of the 7 symptomatic families at T-4, 5 (71%) had been symptomatic at T-3, and 2 (25%) had changed from asymptomatic to symptomatic status in the year between T-3 and T-4 -- a one year incidence rate of 25%. Also, 2 (0081, 0151)) of the 7 families that had been symptomatic at T-3 were asymptomatic at T-4 -- a one year remission rate of 28%. Of the 7 symptomatic families at T-4, 5 (71%) were symptomatic at both times; thus, the one year "chronicity" rate was 71%. Of the total T-4 sample of 17 families, only 7 (41%) were asymptomatic at both times; that 41% was the "continuing well" group.

Stress at T-4

The T-4 stress ratings were based on both the number and type of SLE that occurred and the families' ratings of the severity of the effects on their members. On the stress scale -- rated from 1 (low) to 10 (high stress) -- 4 (24%) families were at high stress, 7 (41%) at mid-stress, and 6 (35%) at low-stress. Between T-3 and T-4, the stress level of 12 (71%) of the 17 families changed: 6 (50%) of the 12 experienced a decrease in stress (1 GLS LF family 2 levels), and another 6 (50%) experienced increased stress (2 GLS HF families 2 levels). The remaining 5 (29%) families had the same stress level at both times. (See notes 3 and 4.)

The Cantril Ladder of Life -- Self-Anchoring Scale

As part of the T-4 evaluation, we included the Hadley Cantril and Lloyd Free Self-Anchoring Scale which had been developed in 1958 in order to find out about the basic hopes and fears of the American People and to examine changes in values and in popular opinion over time. The respondent being evaluated is first asked about his/her wishes and hopes for the future and about what really matters. Then, he/she is also asked about fears and worries and about life in the future.

The second step consisted of showing the respondent a picture of a "symbolic Ladder of Life" (Cantril and Roll, 1978, pg. 16). The top rung represents the entire complex of hopes that the person described and the bottom rung the worst state of affairs. The respondent is asked to indicate where he/she stands on the ladder at present, 5 years ago, and 5 years in the future. Cantril and Roll pointed out that the ratings are self-anchored inasmuch as the respondent defines them in his/her own terms; thus, a mid-rung level of 6 can be considered, for example, to be a middle class New York suburban housewife's psychological equivalent of the rating of 6 given by a Southwestern sharecropper, even though their statuses, hopes, and fears may be markedly different.

The Cantril Ladder of Life-Self Anchoring Scale was used by the Institute for Social Research in 18 different countries between 1958 and 1964 with many different populations. In 1971, the Gallup Organization used it with a nationwide random sample of 1,588 adult Americans that was supplemented 2 months later by an additional 1,446 respondents.

In 1971, the average rung for the present was 6.6, for the past 5.8, and for the future 7.5. Cantril and Associates considered a shift of 0.6 rung to be significant.

The Cantril Questionnaire

The first section consisted of the following questions: "What have been the best things that happened to your family in the past year? What have been the worst things that happened to your family in the past year? What are your greatest wishes and hopes for your family's future?, What are your greatest fears and worries for your family's future?" The responses were categorized as shown in Table 5.15.

During the past year, for "the best things", an Achievement was listed by 8 (47%) of the families, followed by Child-oriented and Financial events, each by 6 (35%), and Family-oriented by 4 (24%). For "the worst things" that happened, Illness was listed by 8 (47%), a Loss by 5 (29%), and a Child-oriented event by 4 (25%). The most common wishes and hopes for the future were Good health 12 (71%) families, a Child- oriented event -- 10 (34%) families, and a Family oriented or Financial event each by 7 (41%) families. The greatest worries and fears were Illness listed by 11 (65%) families, and Child-oriented or Financial events each by 7 (41%) families.

Table 5.15. The Cantril Questionnaire

Events During the Past Year								
Best Things				Worst Things				
Topic	Number of fam.			Topic	Number of fam.			
	n-17	HF	MF	LF		n-17	HF	MF	LF
Achievement	8	4	2	2	Illness	8	4	0	4
Ch.Oriented	6	4	1	1	Loss	5	2	1	2
Financial	6	1	1	4	Ch. Oriented	4	2	0	2
Fam Oriented	4	1	1	2	Troubles	3	1	1	1
Health	4	1	1	2	Financial	3	0	1	2
Misc.	2	1	0	1	Don't know	3	1	2	0

What matters most								
Hopes and Wishes				Greatest Worries and Fears				
Health	12	6	4	2	Illness	11	5	3	3
Ch. Oriented	10	3	3	4	Ch. Oriented	7	1	2	4
Fam.Oriented	7	2	3	2	Financial	7	2	3	2
Financial	7	3	3	1	Loss	4	2	2	0
Achievement	4	4	0	0	Drugs	3	1	1	1
Religious	3	2	1	0	World Events	2	2	0	0
Material	2	1	0	1	Religious	1	0	1	0
Enjoyment	2	1	0	1	Fam.Oriented	1	1	0	0
Drug free	1	0	1	0	Personal Fail.	1	1	0	0
Altruism	1	1	0	0					

Ch. - child Fail. - Failure
Fam. - family

Some of the responses of the various GLS Functioning Groups were:
a)In the GLS HF group, 57% of the 7 families reported an Achievement and Child oriented events as the best things that happened in the past year;

only 1 family (14%) noted a Financial event. As the worst event, Illness was listed by 57% of families, and a Loss and Child-oriented events, each, by 29%. For what matters most, Good Health was listed by 86% of the families, followed by Achievement 57%, and Child-oriented and Financial events by 43% each. In the category, greatest fears or worries, Illness was listed by 71% of the families.

b) The GLS MF group gave many fewer responses to the first 2 questions than either the HF or LF group. An achievement was reported by 2 (40%) of the MF families, and Child-oriented and Financial events each by only 1 (20%) family. For the worst things that had happened, a Loss, Troubles, and Financial events each was listed by 20% of the families; Illness and Child-oriented events were not reported. In response to the third question, what matters most: Good Health was listed by 4 (80%) of the families, and Child-oriented, Family-oriented, and Financial events each by 3 (60%). Their greatest worries and fears were Illness and Financial events, reported by 3 (60%) of the families, and Child-oriented events and a Loss by 2 (40%).

c) In the GLS LF group, 80% of the 5 families reported Financial events as the best thing that happened in the past year. An Achievement, a Family-oriented event, and Health each was reported by 4 (80%) of the families. Illness was reported by 3 (60%). In view of this group's relatively low economic level, we considered it surprising that only 2 (40%) listed Financial events as worries for the future The LF group's greatest worries were about the future of the children.

Examples of Some Responses

We feared that our classification of the responses had resulted in a loss of their "flavor". Some of the best things that happened were "grandparents having spent some time with the grandchildren" and the report by an elderly couple that "they bought a camper and took a long hoped-for trip to Alaska". Some of the worst things reported were deaths of members of extended families. One family that emphasized "love for one another was what really matters", reported as its greatest fear that "grandchildren would become involved with drugs and terrorism".

"A child becoming the best person he/she could be " was a fairly typical Child-oriented family wish and hope. Family-oriented responses were typified by a report (family 0157) that what mattered the most was "family life being good and marriage and children", and its greatest worry was "losing a family member, especially a child'.

Two points we considered interesting were that "World Events" were mentioned 3 times as a "greatest worry" by 2 families, both of which were in the HF group. Also, we were surprised that Family-oriented worries were listed only once, and then by an HF group family that reported fears and worries about "the family falling apart, losing openness".

Comparisons of the 3 GLS Functioning Groups' Responses

The HF group reported Achievement more often than did the MF or LF group, neither of which listed it as a hope or wish. Both the HF and MF groups' greatest concern was for good health, and their greatest fear was of Illness, even though the families in the MF group had experienced no major illnesses during the past year. In contrast, the LF group's greatest hopes for the future were, first, Child concerns and second, Health matters. One of the factors probably contributing to some of these differences could be the number of children in each GLS group; the HF group had an average of only 0.43 child per family, the MF group 1.2, and the LF group 1.8. Although Financial events were noted by the LF group as the best thing that happened in the past year, somewhat paradoxically, Finances were not listed as their greatest concern or hope for their future. Also, Financial events were reported most often by the MF group as "what matters most" and, for the HF group, it was a concern for the future. Although 20% to 40% of families in each of the functioning groups reported that a Loss had occurred, it was a worry for only 29% of the HF families and 40% of those in the MF group, but not for any in the LF group.

We wondered whether the differences in the various functioning groups' ages influenced the report of Loss as their "greatest worry", but the data showed no associations between age and concern about Loss. In the HF group, there were 2 elderly, 3 middle-aged, and 2 young families; ages in both the MF and the LF group a were, 1 elderly and 4 young families.

The Cantril "Ladder of Life"

We used the Ladder of Life to obtain members' views of what had been happening to their families. Also, we considered their positioning themselves on the ladder 3 years in the past, in the present, and 3 years in the future to be an optimism--pessimism index.

For the second section of the Cantril self-anchoring scale, the interviewer presented a picture of the 10 rung ladder to the respondent and stated: "Here is a picture of a ladder. Suppose the top of the ladder represents the best possible life for your family:" Where on the ladder do you feel your family stands at the present time? Where on the ladder would you say your family stood 3 years ago? Where on the ladder would you say your family will stand 3 years from now? Circle the designated rung for each question".

As shown on Table 5.16, on the 10 rung ladder, the 17 families had an average position of 6.64 for 3 years in the past, 7.52 for the present (T-4), and 8.31 for 3 years in the future. Thus, they were generally optimistic. For all 3 times, our respondents' average position in 1991 was 0.8-0.9 rungs higher than the respective 1971 Gallup positions.

a) The GLS HF group average rung on the ladder was 8.6 for the past, 8.6 for the present, and 8.5 for the future. One family showed a decline of 1 rung from past to present, and another family a steady rise of 2 rungs from past to future, but the others showed no change. The 2 symptomatic families in this group showed no changes on the Ladder of Life over the 3 times.

b) The average position of the GLS MF Group on the Ladder of Life was rung 6.8 in the past, 7.6 at present, and 8.6 in the future. Of the 5 GLS MF families, 4 (80%) showed a rise of 1 to 5 rungs from past to future, and the fifth family showed no change. One of those 4 had a steady rise from rung 5 in the past to 8 in the present and to 10 in the future even though their economic ratings and health levels were not optimal and their stress ratings were high; but their T-1--T-3 symptomatic ratings had changed to asymptomatic at T-4. The one symptomatic family in the MF group (0157) had a loss of 1 rung from the past to present, succeeded by a 4 rung rise from present to future, a net gain of 3 rungs.

c) The average position of the GLS LF Group on the Ladder of Life was at rung 3.8 in the past, 6.0 in the present, and 7.4 in the future. A steady rise of 4-7 rungs was shown by 4 families, but 1 elderly family in which the father had major memory problems, showed a steady decline of 4 rungs. All 5 of these LF families were symptomatic at T-4.

Overall, the 3 functioning groups visualized themselves differently on the Ladder of Life. The HF group was remarkably stable; all the families saw themselves at or above rung 8 in the future; 5 had no change in their position from past to future, and only 1 family had a decline. In contrast, the MF group steadily placed themselves even higher (avg. rung 8.6) in the future than did the HF families (avg. rung 8.5). The LF group showed the greatest optimism of all the groups, rising from the average rung of 3.8 in the past to the average of 7.4 in the future.

At least some of the optimism about the future should be put in the context of the level of the economy in the greater Louisville area during the1980's. It was at a significant low in the early to mid-1980s (the time period of the past) but had improved markedly in the following years to T-4, and thus, was possibly associated with the optimism about the future.

Table 5.16. The Cantril Ladder of Life

STUDY I T-4				
Family	Rung on Ladder			
I.D.	Past	Present	Future	
HF Group				
177	8	8	8	no change
151	10	10	DK	(no change)
85	6	7	8	steady rise-2 rungs
127	9	8	8	fall-1 rung
82	9	9	9	no change
S 94	8	8	8	no change
S 111	10	10	10	no change
Average	*8.6*	*8.6*	*8.5*	
MF Group				
81	5	8	10	steady rise-5 rungs
141	8	8	9	future rise 1- rung
S 157	7	6	10	net rise - 3 rungs
121	6	8	8	rise to present - 2 rungs
160	8	8	8	no change
Average	*6.8*	*7.6*	*8.6*	
LF Group				
S 162	2	5	8	steady rise - 6 rungs
108	4	7	8	steady rise - 4 rungs
S 128	3	6	8	steady rise - 5 rungs
S 11	2	6	9	steady rise - 7 rungs
S 8	8	6	4	fall - 4 rungs
Average	*3.8*	*6*	*7.4*	

No. of Families at a particular rung on the Ladder self-placement

Rung No.	1	2	3	4	5	6	7	9	10
Past	0	2	1	1	1	2	1	2	2
Present	0	0	0	0	1	4	2	1	2
Future	0	0	0	1	0	0	0	3	3

S - symptomatic
* 1 family didn't know

As shown in Table 5.16, 7 (42%) of the 17 families considered themselves to be upwardly mobile from the past to the present and projected toward the future, and 6 (36%) families indicated no change; but 2 (12%) families were consistently downwardly mobile, and the remaining 2 (12%)

families fluctuated. From the past to the future, of the 6 families that had the greatest rise of 3 rungs or more on the ladder -- definite upward mobility -- 4 (67%) were symptomatic, whereas all 3 (100%) of those with very small increases of 1 to 2 rungs were asymptomatic. Also, only 2 of the 6 families that indicated no change from the past to the future were symptomatic. Surprisingly, of the 2 (12%) downward mobility families, 1 was symptomatic but the other was asymptomatic.

Table 5.17. The Cantril Ladder and Symptom Status

Symptomatic	Average Rung Position		
	Past	Present	Future
	5.4	7.1	8.2
7 fam.	2-no change, 1- fall, 0-min .rise		
	4-mod. to large rise		
Asymptomatic			
	7.3	7.7	8.4
10 fam.	4-no change, 1- fall, 3- min. rise		
	2-mod to large rise		

The 7 (42%) symptomatic families, as shown in Table 17, had the following average rung positions: 5.4 in the past, 7.1 in the present, and 8.2 in the future. The 10 asymptomatic families had higher average rung positions of 7.2 in the past, 7.7 in the present, and 8.4 in the future. Thus, the asymptomatic group had consistently higher positions on the ladder than the symptomatic in the past, present, and projected future. But, the symptomatic families tended to be about 3 rungs more optimistic about the future than the asymptomatic.

On the Ladder of Life, the GLS HF group had the following changes from past to future: 14% improved, 70% stayed the same, and 14% declined. Their FES scores also were only slightly more optimistic, with 38% improving, 50% staying the same, and 12% declining.

Of the GLS MF families, 80% had higher ladder positions in the future than in the past, 20% saw no change, and none declined. Their FES scores did not change much from T-3 to T-4, they had a slightly higher percentage of high FES subscale scores at T-4 than at T-3 and a lower percentage of normal subscale scores, but about the same percentage of low subscale scores.

Of the GLS LF group, 80% had much higher positions on the ladder in the future than in the past and none had no changes, but 1 family (20%), in which the elderly father had Alzheimer's Disease foresaw a major 4 rung decline in the future. The LF group's FES subscale scores changed somewhat from T-3 to T-4 in that the percentage of high subscale scores rose from 14% to 22% and the percentage of low subscale scores declined from 30% at T-3 to 24% at T-4.

Thus, according to their positions on the "Ladder of Life" and subjective self-report FES subscale scores, on which there was reasonably high concordance, most of the families were genuinely optimistic about their lives. In particular, all but 1 LF family forecast a brighter future.

SECTION C -- LONGITUDINAL ANALYSIS

A) THE T-3 GLS FUNCTIONING GROUPS OVER TIME

Over the 4 time periods, we tracked the families in the 3 GLS Functioning Groups in regard to: 1) Family Composition; 2) Economic level; 3) Physical Health Status; 4) Stress ratings; 5) FES scores and 6) Symptomatic Status. (Table 18.) We had longitudinal data on all of the 19 families except T-4 data on 2 of them (0129,0113).

1) Family Composition Over Time

At T-1, the total sample consisted of 37 adults, 4 adult children, 7 adolescents, and 12 young children. The composition of the families in all 3 GLS Groups was remarkably stable over the almost 4 year period. The only change was that HF family 0111 had a baby born between T-3 and T-4.

The 19 families were distributed among the three GLS groups as follows:

a) The HF group consisted of 8 families (2 elderly couples, 3 middle age couples, 2 young couples, and 1 single parent family). In addition to the 15 parents, the group contained 2 adult children, 1 adolescent, 1 child, and the 1 infant born between T-3 and T-4. Until T-4, there were 4 childless couples.

b) The MF group consisted of 6 families (1 elderly couple, 1 middle age, and 4 young couples). In addition to the 12 parents, the group contained 2 adult children, 4 adolescents, and 3 young children. There was 1 childless couple.

c) The LF group consisted of 5 families (1 elderly couple, 3 young couples, and 1 young single parent). One of them was an African-American family. In addition to the 10 parents, the group contained 2 adolescents and 7 children; there was 1 childless couple.

There were 2 major differences in the composition of the 3 groups. One was that the HF group contained relatively more elderly and middle-aged parents than the MF and LF groups. The second was that the LF group had larger percentage of young families and more children than the other 2 groups.

2) Economic Level Over Time- (See Table 5.18)

At T-1, the families' economic levels were; 3 (16%) excellent, 6 (32%) good, 3 (16%) fair, 3 (16%) poor, and 4 (21%) poverty. Over the course of the study, 7 (36%) of the 19 families had an improvement in their economic level, 9 (48%) had no change, and 3 (16%) had a decline. Two of these 3 were MF families and 1 was an LF family; none of the HF families had a decline.

a) The economic level of 4 (50%) of the 8 HF families improved (poor to fair, fair to excellent, good to excellent, fair to good), and that of the other 4 (50%) remained stationary, 2 at the excellent and 2 at the good level.

b) In the MF group, the economic level of 1 (17%) family improved (good to excellent), 3 (50%) families stayed at the same level (poverty, fair, and poor), and 2 (33%) declined (excellent to good, good to fair) over the period of the study.

c) In the LF group, the economic level of 2 (40%) families improved (poverty to poor or fair); another 2 (40%) had no change in their poverty and poor economic levels, and the remaining 1 (20%) had a major decline of 2 levels (good to poor) over time.

Thus, over the course of the study, the HF group maintained their fair to excellent economic levels, and 4 (50%) families experienced a definite 20-25% improvement. In contrast, the MF group and the LF group tended to stay at relatively low economic levels, only 1 (17%) MF family improved, and 1 (20%) LF family definitely improved. (poverty to fair). Moreover, 2 (33%) of the MF families and 1 (20%) of the LF families had a decline in their economic levels. Thus, during a period of recovery from a severe recession, only the HF group reached higher economic levels.

3) Physical Health Status Over Time

At T-1, on our 4-point scale, of the 19 families, 8 (42%) had a physical health rating of excellent, 2 (10%) were at good, 7 (37%) at fair, and 2 (10%) had ratings of poor. Over the course of the study, 6 (31%) had an improved physical health status at the end of the study, 7 (37%) had no change, and 6 (31%) had a decline.

a) At T-1, of the 8 HF families, 6 (75%) had an excellent physical health rating, 1 (12.5%) had a fair, and the other 1 (12.5%) a rating of poor. As shown in Table 18, 1 (12.5%) of the 8 HF families' physical health status improved over the course of the study, and 3 (37.5%) of them fluctuated but had the same health status at the end as at the beginning. However, 4 (50%) of the families experienced a decline in physical health status; 1 of the elderly (0177) and 1 of the middle-age families (0127) each declined 2 levels (both excellent to fair), and the other 2 middle age families each declined 1 level. Thus, none of the HF families had an improved physical health status and 4 (50%) experienced a decline over the 4 times.

Table 5.18. Longitudinal Data--Study I

Family I.D.	Par. Age	No. of Dependents	Econ Level At Time 1 3 4	Health Rating At Time 1 3 4	Stress Rating At Time 1 2 3 4	Chr. Str. T-3	Symptom Status At Time 1 2 3 4
HF Group							
c 177	E	0	P F F	Ex G F	L L L L	0	As As As As
nc 151	M	16yr.f	Ex Ex Ex	Ex G G	M M M M	0	S S S As
85	Y	1 f ch.	F Ex Ex	G Ex Ex	H H L M	0	S As As As
c 129	M	2f Adult c	Ex Ex --	Ex G --	L M L --	0	As As As --
c 127	M	0	G G G	Ex G F	L M L H	0	As As As As
c 82	M	0	G Ex Ex	Ex G Ex	L L L L	1	As As As As
c 94	E	0	G G G	P Ex P	M M M L	1	As As As S
111	Y	0-inf.T-4	F F G	Ex Ex Ex	M M L H	0	As S S S
MF Group							
c 81	Y	0	Ex F G	F G F	H H M H	0	S S S As
141	Y	2 m ch	P F P	Ex F G	M H L L	0	S As As As
157	E	2 m Adult c	PovPovPov	F F P	H M H M	3	S S S S
c 121	Y	13yr.m	F F F	F G Ex	L L L M	0	As As As As
c 113	M	1 adol	G F --	F F --	M M L --	0	S As As --
nc 160	Y	1 m ch	G Ex Ex	F G G	L L L L	0	As As As As
LF Group							
nc 162	Y	2mch,1mAdol	P P P	F F G	H M H M	4	As As As S
108	Y	3 m ch	Pov P P	F Ex Ex	M L L M	0	S S S As
c 128	Y	1f ch,1f Adol	Pov P F	G P G	H M H M	14	S S S S
11	Y	1 f ch	G P P	Ex F Ex	H M H M	2	S S S S
8	E	0	PovPovPov	P P F	L H H L	5	S S S S

E-Elderly	Pov-Poverty	Stress	Chr-Chronic	Par-Parent
M - Mid-age	P-Poor	H-High	S-Symptomatic	
Y-Young	F-Fair	M-Mid	As-Asymptomatic	
f-female	G-Good	L-Low	c-T-1 Consensus -9 families	
m-male	Ex-Excellent	Str.-Stress	nc-nonconsensus - 3 families	

b) At T-1, 5 (84%) of the 6 MF families had physical health ratings of fair. Most of the families, 4 (67%) of the 6 in this group, experienced considerable physical health changes. At T-4, 2 of them (33%) had improved, another 2 (33%) continued to have a rating of fair; and the remaining 2 (33%) declined. Thus, the MF group maintained their physical health status over the course of the study.

c) At T-1, the physical health status of the LF families varied more than it did in the other groups; 1 (20%) was excellent, another 1 (20%) was good, 2 (40%) were fair, and still another 1 (20%) was poor. Over the course of the study, 3 (60%) had an improved health status at the end of the study; the other 2 families' health fluctuated, but at the end, 1 (20%) had an excellent and the other 1 (20%) had a good health rating. None of the 5 LF families, 4 of which were young, had a decline in health status; in fact, even the 1 elderly family improved from poor to fair physical health.

Thus, we found differences in the 3 GLS groups' health status over the 4 years of the study. In the HF Group, only 1 (12.5%) family had an improved health status in contrast to 2 (33%) of the MF Group and 3 (60%) of the LF Group. Moreover, the health status of 4 (50%) of the HF families declined, in contrast to 2 (33%) in the MF Group, and none of the LF families. Analysis of changes in health status in regard to the families' ages showed that of the 4 elderly families, 2 (50%) had a decline in physical health status as did 3 (60%) of the 5 middle-aged, but only 1 (10%) of 10 young families (0141).

As to be anticipated, the declining health status was associated with advancing age. However, declining health status was not associated with level of functioning.

4) Stress Levels Over Time

At T-1, of the 19 families, 7 (37%) had low stress ratings, another 7 (37%) had mid-stress ratings, and 5 (26%) had high stress ratings. At T-4, 9 (47%) had low, 6 (31%) had mid-level, and 4 (21%) had high stress level ratings. Thus, in the course of the 4 years there was a small, about 10%, shift to lower stress levels.

a) As shown in Table 5.18, the 8 HF families' stress levels at the 4 times showed marked variability; 2 (28%) families that had fluctuated between low and mid-level stress ended at T-4 with a high stress level, but another 1(14%) switched from high to low stress and ended at a mid-stress level. One (14%) mid-stress family at T-1 through T-3 declined to a low stress level at T-4. Three (43%) had no change over time; 2 of them were at low and the other at a mid-stress level.* At T-3, the GLS HF group reported a minimal number of chronic stressors; 4 families reported none, and 3 each reported only 1 chronic stressor.

---

* family 0129 had no T-4 stress data

b) As shown in Table 5.18, 1 (17%) of the 6 MF families had a low level of stress throughout the study, but the others' levels varied. Of them, 2 (33%) fluctuated between mid and high stress levels, a 3rd (17%) dropped to low stress at both T-3 and T-4, and the 4th (17%) changed from low to mid-stress. The 1 family that fluctuated between high and mid-stress reported 3 chronic stressors at T-3; the other families reported none.

c) All 5 LF families' stress levels fluctuated, but they tended, generally, to have a somewhat lower stress level at the end than at the beginning of the study. None of the 3 (60%) that had been at high stress at T-1 was at high stress at T-4. The moderate lowering of the LF families' stress levels was somewhat surprising inasmuch as, at T-3, the group had reported a relatively large number of chronic stressors: in one family 14, another family 5, the third 4, the fourth 2, and only 1 family reported none.

Thus, over the course of the study, 10 (55%) of the 19 families had a change in their stress levels. Of these, 7 (70%) families were at lower and 3 (30%) were at higher stress levels at the end than at the beginning. There were few functioning group differences, except that somewhat more of those in the MF and LF groups than in the HF group changed to lower stress levels and, somewhat unexpectedly, 2 HF families were at high stress at the end. Overall, the greatest difference among the 3 GLS groups probably was that the LF families had many more chronic stressors at T -3 than the others.

The major findings on stress ratings over time were the fairly consistent associations between high stress and symptomatic status. Also, as mentioned, the presence of chronic stressors was consistently associated with being symptomatic and, as to be anticipated, with lower functioning group status.

5) FES Scores Over Time

As shown in Table 5.19, analyses of the families' performance on the FES over the 4 times revealed that when all the scores from the 4 times were combined, the HF group had many more scores indicative of satisfactory relations on the Interpersonal Dimension than the families in the MF group and, particularly, those in the LF group. For example, as shown in Table 5.19, the HF group had twice as many high (satisfying) and many fewer low scores than the MF and LF groups. Also, of the HF group's 32 cohesion scores (4 times combined), 20 (63%) were high; only 1 (3%) was low, and there was only 1 (3%) high conflict score. Of the MF group's 72 Interpersonal Dimension scores, most, 61 (85%), were in the normal range. The exceptions were the few, 5 (28%), high cohesion scores and the 2 (11%) low conflict scores. In contrast, the 5 LF families' interpersonal difficulties were shown by their having only 4 (20%) high, but 9 (45%) low cohesion scores, and 6 (30%) high conflict scores.

Table 5.19. FES Scores (4 times combined) and Functioning Groups

	FES Combined Scores		
	HF Group	MF Group	LF Group
Interpersonal Dimension			
Cohesion	63%-hi, 3%-lo	28%-hi	20%-hi, 45%-lo
Expression			
Conflict	3%-hi	11%-lo	30%-hi
Value Orientation Dimension			
	34%-hi, 2%-lo	17%-hi, 7.6%-lo	15%-hi,19%-lo
Int/Cult	55%-hi, 0-lo	9%-hi, 0-lo	15%-hi, 20%-lo
Achievement	39%-hi,10%-lo	17%-hi, 9-lo	30%-hi, 10%-lo
	51%=nor	74%-nor	60%-nor
Systems/Maintenance Dimension			
Organization	10%-hi, 10%-lo	10%-hi, 10%-lo	10%-hi, 50%-lo
Control	5%-hi, 45%-lo	0%-hi, 10%-lo	25%-hi, 30%-lo
	50%-nor	90%-nor	45%-nor
hi-above norm nor-Louisville norm lo-below norm			

Of the 160 possible Value-Orientation scores, the HF group, again, had a much greater percentage of high (34%) scores, than the MF group's 17% of 120 possible scores, or the LF group's only 15% high of 100 possible scores. In addition, the HF group had few, 4 (2%), low Value-Orientation scores in contrast to the MF group's 9 (7.6%) and the LF group's 19 (19%.). In particular, the HF group had many more, 17 (55%), high Intellectual/Cultural Orientation scores than the MF group's 2 (9%) or the LF group's 3 (15%). Also, the LF group had 4 (20%) low Intellectual/Cultural Orientation scores whereas the other 2 groups had none. There were just a few differences on the Achievement-Oriented subscale: the HF group had 12 (39%) high and 3 (10%) low scores; the MF group had 4 (17%) high and 2 (9%) low scores; and the LF group had 6 (30%) high and 2 (10%) low Achievement scores.

On the Organization subscale of the Systems/Maintenance Dimension, the HF and MF groups had about 10% high and about 10% low scores, most were in the normal range. But, the LF group had, only 2 (10%) high and 10 (50%) low scores, indicative of their difficulties with everyday functioning. Also, there were few differences on the Control subscale scores between the

HF 1 (5%) high and 14 (45%) low and the MF group's. 0 high and 10 (42%) low scores. However, the LF group had 5 (25%) high control scores, 6 (30%) low, and only 9 (45%) in the normal range, a distribution probably indicative of attempts to compensate for difficulties with everyday family functioning.

In summary, the HF families were characterized by their having high scores on Cohesion and very few low Conflict scores. Also, a majority of them had high Intellectual/Cultural scores, reflecting their higher socioeconomic status, and over half of them had low scores on Control. The MF families were characterized by their having many scores in the normal range and very few low Conflict scores; almost half of them had low scores on Control.

In contrast to the two other groups, 45% of the LF families had low Cohesion and 30% had high Conflict scores. Also, 50% had low Organization subscale scores and a tendency toward either high or low Control scores. The LF families' upward striving was shown by their having as large a percentage (30%) of high scores on Achievement as the HF group (39%). The 3 GLS groups had about equal percentages (10%, 8%, 10%) of low Achievement scores.

Examination of the degree of consistency of the families' self-report FES subscale scores showed that, over the 4 times, the HF families' Interpersonal subscale scores, many of which were high on Cohesion, were remarkably stable. Also, they tended to have stable Value-Orientation subscale scores, exceedingly few (2%) of which were low. On the Systems-Maintenance Dimension scores, again, the HF families' Organization and Control scores, high or low, were consistent over the 4 times.

The families in the MF group had predominantly normal Interpersonal subscale scores with a slight trend toward more positive scores over time. Their Value-Orientation subscale scores also tended to become slightly more positive and, on the Systems-Maintenance Dimension, there was a tendency for them to have a few more low Control scores over time.

In contrast, the LF families' Interpersonal subscale scores over time were definitely variable, either higher or, more often, lower, than the HF or MF families' scores; also, the LF families had more high or low scores at T-3 and T-4 than at T-1 and T-2. On the Value-Orientation subscales, there was a trend for the LF families to have higher scores over time, with a noticeable increase in their high Achievement and high Active-Recreational subscale scores. Increasing Active-Recreational subscale scores have recently been reported to be associated with a healthful lowering of expressed emotion (E.E.) in the home (Hibbs, et al., 1993). On their Organization subscale scores, the individual families tended to have fairly stable high or low scores over time.

In general, we concluded that the HF and MF families' self-report FES scores tended to be reasonably consistent over time. However, the LF group showed definite variability that was reflected by their FES scores over time, probably in accord with their problems in functioning that we found on the GLS Assessment.

6) Symptomatic Status Over Time

At T-1, of the 19 families, 10 (53%) were symptomatic, and the remaining 9 (42%) were asymptomatic. From T-1 to T-3, of the original 19 families, 15 (79%) had no change in symptom status; 8 (42%) of them remained asymptomatic and 7(37%) remained symptomatic. Of the 4 (21%) families that had changes, 3 (16%) went from symptomatic to asymptomatic status and only 1 (5%) from asymptomatic to symptomatic status. Thus, at T-3, 8 (42%) of the families were symptomatic and 11 (58%) were asymptomatic. The T-1 to T-3 remission rate of 30% exceeded the incidence rate of 11%.

At the T-4 follow-up of 17 of the original families, 12 (71%) had no change in symptom status from T-3. Of the other 5 (29%), 3 (18%) families changed from symptomatic to asymptomatic status and the remaining 2 (11%) changed from asymptomatic to symptomatic status. Thus, at the end of the study, at T-4, as at the end of T-3, the percentage of symptomatic families was 41%, less than the 57% at the beginning.

a) As shown in Table 5.18, of the 8 HF families, 4 (50%) were asymptomatic throughout the study. Of the 2 others that were asymptomatic at T-1, one family (0111) had fluctuating stress levels and ended symptomatic with a high stress level at T-4; it had been asymptomatic at T-1 but became symptomatic at T-2 and remained so through T-4. The other asymptomatic and T-1 family (0094) was under moderate stress and became symptomatic at T-4 even though it was then at low stress. One family (0151), that had been symptomatic the first 3 times, became asymptomatic at T-4; it had moderate stress ratings throughout the study. Also, family 0085 which was symptomatic at T-1 when it was at high stress, became asymptomatic at T-2 and stayed asymptomatic through the rest of the study; its stress level fluctuated -- high at T-1 and T-2, low at T-3, and at mid-stress level at T-4.

b) The symptom status of the 6 families in the GLS MF group over time was somewhat more variable than that of those in the HF group. Of the 6 MF families, 3 (50%) families (1 symptomatic and 2 asymptomatic) had no change in symptom status, but, the other 3 (50%) families that were symptomatic at T-1 became asymptomatic during the course of the study. The 1 family that was symptomatic throughout the study was elderly, at poverty level, and their physical health status declined from fair to poor. Their stress level, which was high at T-1, fluctuated between high and mid-level of stress over time.   Also, the family had 3 chronic stressors (parenting, family problems, chronic health problems).

Of the 3 families that became asymptomatic, family 0081 which had been at relatively high stress throughout the study, became asymptomatic, possibly as a result of some improvement in finances.   Family 0141 continued at a relatively low economic level but their stress level lowered considerably.   The third family (0113), a middle-aged couple with 3 adolescents, also experienced a lowering of stress from moderate. to low over time, even though they had a decline in their economic status and their physical health status remained only fair; however, their concern about finances lowered.

c) In contrast to the other GLS groups, the LF group was predominantly symptomatic throughout the study. Of the 5 LF families, 3 (60%) were symptomatic all 4 times; the fourth (20%) family (0108) was symptomatic for 3 times but became asymptomatic at T-4, and the 1 (20%) remaining family 0162, which had been asymptomatic T-1--T-3, became symptomatic at T-4. Family 0162 was the only African-American family in the study; it consisted of 2 parents and 3 young children under age 11. The family was poor throughout the course of the study and their stress rating fluctuated from high at T-1 and T-3 to mid-level at T-2 and again at T-4. Also, their improving physical health rating probably contributed to the change to asymptomatic status, even though they had 4 chronic stressors. (finances, housing, occupational role, and mother's low availability)

In summary, 4 (50%) of the 8 HF families were asymptomatic throughout the study compared to 2 (33%) MF families, and none of the LF families; we found that none of the 8 HF families was symptomatic at all 4 times, compared to 1 (17%) family in the MF group, and 3 (60%) of the LF families. Also, as shown in Table 5.18, 4 (50%) of the HF, 3 (50%) of the MF and 2 (40%) of the LF families had changes in symptom status at various times.   Thus, we found a tendency for functioning levels to be associated with symptomatology, and an association over time between persisting symptomatic status and lower levels of functioning. However, there were some exceptions to the association.

Associations Between Symptom Status and Stress

Analyses of the HF group's symptomatic status and stress ratings revealed that over the 4 times, of the 8 families' 30 symptom ratings, 8 (26%) were symptomatic (no data on 1 family at T-4). Of those 8 ratings, 2

(25%) were associated with low stress, 4 (50%) with mid-stress, and the other 2 (25%) with high stress ratings. In contrast, of the 22 (71%) asymptomatic ratings, 13 (59%) were associated with low stress, 7 (32%) with mid-stress, and only 2 (9%) with high stress ratings. There was a tendency for the symptomatic HF families to have about 13% more high stress and 37% fewer low stress ratings than the asymptomatic.

Table 5.20. Symptom Status and Combined Stress Ratings

GLS Group	Stress	Number and Percentages	
	Levels	of Ratings	
		Symptomatic	Asymptomatic
HF Group		8 (29%)	22 (71%)
Stress	High	2 (22%)	2 (9%)
	Mid	4 (56%)	7 (32%)
	Low	2 (22%)	13 (59%)
MF Group		9 (34%)	14 (61%)
Stress	High	4 (45%)	1 (14%)
	Mid	5 (55%)	2 (14%)
	Low	0 (none)	10 (71%)
LF Group		16 (80%)	4 (20%)
Stress	High	6 (37%)	2 (10%)
	Mid	6 (37%)	2 (10%)

Comparisons of the MF group's 23 symptomatic status ratings and their stress ratings over the 4 times revealed that 9 (34%) were symptomatic; none of them was associated with a low stress rating, but 5 (55%) were associated with mid-stress, and the other 4 (45%) with a high stress rating. Of the 14 (61%) asymptomatic ratings, 10 (71%) were associated with low stress ratings, 2 (14%) with mid-stress ratings, and the other 2 (14%) with high stress ratings.

Analyses of the LF group's symptomatic status and 20 stress ratings revealed that of the 16 symptomatic ratings, 4 (25%) were associated with low stress, 6 (37%) with mid-stress, and another 6 (37%) with high stress. Somewhat surprisingly, the family that was asymptomatic at 3 times until T-4 had high stress ratings at T-1 and at T-3, and a mid-stress rating at T-2 and again at T-4 when it became symptomatic. Thus, there was a tendency for most of the LF families to be symptomatic as well as to be at either mid or high stress. Also, at T-3 the LF families had relatively many chronic stressors.

Thus, there was a fairly strong linear relationship between lower stress levels and asymptomatic status over time but a tendency for symptomatic status to be associated mainly with mid-level stress ratings although the distribution was somewhat bi-modal. Also, our look at the families at 4 points in time revealed dynamic associations between stress and symptom status, many of which were not apparent at any one time. Consequently, for clinical and research purposes, it is helpful to obtain a longitudinal perspective on stress, coping and family level of well-being, not just a "snapshot" at one point in time.

Summary

GLS Functioning group status, Symptom status, and Stress Levels

Analyses of the 3 GLS functioning groups' symptomatic status and stress levels revealed that although there were some symptomatic families in each functioning group, there was a trend for the symptomatic, generally, to have lower GLS functioning levels than the asymptomatic. Also, all but one of the LF families and more of the MF than the HF families had symptomatic ratings that persisted over time.

Low stress ratings were definitely associated with higher GLS functioning group levels; there were 48% low stress ratings in the HF group and 40% in the MF group, but about only 20% in the LF group. Also, low stress ratings were strongly associated with asymptomatic status. In both the mid and high stress groups, associations between stress ratings and symptomatic status were about the same. High stress ratings were definitely associated with lower GLS functioning group level: 14% high stress in the HF group, 25% in the MF group, and 40% in the LF group. Thus, there was an association among stress level, symptomatic status, and GLS functioning group level.

There were striking differences in the distribution of the T-3 Chronic stressors among the 3 GLS functioning groups. Only 2 HF and 1 MF family reported any chronic stressors, whereas all but one LF family had a large number of chronic stressors. We think that a comprehensive assessment of Chronic stressors is fundamental to understanding family functioning and wish that we had evaluated Chronic stressors more fully, at all of the 4 times.

Factors Associated with GLS Functioning Group Status

Examination of the various factors associated with the differential functioning of the 3 GLS groups revealed that, over the course of the study, families headed by middle-aged parents tended to be at higher functioning levels than the others, especially the younger families with children. The HF group showed an improvement in its economic level over time even though 50% of those families had a decline in physical health status. Overall, there was a tendency for the HF group's stress levels to decline slightly, but 2 (25%) of the 8 HF families shifted to higher stress levels from T-1 to T-4. Of the 2 HF symptomatic families at the beginning of the study that became asymptomatic, 1 went from high stress to a mid-stress level and also had an improved physical health status and economic levels. The other HF family that became asymptomatic was at mid-stress at all 4 times even though their health status declined from excellent to good and their economic level was consistently excellent.

Two HF families that had been asymptomatic became symptomatic during the course of the study. One changed from low to high stress following the birth of their baby, even though their economic level improved and their physical health was excellent over time. The other that became symptomatic was an elderly family that declined from mid to low stress but had a drastically fluctuating physical health status with a rating of poor at the end of the study. Their economic level was consistently stable.

In the MF group, there was no overall change in the families' economic levels, and although their physical health levels tended to fluctuate, there were no major trends. Also, the MF families had little overall change in their stress levels. But, 3 (50%) of the 6 MF families went from symptomatic to asymptomatic status by the end of the study. Of those 3 families, 2 had lower stress levels at the end than at the beginning of the study even though 2 of the 3 experienced a slight decline in their economic levels. None of the asymptomatic MF families became symptomatic. The 1 (20%) family that was symptomatic over the 4 times was elderly, at poverty level, had a declining health status, and had a fluctuating stress level.

The LF families' economic status did not change markedly over the course of the study. Their health status tended to improve; 3 (60%) of the 5 families had better physical health ratings at the end than at the beginning of the study. Also, none of them had higher stress levels at the end than at the beginning, in fact, 3(60%) had lower stress levels at the end. The 1 (20%) family that changed from asymptomatic to symptomatic status had a fluctuating stress level and their economic level was poor throughout the study. The 1 (20%) family that changed from symptomatic to asymptomatic status had a somewhat improved health rating and lower stress level over the course of the study.

Early in the study, at T-1, we rated 12 families' ability to perform a goal setting task. Later comparisons of their T-1 performance with their T-3 GLS functioning levels showed that of those 12 T-1 families, 5 (55%) of the 9 that had reached consensus about their T-1 goals had ratings on their goal-setting performance that were commensurate with later T-3 GLS functioning levels. However, 4 (44%) of the T-1 consensus families and also the 3 non-consensus families' performance ratings were not congruent with their T-3 GLS family functioning ratings. Generally, the discordant tended to have higher T-1 goal setting ratings than T-3 GLS functioning ratings. Overall, we did not find that an appraisal of family functioning based only on an evaluation of the family's goal-setting abilities and performance provided an adequate assessment of family functioning.

In the next chapter, we present the results of the Study II research with clinic families and their neighborhood controls. Then, we present the consolidated data on the 3 groups -- the 19 random sample families, the 8 clinic families and 9 neighborhood controls. In the last chapter, we look at the limitations of the research and its major findings in terms of GLST subsystem family functioning and such mediating variables as economic level, stress ratings, and mental health symptom status.

Notes

1. (p4)   We had difficulty assessing and rating 2 subsystems--Channel/Net and Association; therefore, we used only 17 of the original 19 subsystems.

2. (p26) The types of goals listed first by families were: health/fitness-by 3 families; closeness/harmony by 2; material acquisitions by 2; success in business by 2; and leisure/travel by 1. We considered the families' first choices to be realistic.

3. (p36) The families were rated on a 10 point scale. In order of decreasing stress, the 3 high stress families were 0081, 0111, and 0127 (rated 7.5). The 8 mid-stress level families, in order of decreasing stress, were families (0011), 0128, and 0151 (tied at 6.5 rating), and families 0157, 0085, 0108, 0162, and 0121 (3.5 rating). The 6 low stress families, in order of decreasing stress, were 0008 (rated 3.0), 0082, 0094, 0141, 0160 and 0177 (families 0141, 0160, and 0177 were all tied with a rating of 1).

4. (p37) Our not having data on chronic stressors at T-4 probably accounted for a few unusual results. For example, family 0008, which had been at high stress at T-3, when we evaluated both their SLE and many chronic stressors, had a low stress rating at T-4 because few SLE had occurred between T-3 and T-4 and we had no new chronic stressors data even though they were still in very poor health and had many problems. In

such an instance, not having information about chronic stressors, for example, at T-4, points to one of the defects of many studies of stress and mental symptomatology.

REFERENCES

Cantril, H. (1965) *The Pattern of Human Concerns.* New Brunswick: NJ: Rutgers University Press.

Gallup (1971) data. Cited in Cantril, H. and Roll, ___, 1978.

Halliday, A., (1828).   State of Lunacy in Scotland and Ireland. In R. Hunter & Ida MacAlpine, (1963) (Eds.) *Three Hundred Years of Psychiatry.* New York: Oxford Univ. Press, pp. 785-789.

Hibbs, E. D., Hamburger, S. D., Markus, J. P., et al., (1993).   Factors affecting expressed emotion in parents of ill and normal children. *Amer J Orthopsychiat, 63(1), Jan. 102-110.*

Jarvis, E., (1971). *Insanity and Idiocy in Massachusetts: Report of the Commission on Lunacy, 1855.* Cambridge, Massachusetts: Harvard Univ. Press.

Keitner, G. I., (Ed)., (1990). *Depressi9n and families: Impact and treatment.* Washington: American Psychiatric Press.

Koos, E. L., (1946). *Families in Trouble.* New York: King's Crown.

Miller, J. G., (1978). *General Living Systems.* New York: McGraw-Hill Book Co.

Miller, J.G., & Miller, J. L., (1980). *The family as a System.* In C. R. Hofling & J. M. Lewis (Eds.), *The Family, Evaluation and Treatment:* New York Brunner/Mazel, pp. 141-184.

Moos, R. H., & Moos, B. S., (1981). *Family Environment Scale Manual.* Palo Alto, CA: Consulting Psychologists Press.

Minuchin, S., Montalvo, B., Guerney, B. G., Jr.,Rosman,B. L.,& Schumer, F., (1967). *Families of the Slums: An exploration of their structure and treatment.* New York: Basic Books.

Schwab, J. J., Stephenson, J. J., & Ice, J. F., (1993). *Evaluating Family Mental Health.* New York: Plenum Press.

Weaver, T. L., Clum, G. H., (1993). Early family environments and traumatic experiences associated with Borderline Personality Disorder. *Journal Cons. and Clin. Psychology, Vol. No. 6, pp. 1068-1078.*

CHAPTER 6
Study II - The Use of the Family Functioning Assessment with A Clinic Population

The next step was to test the applicability of our new GLS family Functioning Assessment Instrument with a clinical population. Inasmuch as funding was limited, we conducted a small case control study to assure that the families we studied would have symptomatic children and adolescents, matched with controls.

The research plan for Study II called for obtaining families with a child or adolescent who was in active treatment for an emotional or behavioral disorder at the Department of Psychiatry's affiliated Bingham Child Guidance Clinic. We selected the first 8 families attending the Clinic that gave their permission and also signed the informed consent for participation. We used the classic "neighborhood" selection method to obtain a matched control group so that the families in the two groups would have about the same socioeconomic status. To do so, the interviewers went to the house in the next block that corresponded with the Clinic family's residence. When that family did not match reasonably well or did not give consent, the interviewers zigzagged back and forth across the street along the block until they found a family that matched and agreed to participate. We made an effort to control for ethnic origin.

METHOD

Each of the families in both the treatment and control groups was interviewed by a team of two or three of the trained interviewers who had taken part in Study I. After explaining the purpose of the study and obtaining signed informed consent from each adult family member, they gathered sociodemographic data about the family. On the next scheduled visit, each family member was interviewed separately for approximately one and one-half hours. We used slightly modified forms of the family, adult and child schedules used in the first study. They included the modified DIS, the CBCL, the CES-D, our SLE inventory, the FES, and an additional new interactional questionnaire that we developed. After the individual interviews were completed, the family, as a group, was videotaped for

197

approximately 1 to 11/2 hours to record their responses to items on the GLS Family Functioning Assessment.

The data were processed and analyzed as had been done at T-3 in Study I. The videotapes were rated for the level of functioning of each subsystem and the number and severity of problems reported for each subsystem by the same three investigators who had rated the families' T-3 videotapes. Then, we rated the families for their ability to deal with the problems. The raters were blind to other information about the families.

SYMPTOMATIC STATUS

Of the original 8 Child Guidance Clinic families, only 6 completed the research; one family did not complete the basic interview schedule and another declined to be videotaped. All of the 6 were symptomatic inasmuch as at least one family member was in treatment. Later, we found evidence of an emotional disturbance in a member of 3 of the 9 neighborhood control families. One had a depressed teen-age daughter who was receiving help from a Psychologist, another had a disturbed foster child who was not in treatment and, in the third, the father had a definite drug problem. Thus, we had a total of 9 symptomatic and 6 asymptomatic families. Comparisons of their sociodemographic characteristics are presented in Table 6.1.

The two groups were reasonably well matched, especially for economic level, adequacy of housing, medical care and insurance coverage. But, compared to the asymptomatic families, the symptomatic contained more middle-aged and elderly parents. In 2 of the 9, grandparents had parental responsibility. The symptomatic group tended to have more rankings of only fair or poor physical health than the asymptomatic.

CLASSIFICATION OF THE GLS FUNCTIONING GROUPS

We used the same procedure as in Study I to rank all the 15 families from the highest to the lowest level of functioning according to ratings of each family's effectiveness in carrying out the subsystem tasks, i.e. 100%, 95-99%, 80-94% etc. We used the frequency distributions, not arbitrary cut-off points, to classify the 15 families into 3 groups: 4 in the high functioning (HF) group; 6 in the mid-functioning (MF) group; and 5 in the low functioning (LF) group.

Characteristics of the HF Group

The 4 HF families consisted of: a) 1 middle-aged couple that had an infant child and was at a poor economic level; b) 1 young couple that had a 10 year old child and was at a fair economic level; c) 1 couple that had a 2 year old child and was at an excellent economic level; and d) 1 young single black mother who had a 5 year old child and was at a poverty level. The following is a case vignette of an HF family:

Family 1016 consisted of a single African American mother, age 28, with a 12th grade education. She had a 5 yr. old son, was on welfare, and lived rent-free in a 5 room apartment with one bath. Her monthly income was $170/mo. from AFDC; she got $145 worth of food stamps monthly. They had no family doctor, Medicare/Medicaid, nor private health insurance. Their physical health status was good as was their mental health rating, although the boy was in need of speech therapy. The mother expressed satisfaction with her life and was able to carry out her duties. She said that she would prefer to go back to work, but could not afford day care for her son.

Characteristics of the MF Group

The 6 MF families consisted of: a) 1 elderly couple at a good economic level, with 2 children ages 11 and 5 years; b) 2 middle-aged couples, 1 at an excellent economic level that had a 17 year old daughter at home, and 1 African American couple at the poverty level with 2 children ages 13 and 10 years, and c) 3 young couples, 1 at a good economic level with 2 young children, 1 at poverty level with a 9 year old child and an infant, and the third that was at a good economic level and had a young child. The following is a case vignette of an MF family:

Family 1001 consisted of 2 grandparents whose physical and mental health were good. They were fighting for the custody of 2 granddaughters, ages 11 and 8 yrs., who lived with them. The grandmother, age 66, had a 10th grade education; she had a previous marriage that lasted 14 yrs. and ended in divorce. There were 9 living children from that marriage, none of whom were living in the home; the 10th child had died.

They owned a 6 room, 1 bathroom single-family dwelling. Everything in and outside the residence was spotlessly clean and in excellent condition. The grandfather worked part-time but had problems of uncertainty about his employment. Monthly income was $1500/mo. -- from Social Security, alimony, pension, and child support. The family was in a negative financial balance because the grandfather had lost his job and they had no savings or food stamps. Their physical and mental health were good, but the 8 yr. old granddaughter was doing poorly in school because of a learning disorder; the 11 yr. old's performance was fair. Members of the family were able to carry out their duties and felt satisfied despite their problems.

Characteristics of the LF Group

The 5 families in the LF group included: a) 2 middle-aged African American couples, 1 of which was a grandparent couple at a poor economic level with 3 grandbabies, and the other was a 3-generation family at a poverty level that contained 10 members: 2 grandparents, 2 adult children, 2 teen-age children, a teen-age foster child, and 3 grandbabies; and b) 3 young couples, 1 at a poor economic level that had an autistic child; another at a good economic level, with 2 children ages 12 and 5 years, and a third that was at a fair economic level and had 3 children ages 6, 2, and 1 year. The following is a case vignette of an LF family:

Family 1006 consisted of a couple with 3 children. Also, the wife's sister, her husband, and their two children lived with them. The 27 year old mother was a sophomore in college. She had a 6 yr. old child from a previous marriage. The 1 and 2 yr. old children were Hispanic. The family was renting a 10 room house with one bath. The home was not well kept. Their income was $2500/mo. from wages and dividends. The father earned $18,000, and the mother $10,000 annually; they had savings of $50/mo. They had no family M.D., and no Medicare/Medicaid or private health insurance. The family's physical health status was fair and their mental health status poor to fair. The 6 yr. old was hyperactive and had behavior problems.

THE THREE FUNCTIONING GROUPS' SOCIOECONOMIC DATA

As can be seen in Table 6.1, the functioning groups did not differ greatly in age of parents or family size except that the LF group, generally, contained larger families, an average of 5.4 persons per household, compared to the MF group that contained 3.5 persons and to the HF group with 2.75 persons per household. There were no differences between the three groups' economic status; each contained families at the poverty level. The physical health ratings declined according to functioning group level:

the HF group had 1 excellent and 3 good health ratings; the MF group 1 excellent, 1 good, 2 fair, and 1 poor rating; and the LF group had no excellent, 1 good, 2 fair and 3 poor ratings.

Table 6.1. Symptomatic/Asymptomatic Comparative Data

STUDY II					
Family I.D.	Par. Age	Family Comp.	Econ. Level	Health Status	GLS Group
Symptomatic					
B 1002	M	13y f & 10y m	Pov.	Poor	Mid
1010	Y	male ch.	Good	Good	Mid
gps 1001	E	11y f & 5y f	Good	Fair	Mid
1015	M	17. f	Ex	Good	Mid
gps B 1005	M	3 presch.	Poor	Poor	Low
1006	Y	6y m,1& 2y f	Fair	Fair	Low
1003	Y	6y m-autistic	Poor	Poor	Low
1014	Y	12y m & 5y m	Fair	Poor	Low
gps B 1017	M	21y m 18y f 15y m 14y f 14y f foster 3 presch.	Pov.	Fair	Low
Asymptomatic					
1013	Y	12f & 2yr.f	Good	Fair	Mid
1011	Y	10y m	Good	Good	High
1019	M	1y	Poor	Good	High
1018	Y	2y	Ex	Ex	High
B 1016	Y	Sgl Par & 5y m	Pov	Good	High
1012	Y	9y m & inf	Pov	Ex	Mid

1004 - no video	m-male	Ex-Excellent
1009 - incomplete data	f- female	Pov-Poverty
Par.-Parental	presch -preschool	
Sgl-Single	inf-infant	
Comp-Composition	B-Black	
y-year	gps-Grandparents	

PROBLEM/SEVERITY RANKINGS OF THE FUNCTIONING LEVELS

The average number of subsystem functioning problems per family and their severity increased progressively from the HF to the LF group. The HF group had 2.5 problems per family with an average rated severity of 21.02; the MF group had 3.95 problems per family with an average rated severity of 22.17; and the LF group had 5.36 problems per family with an average severity of 26.51.

A comparison of the ranking of the families' functioning levels with their problem/severity (P/S) rankings is shown in Table 6.2. In the HF group, there were reasonably consistent correlations between the families' overall functioning and their P/S rankings; specifically, families that had been ranked 1,2,3,4 for functioning had corresponding P/S rankings of 2.5, 4.0, 7.0, and 2.5. The one discrepancy was that the family that ranked 3 on functioning had a P/S ranking of 7.0 indicative of mid-level P/S status.

Table 6.2. Family Ranking According to Subsystem Problem/Severity

Family I.D.	Symp. Status	Age of Par	No. in Fam.	Econ Level	Total Prob	Severity Weight	P/S Rank	GLS Rank
HF Group								
1011	As	Y	3	Fair	1.6	18.6	2.5	1
1019	As	M	3	Poor	2.7	21.6	4	2
1018	As	Y	3	Ex	4.2	21.9	7	3
1016	As	Y	2	Pov.	1.5	20	2.5	4
MF Group								
1015	S	M	3	Ex	7.7	25.6	13	5
1013	As	Y	3	Poor	6.4	23.1	11	6
1012	As	Y	4	Pov.	3.3	20.3	5	7
1001	S	E	4	Good	3.7	20	6	8.5
1002	S	M	4	Pov.	1.2	19.5	1	8.5
1010	S	Y	3	Good	8.4	24.5	14	10
LF Group								
1005	S	M	5	Poor	4	27.3	8	11
1017	S	M	10	Pov.	5.6	23.3	10	12
1014	S	Y	4	Good	4.6	22.1	9	13.5
1006	S	Y	5	Fair	15.3	31	15	13.5
1003	S	T	3	Poor	6.3	29	12	15

As - Asymptomatic   E - Elderly   Econ. - Economic
Prob - Problems   P/S - Problem/Severity   Pov. - Poverty
S - Symptomatic   M - Mid-Age
Par. - Parental   Y - Young

Of the 6 families in the MF group, however, only 2 had reasonably consistent correlations between their functioning ratings and their P/S rankings; 4 (67%) had discrepancies between those two rankings. Three of those 4 MF families had lower (more negative) rankings on Family Functioning than on their P/S rankings, but, 1 had a mid-level functioning rank of 8.5, and a surprisingly high P/S ranking of 1 (the least number of problems).

In the LF group, 2 (40%) of the 5 families had functioning levels that corresponded with their P/S rankings. The other 3 (60%) had lower (better) family functioning rankings indicative of MF group status, than their P/S rankings.

Thus, there were differences in the 3 functioning groups' percentages of inconsistencies between functioning levels and number/severity of problems, HF 25%, MF 67%, and LF 68%, respectively. Rating families' functioning levels solely on the basis of the number and severity of their problems appears to be insufficient because it does not take into account the families' resilience and their ability to cope.

SUBSYSTEM ANALYSIS

Overall, many fewer of the subsystems, 8 (46%) were reported as producing problems for the HF families than the 15 (89%) for the MF families or the 13 (76%) for the LF families. Of the 17 subsystems, 3 -- *Storage, Internal Transducer,* and *Producer* -- were reported as giving problems to at least two-thirds of the 15 families. Two of those 3 subsystems deal with the activities of everyday living; *the Storage* refers to the adequacy of storage space and the *Producer* refers to the upkeep of the home and yard. In contrast, the third, the *Internal Transducer,* refers almost exclusively to major interpersonal issues: how members convey, deal with, and understand feelings within the family.

An additional 4 subsystems that gave problems to at least 50%-60% of the families are seen by many researchers as being critical aspects of family functioning. They are: 1) the *Decider* that refers to decision making within the family; 2) the *Reproducer* that refers mainly to the transmission of values; 3) the *Boundary* subsystem that refers to both family and intergenerational boundaries; and 4) the *Supporter* subsystem that refers to the adequacy of living space which, surprisingly, is not evaluated in many studies, although crowding has been linked to mental disorder as well as to poor family functioning (Schwab, et al., 1979) (Minuchin, et al., 1967).

In contrast, 5 subsystems -- the *Decoder, Encoder, Extruder, Motor,* and *Memory* -- were reported by only 3-4 (20-28%) of the 15 families as giving problems. An additional 5 subsystems were reported as giving problems to only 1 (7%) family each; they were the *Converter*, *Distributor*, *Input Transducer*, *Ingestor*, and *Output Transducer*.

Analysis Of Subsystem Performance At The Different Functioning Level

Of the subsystems, 7 gave problems to at least 8 of the 15 families, but 5 subsystems each gave problems to only 1 family. As we had found in Study I, the *Storage* subsystem gave problems to most of the families. We were surprised that the *Internal Transducer* subsystem gave problems to 100% of the 4 HF families, as well as to 50% of the 6 MF, and to 80% of the 5 LF families. But, 9 of the 17 subsystems gave no problems to the 4 families in the HF group, whereas only 2 subsystems gave no problems to the MF families and 4 subsystems gave no problems to the LF families.

The 4 HF families gave 14 reports of problems with the 17 subsystems (avg. 3.5 per family). The 6 MF families gave 39 (avg. 6.5 per family); and the 4 LF families reported problems with 36 (avg. 7.2 per family).

Thus, we can see that a much smaller percentage of the families in the HF group reported problems with the subsystems than the families in either the MF or LF groups, both of which reported problems with the majority of the subsystems. The difference between the MF and LF groups was small, not as large as we had anticipated.

Subsystems Differentiating the Functioning Groups

The number of families reporting problems with the following 5 (30%) of the 17 subsystems differentiated the 3 GLS functioning groups. They were the *Storage*, *Producer*, *Reproducer*, *Boundary* and *Supporter* subsystems.

Ranking of Subsystems with Problems

1. *The Storage Subsystem*

Only 2 (50%), of the HF families, in contrast to 5 (84%) of the MF, and all 5 (100%) of the LF families, reported problems with the *Storage* subsystem. However, per family, there were practically no differences in the average number of problems reported with the *Storage* subsystem by the different functioning groups: avs. 1.0 for the HF group; 0.9 for the MF group; and 0.86 for the LF group. We then looked for possible associations between the various economic levels and the number and severity of problems reported with this subsystem; surprisingly, there was a slight trend for an increasing number and severity of problems to be associated with increasingly higher economic levels. As to be anticipated, there was a tendency for families with small children to have problems with storage. In the HF group, 1 of the 3 families with small children had a problem with storage; in the MF group 2 of the 3 families with children had problems; and, in the LF group, 3 of the 5 families with small children had problems with the *Storage* subsystem.

2. *Producer Subsystem*

The percentage of families in each functioning group reporting problems with the *Producer* subsystem differed markedly, from 25% of the HF families to 85% of the MF, and 80% of the LF families. Also, 1 HF family reported a minimal number of problems (av. 0.3 per family), whereas, the families in both the MF and LF groups reported a low to moderate number of problems (av. 0.8 and 1.0 per family respectively). Inasmuch as the *Producer* subsystem deals with house repairs and upkeep, house cleaning, and health care, it is a critical aspect of family functioning and problems with it often are indicators of how well the family is handling the everyday activities necessary for well-being and orderly living.

3. *The Reproducer Subsystem*

The *Reproducer* subsystem, which deals with the transmission of family values and with discipline and rules within the home, obviously is a critical one, especially for families with children. Again, only 1 (25%) HF family reported problems with the *Reproducer* subsystem, in contrast to 4 (67%) of the 6 MF families and 4 (80%) of the 5 LF families. Both the HF (av.0.7 per family) and the MF groups (av. 0.7 per family) reported a small number of problems, and the number reported by the LF group was only slightly greater (av.1.0 per family). One LF family reported a relatively large number of 2.3 problems, more than any other family in the study; it consisted of two young parents with a fair income and 3 children under the age of 6.

4. *The Boundary Subsystem*

The *Boundary* subsystem, which deals with both family and intergenerational boundaries, concerns persons entering or leaving the house and the use of the telephone and television. None of the HF families reported problems with the *Boundary* subsystem in contrast to 5 (84%) of the MF families and 3 (60%) of the LF families. The number of problems reported by families was small (0.7 per family). However, MF family 1013 reported a relatively large number (1.7) of problems; it was a young family consisting of 2 parents who had a good income, and 2 chidlren, a 12 yr. old daughter and a 2 yr. old son. Also, the number of problems reported in the LF group was relatively low (0.8 per family); no family had more than 1 definite problem.

5. *The Supporter Subsystem*

In the HF group, 2 (50%) of the 4 families reported a minimum number of problems (av. 0.3 per family) with this subsystem which deals with adequacy of the living space, but 1 (17%) MF family reported a relatively large number of problems (1.7). In contrast, all 5 (100%) of the LF families reported problems (av. 1.2 per family) with the exception of family 1006 that reported a large number (2.0).

Summary

In summary, there were functioning group differences in the number of families having problems with the top 7 of the 17 subsystems. The relatively few in the HF group sharply differentiated it from both the MF and LF groups, each of with had considerably more problems per families. One exception was that for the *Supporter* subsystem, 50% of the HF families reported problems compared to 17% of the MF and 100% of the LF families.

Subsystem Functioning and Symptomatic Status

Of the 15 families, 9 (60%) were symptomatic and 6 (40%) were asymptomatic. We found a strong association between functioning group level and symptom status. None of the 9 symptomatic families was in the HF group. In contrast, 4 (67%) of the 6 MF families were symptomatic, as were 5 (100%) of those in the LF group. Thus, there was a definite association between lower level of functioning and symptomatology, especially in the LF group.

The subsystems that gave problems to at least twice as many symptomatic as asymptomatic families were the *Encoder*, *Supporter*, *Reproducer*, *Storage*, *Producer*, *Decoder*, and *Decider*. The two subsystems that gave about an equal number of problems to both the symptomatic and asymptomatic families were the *Internal Transducer* and the *Motor*. The 4 subsystems that did not give any problems to families in either group were the *Converter*, *Extruder*, *Distributor*, and *Input Transducer*.

We were surprised to find that the *Internal Transducer* subsystem, which deals with how the family keeps up to date with what is going on within it and how the family deals with members' feelings, gave problems to a majority of both the symptomatic and asymptomatic families. In particular, even 3 of the 4 asymptomatic HF families had problems with that subsystem.

Thus, of the 17 subsystems, only 4 (the *Storage, Motor, Producer Internal Transducer*) gave problems to the asymptomatic families, definitely fewer than the 13 subsystems that gave problems to the symptomatic group.

Table 6.3. Symptom Status - Subsystem Problems

STUDY II	
Frequency of Subsystem Giving Problems	
No. of Families	Subsystem
Symptomatic - n- 9	
7 families	Internal Transducer
6 families	Reproducer, Decoder
5 families	Encoder, Supporter
4 families	Memory, Storage
	Decider
3 families	Producer
2 families	Output Transducer
	Boundary
1 family	Ingestor, Motor
Asymptomatic - n- 6	
4 families	Internal Transducer
3 families	Storage
1 family	Motor, Producer

Problems - Problem/Severity (P/S) Rankings, and Symptom Status

As shown in Table 6.3, there was a definite difference in the number of problems reported by the symptomatic and the asymptomatic groups; the 9 symptomatic families had a total of 56.8 problems (avg. 6.3 per family), whereas the 6 asymptomatic families had a total of 19.7 problems (avg. 3.3 per family). The families were ranked according to the number of problems weighted for severity, the family with the lowest score (few problems/little severity) ranked 1 on the P/S scale and the family with the highest (many problems/great severity) ranked 15. On the scale, 1 symptomatic family (11%) was in the upper third (1-5) of the P/S scale, 4 families (44%) ranked in the middle third (6-10), and another 4 (44%) were in the lowest third (11-15). Thus, the distribution showed a fairly strong association between a larger number of problems with greater severity and being symptomatic.

Of the 6 asymptomatic families, 4 (66%) ranked in the upper third of the P/S scale; 1 (16%) was in the middle third; and 1 (16%) was in the lowest third. Thus, the distribution of the asymptomatic families on the P/S scale was the converse of that of the symptomatic.

Examination of the P/S rankings and the symptomatic status of the families in each of the 3 functioning groups revealed that within the HF group, all of the 4 families were asymptomatic; 3 of those 4 (75%) were in the upper third of the P/S scale, 1 (25%) was in the middle third, and none was in the lowest third.

In the MF group, 1 (25%) of the 4 symptomatic families ranked in the upper third of the P/S scale, another 1 (25%) ranked in the middle third, and 2 (50%) ranked in the lower third of the scale. Of the 2 asymptomatic families, 1 ranked in the upper third and the other ranked in the lowest third of the P/S scale.

In the LF group, however, none of the 5 symptomatic families was in the upper third of the P/S scale; 3 (60%) were in the middle third, and 2 (40%) were in the lowest third of the P/S scale.

Thus, we found an association between functioning group level, symptomatic status, and P/S ranking, particularly for the HF and LF groups. As anticipated, the HF families were mainly asymptomatic and in the upper third of the P/S rankings. In contrast, all of the LF families were symptomatic and were in the middle and lowest thirds of the P/S rankings. For the MF group, the distribution according to symptom status and the P/S ranking was mixed.

Then, we examined the question: was the association between the P/S rankings and functioning group level stronger than the association between the P/S rankings and symptom status? There were no meaningful differences. But, we found the anticipated overall positive association between higher functioning group level and being asymptomatic, and a strong positive association between P/S rankings and symptomatic status with more problems of moderate or marked severity associated with being symptomatic.

GLS Functioning Levels and Stress Ratings

Analyses of the number of stressful life events (SLE) weighted for their effects on the families enabled us to categorize them into high, mid, and low stress groups. Of the 14 families on which we had complete stress data, 6 (43%) were at a high stress level, 5 (36%) at mid stress, and 3 (22%) low stress.

Stress Groups and Functioning Level

The distribution of the stress ratings in the three GLS functioning groups showed that of the 3 families (data on the 4th family were incomplete) in the HF group, 2 (67%) were in the high, none was in the mid, and 1 was in the low stress group. Of the 6 families in the MF group, 2 (33%) were high stress, 2 (33%) mid-level stress, and still another 2 (33%) low stress. And, of the 5 families in the LF group, 2 (40%) were high stress, 3 (60%) mid- stress, and none was low stress. Thus, 66% of the HF families, 33% of MF families and 40% of LF families were at high stress. At low stress, there was only 1 (33%) HF family and 2 (33%) MF families, but none of the LF families. Thus, there was a larger percentage of high stress families in the HF than the other groups, which had equal percentages of high stress families. All 3 of the low stress families were in either the HF or MF group.

Symptomatic Status and Stress Ratings

Overall, as shown in Table 6.4 there were few differences in the distribution of the stress ratings according to the families' symptomatic status.

Table 6.4. Stress Levels and Symptom Status

Study II			
Symptom Status	Stress Level		
No. of Families	High	Mid	Low
Symptomatic - n=9	4 (44%)	4 (44%)	1 (11%)
Asymptomatic- n=5*	2 (40%)	1 (20%)	2 (40%)
* 1 data incomplete			

The symptomatic had a slightly larger percentage (44%) of families at high stress and a definitely larger percentage (44%) at mid-level stress than the asymptomatic of which 40% and 20% respectively were at the high and mid-stress levels. At low stress, there were 1 (11%) symptomatic and 2 (40%) asymptomatic families.

FES Scores and Functioning Levels

As shown in Table 6.5, comparisons of the subscale scores on the FES Interpersonal Dimension subscales -- *Cohesion*, *Expressiveness*, and *Conflict* -- and the GLS functioning group levels showed some striking trends. One was that there were few functioning group differences in the clinically important *Cohesion* subscale scores. Another was that 1 family in the MF group and 2 in the LF group had high *Conflict* scores, indicative of family difficulties. A second trend was that the pattern of the high and low scores in the LF group signified family difficulties.

Comparisons of the 3 GLS functioning groups' Interpersonal Dimension subscale scores showed a weak association between lower functioning levels and lower subscale scores. Of the HF group's 9 scores, only 2 (22%) were low, as were only 2 (11%) of the MF group's 18 scores and 4 (27%) of the LF group's 15 scores. In particular, the percentage of high *Conflict* scores, indicative of serious interpersonal difficulties, which ranged from 0 in the HF group, to 1 (17%) in the MF group, to 4 (80%) in the LF group, pointed to a definite association between a high level of *Conflict* and a relatively low level of functioning.

On the Systems/Maintenance Dimension, we were surprised to find that 2 (67%) of the 3 HF families had low *Organization* subscale scores, in contrast to only 1 (17%) of the MF families, and only 1 (20%) in the LF group. Generally, low scores on *Organization* have indicated difficulties in everyday living.

The 1 LF family that had a high *Control* subscale score consisted of a young couple with 2 boys, ages 13 and 5 yrs. The family had a mid-level economic rating and were at high stress. The father had a drug problem and the mother had depressive symptoms. It appeared that the high *Control* score represented attempts to lessen distress in this obviously troubled family.

Comparisons of the 3 functioning groups' scores on the Value/ Orientation subscales -- *Independence, Achievement, Intellectual/Cultural, Orientation, Active Recreational Orientation,* and *Moral/Religious Emphasis* -- revealed few functioning group differences. Of the HF group's 15 scores, only 2 (13%) were high as were 4 (13%) of the 6 MF families' 30 scores, and 2 (8%) of the 5 LF families' 25 scores. However, the HF group had 5 (33%) low Value/Orientation scores, the MF group had 5 (17%) low scores, and the LF group, 3 (12%), low scores. All the other scores were in the normal range. We could not explain why, contrary to expectations, the HF group had a somewhat larger percentage of low Value/Orientation subscale scores than the other 2 groups, especially the LF group.

On the Value/Orientation dimension, the scores on two subscales deserve attention. The HF group had 2 (67%) families with low *Moral/Religious Emphasis* scores as did 2 (33%) in the MF group, but only 1 (20%) in the LF group. We had not anticipated that all of the 5 families with low *Moral/Religious Emphasis* subscale scores would have young children, inasmuch as, historically, the greater Louisville community has

Table 6.5. FES Scores, Stress and Symptom Status

Study II	FES Scores										
Family I.D.	Interpersonal Dimension			Value/Orientation Dimension					Sys/Main Dimension		Stress
	Coh	Exp	Con	Ind	Ach	I/C	Rec	M/R	Org	Ctrl	
HF Group											
1011	no data			no data					no data		
1019	n	n	n	n	n	n	lo	lo	lo	n	Low
1018	lo	lo	n	n	lo	n	n	lo	lo	lo	High
B 1016	hi	n	n	hi	hi	n	lo	n	n	n	High
MF Group											
1012	n	hi	n	hi	n	n	lo	n	n	lo	Mid
S 1010	hi	n	n	n	n	hi	n	lo	n	lo	High
1013	n	n	n	n	n	n	n	lo	lo	n	Low
B, S 1002	n	n	n	n	hi	n	lo	n	n	n	Low
S 1001	lo	n	n	n	n	n	lo	n	n	n	High
S 1015	lo	n	hi	n	n	n	hi	n	n	n	Mid
LF Group											
S 1014	n	n	hi	n	n	hi	n	n	n	hi	High
B, S 1005	n	n	n	n	n	n	n	n	n	n	Mid
S 1006	hi	lo	hi	n	n	n	n	hi	n	n	High
S 1003	lo	lo	hi	n	n	n	lo	lo	n	n	Mid
B, S 1017	lo	no	hi	n	n	n	lo	n	lo	n	Mid

1004 - No Video   Ach - Achievement   B - Black
1009 - Incomplete Data   I/C - Intellectual/Cultural   S - Symptomatic
Coh - Cohesion   Rec - Recreational
Exp - Expressiveness   M/R - Moral/Religious
Con - Conflict   Org - Organization
Ind - Independence   Ctrl - Control
n - Normal
hi - Above Louisville Norms
lo - Below Louisville Norms

been known for its religious institutions and intensity of involvement with the number and variety of churches and other houses of worship in the community (See Ch 1, Pg. 19). We saw our finding as evidence of drastic social change inasmuch as, traditionally, families with young children have usually been involved with their religions. Also, 7 (50%) of the families (almost equally distributed among the 3 functioning groups) had low *Active Recreational Orientation* scores indicative of some disregard for healthful living and possible "addiction" to television and computers (Weaver & Clum, 1993; Hibbs, et al, 1993).

FES Subscale Scores and Symptom Status

There were some differences between the number of the symptomatic and asymptomatic groups' high and low FES scores. Of the 9 symptomatic families, 4 (48%) had low *Cohesion*, 2 (22%) had low *Expressiveness*, and 5 (55%) had high *Conflict* subscale scores. In contrast, of the 6 asymptomatic families, only 1 (17%) had a low Cohesion and also a low *Expressiveness score*, 1 (17%) had high *Expressiveness*, and. none had a high *Conflict* subscale score. Thus, 7 (78%) of the 9 symptomatic families had abnormal FES Interpersonal subscale scores in contrast to 3 (50%) of the 6 asymptomatic families.

On the Value/Orientation dimension, we found practically no difference between the symptomatic and the asymptomatic groups' number of high or low subscale scores.

On the *Organization* subscale of the Systems/Maintenance Dimension, the symptomatic group had 1 (11%) low score, but the asymptomatic group had 2 (33%). On the *Control* subscale, there was 1 (11%) low and 1 (11%) high score in the symptomatic group compared to 2 (33%) low scores in the asymptomatic group.

Overall, the FES scores on the Interpersonal Dimension showed a tendency toward comparatively high *Conflict* scores in the LF group and low *Cohesion* scores in the symptomatic families. On the Value/Orientation subscale scores, most of the families in all 3 functioning groups had scores in the normal range. On the System/Maintenance Dimension, the HF group's low *Organization* scores were somewhat contradictory to their high functioning level.

FAMILY MEMBERS' ACTIVITIES TOGETHER

In this second study, we introduced an assessment of everyday family activities to ascertain their possible associations with differing levels of family functioning. We obtained data by asking each member about how often the family had meals together? talked together? attended church together? took part in sports together ? visited friends together? or went to recreational activities together? Their responses were tabulated and averaged to obtain a family score. Those scores ranged from 15 to 35, but clustered around the mean of 25.6.per family. Table 6.6 shows the families' levels of activity: 5 (33%) had high family activity scores; 7 (47%) had mid-level; and 3 (20%) had low activity scores.

GLS Functioning Level, Activity Level, and Symptom Status

As shown in Table 6.6, in the GLS HF group, 1 (25%) family had a high family activity score, 2 (50%) had mid, and 1 (25%) had a low score, while the MF group had 3 (50%) high, 2 (33%) mid, and 1 (17%) low scores. The LF families, had a relatively high percentage of mid-level activities 1 (20%) had a high score, 3 (60%) had mid level scores, and 1 (20%) had low family activity scores. Thus, each of the 3 functioning groups had about the same percentage of combined high and mid level activity scores, and each functioning group had 1 family with a low activity score.

Table 6.6. Level of Family Activities-Comparative Data

Family I.D.	Symp Status	Level Act. Tog.	Family Size	Econ. Level
HF Group				
1011	As	Low	3	Fair
1019	As	Mid	3	Poor
1018	As	Mid	3	Ex
1016	As	High	2	Pov.
MF Group				
1015	S	Mid	3	Ex
1013	As	High	3	Poor
1012	As	Mid	4	Pov.
1001	S	Low	4	Good
1002	S	High	4	Pov.
1010	S	High	3	Good
LF Group				
1005	S	Mid	5	Poor
1017	S	Mid	10	Pov.
1014	S	Mid	4	Good
1006	S	High	5	Fair
1003	S	Low	3	Poor

S-Symptomatic Ex-Excellent
As-Asymptomatic Act.-Activities
Econ.-Economic Tog.-Together
Pov.-Poverty

Of the 9 symptomatic families, 3 (33%) were in the high activity group, 4 (44%) were in the mid, and 2 (22%) were in the low activity group. Of the 6 asymptomatic families, 2 (33%) were in the high activity group, 3 (50%) were in the mid activity group, and 1 (17%) was in the low activity group. Thus, in this small number of families, there were no outstanding differences in the 3 functioning groups' level of family activities. There was only a weak trend for the asymptomatic group to have a higher level of family group activities than the symptomatic group (H-33%, Mid-50%, Low-17% vs. H-33%, Mid-44%, Low-22%) confirming general opinions about family health groups and well-being.

The analysis of family activity level according to economic status revealed the tendency for the families at lower economic levels, especially the poverty level families, to have higher "family togetherness" activity ratings than the families at higher economic levels. Also, there was a tendency for the "family togetherness" activity level to be less frequent in the smaller than in the larger families. There was no association between the age of the children in the family and the level of family activity.

Conclusion

In conclusion, we found that we could use the GLS Assessment Instrument successfully with a family mental health clinic population. Also, we were pleased that we could obtain a "neighborhood" control group. In the next Chapter, we present a comparison and summary of the major findings from the research with the different groups, the random sample from the community, the clinic families, and their matched neighborhood controls.

References

Schwab, J. J., Warheit, G. J., Nadeau, S. E., (1978). Crowding and mental health. *Pavlovian J. Biol Sci.,* 14(4):226-233.

Minuchin, S. Montalvo, B., Guerney, B. G, Jr., et al., (1967). *Families of the slums: An exploration of their structure and treatment.* New York: Basic Books.

Hibbs, E. D., Hamburger, S. C. Markus, J. P., et al., (1993). Factors affecting expressed emotion in parents of ill and normal children. *Amer J Orthopsychiat, 63(1), Jan., 103-110.*

Weaver, T. L & Clum, G. A., (1993). Early family environments and traumatic experiences associated with borderline personality disorder. *J Consult and Clin Psychology, 61(6), 1068-1075.*

CHAPTER 7
The Applicability of the GLS Model and Assessment Instrument to Different Populations

In this chapter, we present the similarities and differences between the results of the use of the GLS family functioning assessment instrument with the 3 different populations, the Study I random sample of 19 families and in Study II the 8 clinic and 9 neighborhood families described in Chapters V and VI. We were especially interested in determining the applicability of the GLS assessment to a variety of families, particularly those in which there were young persons receiving treatment for some type of emotional or behavioral disorder. Therefore, the Study II population consisted of 2 groups of families, one with children in treatment at the Bingham Child Guidance Clinic and the other, their neighborhood matched controls. We recognized that the neighborhood control group for Study II would be somewhat more homogeneous than the Study I random sample; however, this selection enabled us to test the GLS assessment instrument with two populations (clinic and neighborhood controls) different from the true random sample.

Table 7.1 shows the demographic characteristics of the 2 Study populations. They differed in that the 19 families in the Study I population contained 18 children and 4 adolescents, 6 childless couples, 2 families with 2 adult children each, and 1 African-American family, whereas, the Study II populations contained 15 families with 26 children and 3 adolescents, no childless couples, only 1 family with 2 adult children, 4 (27%) African-American families, and 1 mixed Caucasian-Hispanic family. The composition of the populations differed in that there was a higher percentage of elderly families in the Study I than in the Study II samples with the 3 families in which grandparents were raising the children. The Study I population also contained a higher percentage of families at the excellent economic level than the Study II population with its higher percentage of families at the poverty level. Compared to the Study I population, Study II had a higher percentage of families with poor physical health even though there was only 1 family with elderly parents. Still another difference was that the Study I population had a much larger percentage of low stress families than the Study II population, which had a much larger percentage of high stress families. Despite those differences, the percentages of the two populations in the three GLS functioning levels differed only slightly.

Table 7.1. Study I and Study II Comparisons

	Study I	Study II
	No. of Fam.	No. of Fam.
Total No. of Families	19	15
With Adult Children	2 with 4	1 with 2
With children	11	15
Under age 18	19	29
Adolescents	7	5
Under age 13	12	24
With no children	6	0
Age of Parents		
Elderly	4 (21%)	1 (7%)
Mid-Age	5 (26%)	5 (33%)
Young	10 (53%)	9 (60%)
GP raising children	6	0
African American	1	4
Economic Level		
Excellent	5 (26%)	2 (13%)
Good	2 (10.5%)	4 (27%)
Fair	6 (32%)	2 (13%)
Poor	4 (21%)	3 (20%)
Poverty	2 (10.5%)	4 (27%)
Health Status		
Excellent	4 (21%)	3 (20%)
Good	8 (42%)	5 (33%)
Fair	5 (26%)	3 (20%)
Poor	2 (11%)	4 (27%)
Stress		
Low	10 (55%)	3 (21%)
Mid	4 (22%)	5 (36%)
High	4 (22%)	6 (43%)
GLS Functioning Level		
High	8 (42%)	4 (27%)
Mid	6 (32%)	6 (40%)
Low	5 (26%)	5 (33%)

Compared to the Study II populations, a larger percentage of Study I families was at the high functioning (HF) level (42% vs. 27%) and a slightly smaller percentage was at the mid (MF) level (32%vs.40%) and at the low functioning (LF) level (20%vs.33%). (See Table 7.1)

Number of Problems

There was only a slight difference between the 2 Study populations in the number of problems with subsystem functioning per family. In Study I, the number of problems ranged from 0.3 to 20.8 (av.5.5) per family, whereas in Study II the range was narrower, from 1.3 to 15.3 (av.5.1). The average number of problems reported by the 2 HF groups was about the same, 2.3 for the 8 Study II HF families and 2.1 for the 4 Study II HF families. However, the average number of problems reported by the MF and LF families in the 2 studies differed: av. 4.3 per family for the 6 Study I MF families, somewhat less than the 5.2 per family for the 6 Study II MF families; but, for the LF groups, the 5 Study I LF families had a considerably larger average number of problems, 12 per family, than the 5 Study II LF families, 7.4 per family.

Table 7.2. Number of Subsystem Problems in the Two Study Populations

	Study I		Study II	
	Av. No. Probs.	Av Sev Wt	Av. No. Probs.	Av Sev Wt
HF Group	2.26	23.8	2.13	18
MF Group	4.3	7.3	5.2	11.4
LF Group	12	4.9	7.4	7.8
Range	0.3 - 20.8	0 - 36.9	1.3 - 15.3	4.6 - 24
Total av	5.5	10.6	5.1	12.6

Probs. - Problems   Av. - Average per family
Sev Wt - Severity Weight   No. - Number

We looked at the variables possibly associated with the marked difference in the average number of subsystem problems reported by the LF families in the 2 studies and found that the 2 LF groups tended to be similar in regard to age, health status, financial status, stress levels, and even symptomatic status. A major difference was that the 5 Study I LF families had a total of only 8 children, whereas the 5 Study II LF families had a total of 15 children. We had anticipated that having more children would be associated with more problems; however, the Study I LF group with only about one-half as many children as the Study II LF group, had about 50% more problems. Consequently, we looked at possible differences in the severity of the 2 different LF groups' problems.

As shown in Table 7.2, the severity weight of the families' subsystem problems varied in that the range and average per family in Study I was from 0 to 36.9 (avg. 10.6 per family), compared to the range of 4.6 to 24 (avg.12.6 per family) in Study II. The comparative severity weights for the Study I HF, MF, and LF groups were 23.8, 7.3, and 4.9, in contrast to 18.0, 11.4, and 7.8 respectively for the Study II functioning groups. Examination of the clinical and the demographic variables suggested that the Study I HF group's high severity rating possibly could be attributed to its containing 2 (25%) symptomatic families whereas there were none in the Study II HF group. However, for the MF and LF Study II groups, the average severity weight was about 50% greater than for their Study I counterparts. The relatively large percentage, 67%, of Study II MF families that were symptomatic differentiated it from the 33% in Study I. Those findings point to the associations between problems with family functioning and increased symptomatology.

Ranking of the Subsystems

The ranking of the 17 subsystems according to the number of families having problems revealed that in Study I, the 5 most frequently reported by at least 8 (42%) of the families, in order of decreasing number of families, were: *Storage, Producer, Decider, Boundary*, and *Internal Transducer*. For the Study II families, the 5 most frequently reported subsystems that gave problems to each of at least 9 (60%) families were: *Storage, Internal Transducer, Producer, Decider*, and *Reproducer*. Thus, 4 of the 5 subsystems giving the families the most problems were the same in the 2 different studies.

Moreover, the *Boundary* subsystem, one of the top 5 that gave problems to 9 (46%) Study I families, ranked 6th among the subsystems in that it gave problems to 8 (53%) Study II families. For the Study I population, the Reproducer subsystem gave problems to 6 (32%) of the families and ranked 7th among the subsystems giving problems. But, for the Study II population, it ranked 5th, giving problems to 9 (60%) of the families. The difference in the percentage of families having problems with the *Reproducer* subsystem may be attributable to the larger number of children in the Study II population.

Thus, 80% of the first 5, or 86% of the first 7 subsystems (the ones reported most often as troublesome) were the same in the 2 different populations. Moreover, those subsystems tap fundamental aspects of family functioning in everyday life. Such findings support the applicability and utility of the GLS Assessment Instrument with various populations.

Number of Subsystems Giving Problems

We were interested in the possible number of subsystems that gave problems to families in each Study. As shown in Table 7.3, 10 (55%) of the 19 families in Study I had all of the subsystems functioning at a 90% or better level, in contrast to only 1 (7%) of the Study II families. Also, 3 (16%) Study I families had only 1 subsystem rated below 90% functioning effectiveness, and only 4 (22%) of the families had difficulties with 2 or more subsystems. However, 1 (5% of the 19 Study I families) reported functioning difficulties with 11 subsystems and another with 14.

Of the Study II families 3 (20%) had difficulty with only 1 subsystem rated as functioning at less than 90% effectiveness; another 3 families had such difficulties with 2 subsystems and, generally, definitely larger percentages of the Study II than Study I families reported difficulties with subsystem functioning. In fact, 1 family had difficulties with 8, another with 9, and still another with 10 subsystems rated as functioning at a less than 90% level of effectiveness.

Table 7.3. Comparisons of Subsystem Functioning

	STUDY I	STUDY II
Subsystem	No. of families	
Functioning Level	n-19	n-15
all at 90% or better	10	1
with only 1 below 90%	3	3
with 2 or more below 90%	6	11
8 subsystems below 90%		1
9 subsystems below 90%		1
10 subsystems below 90%		1
11subsystems below 90%	1	
14 subsystems below 90%	1	
subsystem below 60%	2	7

Thus, we had marked Study I--Study II differences between the number of subsystems reported as giving problems to the families. In particular, more of the Study I than Study II families had all subsystems functioning at a better than a 90% level of effectiveness, and a relatively large number of families in Study II had difficulties with subsystems functioning below the 90% level of effectiveness.

We then looked at whether the number of subsystems reported as giving problems differentiated the 3 GLS functioning groups in the two studies. In the Study I population, 6 subsystems did so, as did 5 subsystems for the Study II population. Of those subsystems, 3 -- *Reproducer, Boundary*, and *Supporter* -- distinguished the GLS functioning groups in both studies. For the random sample composing the Study I population, an additional 3 subsystems -- the *Decider, Internal Transducer*, and *Converter* -- distinguished the 3 GLS functioning groups, and, in the Study II clinic/neighborhood control populations, 2 additional subsystems -- the *Storage* and the *Producer* differentiated the GLS groups. Thus, the differences in the number of families having problems with the same 8 subsystems distinguished the functioning groups in these reasonably diverse non-clinical and clinical populations. The results suggest that a shortened version of the Family Functioning Assessment Instrument that focuses on those 8 subsystems would yield most of the information needed to identify and delineate the functioning levels.

Comparisons of Study I and Study II Subsystem Functioning, Sociodemographic Data, and Health Variables

As shown in Table 5.1, in Chapter 5, the analyses according to Parental Age showed that there were relatively more young families reporting a large number of subsystems with functioning below the 90% level of effectiveness than the mid-age or elderly families, with the exception of 1 elderly family in which a parent had Alzheimer's Disease. The analyses indicated that the 3 different age groups had almost the same average number of problems with the subsystems.

Analyses of the associations between Family Size and subsystem functioning revealed a definite pattern. In Study I, of the 7 childless families and the 5 with only one child, 9 (75%) had all subsystems functioning at a 90% or better level of effectiveness. But, of the 7 families, each with 2 or more children, 6 (85%) had difficulties with 1 to 5 subsystems functioning at less than 90% effectiveness. In Study II, although there were practically no differences in the number of subsystems giving problems to families with either 1 or 2 children, the 3 families with 3 or more children had many problems with subsystem functioning; for example, in 2 of those families, 9 and 10 subsystems respectively were rated as functioning at less than 90% level of effectiveness.

Examination of the associations between Economic Levels and subsystem functioning showed that in the Study I population there was a marked association between higher economic level and excellent subsystem functioning. However, in the Study II populations, there were no distinctive differences between Economic Levels and percentages of families having difficulties with subsystem functioning rated below the 90% level of effectiveness; in fact, the percentages were 31% for the excellent and good economic levels, 32% for the mid-economic level, and, again, 32% for the poverty and poor. Thus, there were fairly definite Study I -- Study II differences as evidenced by the strong positive relationship between higher Economic Levels and excellent functioning in the Study I population.

Examination of possible associations between Physical Health Status and subsystem functioning showed that in the Study I population there was a definite positive relationship between both excellent and good physical health statuses and effective subsystem functioning. In fact, 10 (82%) of the 12 families with excellent and good physical health were rated as functioning at a 90% level or better on all the subsystems but, there was a linear increase in the number of subsystems reported as causing difficulties to the 7 families with either fair or poor physical health; for example, 1 of the 2 families with poor health reported difficulties in functioning with 11 subsystems, and the other with 14 subsystems. The Study II families had a definite linear relationship between better Health levels and better subsystem functioning.

In Study I, analyses of possible associations between Stress Levels and subsystem functioning showed a strong relationship between low stress and excellent subsystem functioning and, again, a linear relationship between increasing stress levels and a larger number of subsystems rated as functioning below 90% level of effectiveness. In contrast, in Study II relatively more families reported difficulties with subsystem functioning than in Study I and the relationship between stress levels and number of subsystems giving problems was not linear; in particular, the mid-stress level Study II families had an unusually large number of subsystems rated as functioning at a less than 90% level of effectiveness compared to those at either high or low stress.

Comparative analyses of the associations between Symptomatic Status and subsystem functioning revealed that in Study I both the asymptomatic and the symptomatic families had definitely fewer subsystems with functioning difficulties than the asymptomatic and symptomatic Study II families. In the Study I population, there were 11 (58%) asymptomatic families, 8 (73%) of which had no difficulties with subsystem functioning, and of the remaining 3 (27%) families, 1 had only 1 subsystem, another had 3 subsystems, and the third had 5 subsystems rated below 90% functioning effectiveness. In contrast, of the 8 (42%) symptomatic in Study I families, only 2 (25%) had no difficulties with subsystem functioning; of the other 6 families, 2 (33%) functioned below the 90% level of effectiveness on only 1 or 2 subsystems and the remaining 4 (67%) did so on 5, 9, 11 and 14 subsystems respectively.

In Study II, there were 6 (40%) asymptomatic families, only 1 (17%) had no difficulties with subsystem functioning and, of the remaining 5, 4 (80%) had difficulties with only 1 or 2 subsystems, but the 5th family had 3 subsystems functioning below the 90% level. However, all of the 9 (60%) symptomatic families had at least 1 subsystem rated as functioning at less than the 90% level of effectiveness, and 4 (44%) families functioned at a relatively low level on 6 or more subsystems. We noted that in Study I none of the asymptomatic families had difficulties with the *Internal Transducer* subsystem, but in Study II, 4 (67%) of the 6 asymptomatic families had difficulties with it.

The 19 Study I families at T-3 had 190 FES subscale scores of which 35 (18%) were high, 13 (64%) were in the normal range, and 30 (16%) were low scores. The GLS HF group had more, 23 (80%) high scores and fewer 9 (11%) low scores than the LF group which had only 7 (14%) high, but 15 (30%) low scores. Almost all of the MF group's scores, 49 (82%), were in the normal range. The HF group's high level of functioning was associated with high *Cohesion,* normal *Expressiveness,* and normal *Conflict* scores whereas the LF families had disproportionately more low *Cohesion,* low *Expressiveness,* and high *Conflict* scores. The functioning groups' system maintenance scores differed -- the HF group tended to have *Organization* and *Control* scores in the normal range, but the LF group tended to have low *Organization* scores and high *Control* scores. Also, the HF group had more 10 (25%) high Value Orientation and a few more 4 (15%) low scores than in the families the MF or LF groups.

The 14 Study II families (date incomplete on the 15th family) had 140 FES scores of which, compared to Study I, fewer, 19 (13%) were high, and a few more, 28 (20%) were low; 93 (67%) were in the normal range. In Study II, there were few functioning group differences in their clinically important *Cohesion* subscale scores. However, there were relatively more high *Conflict* scores, especially in the LF group, than in their Study I counterparts. Also, there were disproportionately more low *Organization* subscale scores in the Study II HF group than in the Study I HF group. The Study II group's Value Orientation subscale scores revealed relatively few functioning group differences, fewer than in the Study I sample.

In the Study II populations, the scores on their FES Interpersonal subscale -- *Cohesion, Expressiveness,* and *Conflict* -- clearly differentiated the symptomatic from the asymptomatic families. For example, of the 9 symptomatic families, 4 (44%) had low *Cohesion* scores and 5 (55%) had high conflict scores. In contrast, of the 6 asymptomatic families, only 1 (17%) had a low *Cohesion* score and none had a high *Conflict* score.

Thus, the variables associated with differences in subsystem functioning in the 2 Study populations were: 1) Compared to the Study I population, in the Study II population, there was a trend toward larger Family Size, especially a larger number of children, to be associated with increased subsystem problems; 2) In Study I, high Economic Level was more strongly associated with excellent subsystem functioning than in Study II; 3) The anticipated linear increasing Stress--increasing number of subsystem problems relationship was found in the Study I population but, in Study II, the mid-level stress families had a disproportionately large number of families with subsystem problems; and 4) In booth studies, the Symptomatic families had more subsystem functioning problems than the Asysmptomatic, and both the Symptomatic and Asymptomatic Study I families tended to have fewer subsystem problems than their Study II counterparts.

A Look at the Combined Populations

To evaluate the applicability of the GLS Family Functioning Model and Assessment Instrument as fully as we could, we examined possible associations between the various demographic and clinical variables and subsystem functioning in all 34 families in the combined populations of the 2 studies (see Tables 7.4 Parts 1 and 2).

Examination of the first variable, Parental Age (Table 7.4 Part 1) showed that as the age of the parents increased, the percentages of families having problems with the subsystems decreased from 74% of the young to 60% of those in the middle-age and elderly categories. In particular, difficulties with the *Internal Transducer* subsystem decreased from 53% of the young to 40% of the mid-aged and none for the elderly. But, we found a number of minor exceptions to the age--difficulty with subsystem functioning relationship. One was that the percentages of families having difficulties with the *Reproducer* subsystem increased from 21% of the young to 40% of the mid-aged and 40% of the elderly. We had assumed that in modern America, the complexities of transmitting values and maintaining rules and discipline with adolescent and young adult children by their mid-aged and elderly parents would be greater than for young parents with young children. Another was that the *Boundary* subsystem gave problems to only 5% of the families in the young category, many of whom had small children, compared to 10% of the mid-aged and 40% of the elderly families. But, as to be anticipated, problems with the *Memory* subsystem were reported by 11% of the young, 20% of the mid-aged, and by 60% of the elderly.

As shown in Table 7.4 Part 2, analyses of the next variable, Family Size, revealed a definite trend toward an increasing number of subsystems giving problems as the number of children in the family increased. Of the 9 families with no young children in the home, 5 (55%) reported no problems with subsystem functioning, as did 5 (42%) than those with 1 child, but only 1 (7.7%) of 13 with 2 or more children. All three of the families with adult children in the home reported subsystem problems. Also, the percentages of families that had problems with the *Producer* subsystem (maintenance and cleaning of the home) increased from 25% of the childless families to 40% of the families with 3 or more children. The percentages that had difficulties with the *Reproducer* subsystem (transmission of family values to the children, discipline, and rules) rose from 9% to 80% with an increasing number of children, and with the *Encoder* subsystem (sharing information about the family with outsiders), the percentages rose from 8% of those with 1-child to 22% of the 2-children families and 80% of the 3-children families. An exception to the linear relationship between larger family size and an increasing number of difficulties with subsystem functioning was that for the *Internal Transducer* subsystem (handling of members' feelings, keeping up with activities, and health); the percentages having problems varied from 58% of those with 1 child to 33% of the 2 children families and 40% of the 3 children families.

We wondered whether Symptom Status would explain the exception with the *Internal Transducer* subsystem. However, only a slightly larger percentage, 48%, of the families with 2 or more children was symptomatic, compared to 39% of the families with 1 child and 42% of the childless couples. Therefore, symptomatic status was not associated with the *Internal Transducer* subsystem exception that we noted.

Analysis of the third variable, Economic Level, (Table 7.4 Part 1) revealed that only 2 (29%) of the families with excellent incomes, and 3 (60%) and 4 (50%) of those with good and fair incomes reported difficulties with subsystem functioning in contrast to all 14 (100%) of the families with poor and poverty level incomes. Furthermore, although each of the top 3 income groups reported difficulties with 7 (41%) or 8 (47%) of the 17 subsystems, those at either the poor or poverty level had difficulties with 15 (88%) subsystems.

Many of the families in the poor and poverty level categories had problems with certain subsystems. In particular, the *Producer*, which deals with house repair and cleaning the house, gave difficulty to only 1 (5%) family in each of the 3 higher economic levels, but to 8 (58%) of the 14 families in the poor and poverty level categories. The *Internal Transducer* subsystem (dealing with information about family members and their feelings and coping with health and illness) presented difficulties to 30% of those in the higher income groups, but to 65% of the poor and poverty level families. For the families in the poor category, 2 subsystems were especially troublesome; the *Storage* subsystem was reported as giving problems to 75% of them, and the *Extruder*, which involves removal of garbage and trash, gave problems to 50% of them, although, none of the other 4 income groups had problems with the *Extruder* subsystem.

Table 7.4 Variables and Subsystem Functioning - Part 1

Variable	Par. Age			Economic Level					Health Status			
	E	M	Y	Ex	G	F	P	Pov.	Ex	G	F	P
Subsytem												
Ingestor	0	0	1	0	0	0	1	1	0	0	0	2
Converter	0	0	2	0	0	0	0	1	0	0	1	2
Extruder	0	0	2	0	0	0	4	0	1	0	2	0
Motor	0	0	3	0	0	0	3	1	0	0	2	2
Supporter	0	0	0	0	1	0	3	2	0	1	2	4
Storage	0	0	8	2	0	2	6	1	2	1	5	3
Producer	2	2	4	1	0	0	5	3	1	1	3	4
Distributor	0	0	1	0	0	0	1	1	0	0	0	2
Boundary	2	1	1	0	1	0	1	2	1	0	1	2
Input Trans.	0	0	0	0	0	0	0	0	0	0	0	2
Internal Trans.	0	4	10	2	2	2	6	3	1	5	4	4
Memory	3	2	2	1	1	1	2	2	1	1	3	2
Decider	0	2	4	1	1	1	3	1	0	1	2	4
Decoder	2	3	2	1	2	1	1	2	1	1	0	3
Encoder	0	5	2	1	0	2	2	2	0	1	4	2
Output Trans.	0	1	4	0	0	2	3	1	0	0	7	0
Reproducer	2	4	0	1	2	2	3	2	1	1	4	4
No problems	2	4	5	5	2	4	0	0	3	8	0	0
Total No. Fam. (34)	5	10	19	7	5	8	8	6	7	13	8	6

E-Elderly   Ex- Excellent   Ex.-Excellent
M-Mid Age   G-Good   G -Good
Y-Young   F- Fair   F-Fair
                 P-Poor   P-Poor
                 Pov-Poverty

Analyses of the Physical Health ratings (Table 7.4 Part I) showed that fewer, 4 (56%), families with excellent and 5 (38%) with good physical health ratings reported difficulties with subsystem functioning than the 8

(100%) of those with fair health ratings or, the 6 (100%) with poor health ratings. Difficulties with the *Internal Transducer* subsystem were reported by families in all 4 health categories, but only 1 (14%) family with an excellent physical health rating and 5 (39%) of those with good health ratings did so, in contrast to 4 (50%) of families with ratings of fair health and 4 (67%) of those with health ratings of poor.

Table 7.4. Variables and Subsystem Functioning Combined Populations- Part 2

Variable	Number of Families with Problems					
	No. of Ch. per Family	Families with	Sym. Sta		Stress	
	0. 1. 2. 3. 6 .	Adult Ch.	As S		L M H	
Subsystem						
Ingestor	1 0 0 0 0	0	0	2	0 1 1	
Converter	1 1 1 0 0	0	0	3	0 0 3	
Extruder	0 1 1 2 0	0	1	3	1 0 3	
Motor	1 2 1 0 0	0	1	3	1 1 2	
Supporter	1 2 1 2 1	1	0	7	3 3 4	
Storage	1 5 3 4 0	0	5	6	2 4 5	
Producer	1 3 2 2 0	1	2	7	0 4 5	
Distributor	0 0 0 0 0	0	0	2	0 0 2	
Boundary	1 0 2 0 1	1	0	4	0 1 3	
Input Trans.	1 0 0 0 0	0	0	1	0 0 2	
Internal Trans.	2 7 3 2 1	1	5	10	2 5 7	
Memory	1 2 1 2 0	1	0	7	0 0 5	
Decider	1 2 2 2 0	0	1	6	0 2 5	
Decoder	1 1 2 2 1	1	1	6	0 3 4	
Encoder	0 1 2 4 1	1	2	5	2 3 2	
Output Trans.	1 1 2 2 0	0	1	0	0 1 5	
Reproducer	1 1 3 4 1	1	3	7	1 3 6	
no problems	5 5 1 0 0	0	9	2	8 2 0	
Total Fam.	7 12 7 5 1	3	18	16	13 8 12	
N = 34						

Ch-children
Fam-Family
Trans.-Transducer

Sym Sta-Symptom Status
S-Symptomatic
As-Asymptomatic

Thus, as to be anticipated, there was a strong association between poorer health ratings and difficulties with subsystem functioning. These functioning difficulties covered many aspects of family life, such as dealing with feelings, decision-making, transmission of values, and even space in the home.

We next looked at the 5th variable, family Stress ratings (Table 7.4-Part 2). There was a slight tendency for those with either 2 or more children to be at somewhat higher stress levels, than the smaller families. But, there were no clear-cut associations between stress levels, family size, and reports of problems with the Internal Transducer subsystem.

Symptom Status and Subsystem Functioning

We found a strong association between Symptomatic Status and subsystem functioning. Of the 17 asymptomatic families, 9 (53%) reported no difficulties with any subsystem functioning, in contrast to only 2 (12%) of the 17 symptomatic families. In particular, comparatively large percentages of the symptomatic families had difficulties with *Decision-making* (41%), *Internal Transducer* (handling of information and dealing with feelings in the family) (65%), *Memory* (43%), *Producer* (40%) (upkeep of home and housework), *Reproducer* (47%) (transmission of values, rules and discipline.), and *Supporter* (41%) (allocation of space in the home) subsystems. We noted that the *Boundary* subsystem was reported as giving difficulties to 17 (50%) of the families, in particular, to the elderly families with adult children in the home; and to 4 (24%) of the 17 symptomatic families but to none of the asymptomatic.

The Subsystem Analysis of a Family

In addition to its research value and the data about functioning groups, the following detailed analysis of a GLS assessment reveals the family interactions that can deepen interviewers and family members' understanding of the family. A senior Child Psychiatrist, who had independently evaluated the family functioning videotapes of all the families in Study I, analyzed the family's problems with each subsystem, proposed solutions, and also evaluated the parental roles. The following is an example of such an assessment.

The father was a 34-year-old Caucasian contractor who remodeled houses. The mother was a 33 year old Caucasian who was employed outside the home. Their only child was an 8-year-old girl who was an excellent student. The family's financial rating was 4 (poor) on a 5-point (excellent to poverty level) scale; their overall physical health rating was 3 (fair) on the 4-point (excellent to poor) scale; and, the family was symptomatic on the basis of the mother's high CES-D scores. On the 3-point (high-mid-low) stress rating, they had a rating of high stress inasmuch as they had 2 chronic stressors: extended family members' poor physical health and financial insecurity.

Some of the problems appeared at the beginning of the assessment with the question regarding the *Ingestor* subsystem (one of the 8 matter-energy subsystems); the mother stated that she did not like grocery shopping and did it quickly to limit her husband's overbuying of "goodies". Also, on the *Converter* subsystem, a conflict was evident inasmuch as the father did not like meat, and the mother "fixes what she wants". When she works, they eat "lots of sandwiches". The *Extruder* subsystem also was a source of irritation in that the husband "hates to do it" and the mother constantly reminded him to carry out the garbage, but dismissed the importance of the conflict by saying "its not a big problem."

The problems with the *Storage* subsystem illustrated some of the parent-child conflicts. The daughter "cannot find things" and repeatedly asked her mother who stated: "I spoiled her rotten, get upset and lose my temper, and then I get her to help."

There were no problems with the *Producer*, the *Supporter*, or the *Distributor* subsystems, but there were problems with the *Motor* subsystem. The husband did not trust his wife's driving and did all of it when the three were together; however, she did devote 2-3 hours per week to driving her daughter and herself.

For the subsystems that process information, some of the major points are: for the *Internal Transducer* subsystem that deals with feelings, the family reported no problems, but the mother was more talkative than the father and she "also had a temper and is emotional". The evaluator noted succinctly that, in the family, "there was no good communication." For the *Output Transducer* subsystem, the mother dealt with the daughter's school, paid the bills, kept the checkbook, which she perfectionistically "balanced to the penny", and monitored her husband's expenditures.

The parents had ongoing differences with the functioning of the *Encoder* subsystem -- how family members talked to others about their activities. The father was "a more private person"; he indicated that his wife talks too much. With the *Decoder* subsystem, which refers to the family's "private code of communication", the family members emphasized that they kept things to themselves but shared everything with the wife's parents.

Responses to questions about the functioning of the important *Decider* subsystem revealed even more differences. They reported that they made mutual decisions, but the mother stated that after the decision was made "I get hyper, I'm real nervous, it depends on my mood, and I handle it by yelling, screaming, or going to bed".

Analysis of the functioning of the 2 subsystems that deal with both matter-energy and information showed that for the *Boundary* subsystem that deals with visitors and the regulation of the use of the telephone and television, the family reported no problems even though the mother apparently was "afraid of all strangers". For the *Reproducer* subsystem that deals with family values, the parents stated that their daughter shared their values and that both of them were involved with her even though, when they were children, their families of origin had not shared values.

We can see that this analysis of a family's subsystem functioning surfaced many of their problems in living as well as their LF group status. The mother's symptomatology was manifested by her descriptions of their daily activities and their interactions. Moreover, their scores on the FES Cohesion and Expression scales were low, in the pathological range, and were in accord with the observations of low functioning on our GLS assessment. Also, that they had low scores on both the *Organization* and *Control* subscales that constitute the Systems/Maintenance Dimension.

Thus, the GLS Assessment can provide a profile, if not a graphic description, of how a family functions in daily life. In addition, the analysis highlights emotional and interpersonal difficulties within the family and also points to strengths that can be mobilized for coping and for enhancing well-being.

In summary, the findings from Study I and Study II showed that the GLS model of family functioning and the GLS Assessment Instrument could be used with the general population and also with Clinic groups to evaluate families. The assessment identified specific difficulties in family functioning associated with such major demographic variables as family size, age of parents, economic level, physical health status, stress level, and, especially, mental health status. Moreover, the results of the research studies are in accord with our clinical experiences. We think that identifying families' specific difficulties and strengths in functioning has significant therapeutic potential that is bolstered by the in-depth picture of day to day living that the GLS Assessment of family functioning provides.

CHAPTER 8
Critique and Recommendations

The GLS model of assessment of family functioning gives researchers and clinicians a tested method to evaluate the multifaceted aspects of family life. The assessment, therefore, addresses specifically how and how well the family functions in daily life, not symptoms of mental disorder or substance abuse problems. Thus, it voids the circularity of the functioning-illness tautology that often limits approaches to the serious problem: what are the associations between family functioning and the mental illness-substance abuse disorders. We have used the GLS assessment effectively with about 50 families in our 3 different studies and an additional 10 families in outpatient clinical practice. During the assessment, its focus on daily activities was non-threatening to both the young and the older family members, and thus it was possible to include the whole family in the GLS assessment. Inasmuch as it measures the ability of the family to carry out the subsystem functioning essential to all levels of biosocial organization described by Miller (1978), it addresses the activities and interactions that are the fundamentals of family functioning.

In their discussion of "The Family as a System," Miller and Miller (1980) presented a description and critique of the applicability of GLS concepts to families and emphasized that both the concepts and terminology were neutral. In many ways, the use of the GLS Assessment, rooted in 20th century general systems theory, enables researchers and clinicians to organize efficiently the information obtained from families into a meaningful framework. Moreover, the explicit organization allows for comparisons of family functioning across cultures and over time. Consequently, the GLS assessment of families should be applicable to those in any population selected for study, and in view of the almost universal breakdown in family cohesion (Bruce, et al., 1995), the use of this instrument with families in different cultures can identify weaknesses in family functioning and related structure that might benefit from interventions.

The emphasis on the realities of everyday living can lead to identification of patterns of family interaction, especially those associated with children's development, motherhood, and parents' healthful and maladaptive behaviors. Furthermore, the GLS conceptualization of family functioning, method of assessment, and the ease of organization of the material obtained have the potential to enlarge researchers' evaluations of some of the dynamic aspects of family life other than the more strictly defined family functions. For example, the data could be used to develop a typology of families on an authoritarian/egalitarian axis according to delineation of roles, determination of the hierarchical arrangement of the family structure, level and type of family activities, and the patterns of family interaction. Researchers could ascertain whether and in what ways families' various positions on the axis were linked to children's social development and their healthful/maladaptive behaviors in order make necessary interventions.

We found that videotaping the GLS family functioning assessment can be valuable. The videotape shows details of interactions that may not be noted by interviewers. Also, a tape can be used by independent observers for research and teaching purposes. Importantly, it supplies the family as well as therapists and investigators with a baseline record -- a picture of family functioning.

Clinical Utility

During the GLS assessment of couples and of families in ongoing outpatient treatment, many spontaneously and repeatedly told us that they considered the assessment to be important and helpful. In particular, they emphasized that it surfaced difficulties in functioning and, especially, helped them focus their thinking on aspects of their relationship that they had not recognized as pertinent or had overlooked. Also, as a process, the assessment stimulated their thoughts about problem solving and thus facilitated treatment.

Historically, therapy has often been so involved with complaints and problems that it did not address strengths that could lead to enhanced cohesion and coping. However, the comprehensive GLS assessment led to thoughts about and a discussion of aspects of family functioning not usually surfaced by therapists during the customary clinical interview, nor brought into the treatment process by patients. Just as the omission, for many years, of therapists' direct questions about sexual abuse and its effects on both the family and the individual involved resulted in the neglect of that problem, the weakness in the functioning of particular subsystems, evidenced by the GLS assessment, sometimes turned out to have fairly serious ramifications in regard to roles, decisions, money, and other family activities and responsibilities. In those respects, overall, therapists were impressed by the GLS Assessment's ability to identify strengths in family functioning that could be emphasized and further developed to enable the couple or family to cope more effectively and thereby reduce the apparent dominance of the stresses and problems.

Synopsis of a Clinical Case

The reasonably successful use of the GLS assessment instrument is illustrated by the following case history.

An upper middle socioeconomic status Caucasian family consisted of a 41 year old husband/father (J) who was an attorney in private practice in a small suburb of a middle western city, the 38 yr. old wife/mother (M), who was a CPA with a large accounting firm, a 6 year old son, and 2 year old twin daughters. The husband had sought treatment about 15 years earlier, at the beginning of his last year of law school, because of chronic depression, a tendency toward excessive drinking, and ambivalence about his career choice. As the only young male in a fairly large prosperous family, he told that, as a child, he had been "spoiled" and had seldom been held responsible for his behavior or for his marginal academic performance. He had become the master of the art of "just skimming by". His ambivalence and indecisiveness involved his many pre-marital affairs with young, usually poorly educated women. He had been in and out of therapy for about 8 years and, especially, needed a great deal of supportive therapy after his father had died suddenly of a myocardial infarction, about the time that J. opened an office for a small general law practice. He had completed law school only after he had been placed on probation two times for barely passing, and was warned that he would be dismissed for any future failures to meet the requisite grade level satisfactorily. He chafed about not having a field of special interest and expertise.

M, in contrast, had been an excellent mathematician and after receiving her bachelor's degree in business and accounting, she accepted a position with a large accounting firm. She had been studious and serious and was considered to be a potential partner. In her early and mid-twenties, she had had 2 significant relationships. She had lived with one man her age for 2 years and later with a somewhat older divorced man for about 4 years. Each had wanted to marry her but she had declined, the first time because she thought they were too young, and the second time, because of his lack of spontaneity.

M and J began dating and continued to date, sometimes intermittently, for 4 years, but when she became

31, she gave him an ultimatum about marriage. Although they had talked of marriage, he had never acted as if he would follow through. After she stopped seeing him, however, he began to pursue her and expressed willingness to make a commitment. They married a few months later.

Their first 2 years of marriage were characterized by his somewhat increased dedication to work and her continuing success. She then began to worry about "the biological clock" and about having children. After considerable persuasion, he agreed and she became pregnant shortly after she stopped taking "the pill". Throughout their marriage, their level of sexual activity was low; they had intercourse only about once or twice a month and after she became pregnant, he began to frequent bars in working class districts where he thought he would not be recognized. Also, he resorted to reading porno magazines and masturbating. Often, he slept in the basement, ostensibly so that he could watch sports late at night.

Even after their first child was born, they continued to lead somewhat separate lives. She had tolerated his highly individualistic, somewhat narcissistic, life style that was punctuated by occasional good moments when his spontaneity and humor enlivened an evening or a weekend. Generally, however, each had her or his own interests and activities. They had occasionally bickered but had done little definite quarreling. After the birth of the twins, however, they were overburdened by the care of 3 small children, concerns about work, and the chores of everyday life. Their existence was drab. Also he began to suffer from chronic anxiety and low grade depression and withdrew increasingly from the family and the household by staying out in the evening after work, and also by oversleeping on weekends when possible. She became increasingly overwhelmed by the many responsibilities of children, work and the home and, for the first time, developed anxiety symptoms. She insisted that they seek psychiatric care and came to the senior author (JJS) inasmuch as J. had known him and benefited from treatment previously.

The first interview was devoted largely to eliciting complaints, descriptions of their problems, and ventilation of feelings, generally of blame and anger. They were told that a comprehensive evaluation was necessary and plans were made for a one and one-half hour GLS assessment at the next session. The GLS assessment was described briefly: they would be asked about their day-to-day activities, those dealing with both matter-energy and information. For each of the 15 subsystems they would be asked a specific panel of questions: How is the function (i.e. buying food) carried out? Who does it? How is it decided who does it? How much time does it take? What problems (issues) does your family have with it? How does your family deal with the problems (issues)?, and What is their degree of satisfaction with the function or activity?

Even at the beginning of the GLS assessment, when the matter-energy subsystems were assessed, the problems of their haphazard style of living quickly became apparent. For the *Ingestor* subsystem, M shopped once a week and, increasingly, relied almost completely on prepared frozen foods that could be put in the microwave. Also, she bought as many prepared foods as possible for the children. The couple, especially the husband, relied on many snack foods and had been gaining weight. The major problems were that the burden of the *Ingestor* function was almost completely on her shoulders and was not shared. The *Converter* function also was almost completely carried out by her. The *Extruder* function was largely neglected; wastes piled up in the kitchen and hallway and she nagged her husband, sometimes bitterly, about his not accepting responsibility for taking it to the garbage can in the alley behind their home.

The *Motor* function was not a significant problem; each had an automobile. When they went out together, generally, he did the driving; but she did so when he was drinking. Also, the *Supporter* subsystem presented no significant problems. Their 6-room house was moderately large and had an attic for storage and a finished basement. However, the *Producer* function was largely ignored or carried out by others. A maid service came to the home once a week for 4 hours and the neighborhood lawn service cut the grass regularly. However, J. and M. described their house as "usually being a mess;" she blamed him for being both "sloppy and disinterested." He responded with a passive shrug of the shoulders. The *Encoder* and *Decoder* subsystems functioned fairly well inasmuch as J and M were intelligent, articulate, and could handle information processing very well. In contrast, their responses to questions about the *Internal Transducer* subsystem, especially, about how they handled feelings, quickly brought to light both problems and dissatisfactions. M accused J of never wanting to discuss feelings and J either looked bored, or on one occasion, stated dryly that he was tired of her complaining. The problems with the *Boundary* subsystem were allied with those of the *Internal Transducer* and with J's personal problems. He devoted many hours each week to T.V. sports and was noncommunicative. In addition, he almost never answered the telephone because that "would just be about work," to which his level of commitment was low. The *Distributor* subsystem functioning presented no difficulties despite their living somewhat independent lives prior to the birth of the children, especially the twins. However, the *Output Transducer* subsystem was barely functioning -- M was so overwhelmed by the responsibilities and care of the children and her work that she did not have time to pay bills or attend to such functions as parents' meetings at day care, and J was so lackadaisical that he did little or nothing. The questions about the problems with that subsystem led to a discussion of the amount of money wasted each month by not paying household bills on time.

The questions about two vital subsystems, the *Decider* and the *Reproducer*, along with the *Internal Transducer*, brought their problems to the fore and also led to their realizing that their family life was dysfunctional and had the potential to be deleterious to their children. There was very little actual decision-making; often actions or decisions were made by default -- or things just happened. This was so appalling that it gave the psychiatrist (JJS) the appropriate opening to ask directly what all of that would mean for the children. They looked startled. J said, "This is serious". Later, when the questions about the *Reproducer* subsystem were presented, he stated spontaneously that they tied into the problems, implicit and explicit, that had been brought to light in the discussion of the *Decider* subsystem. Both J and M then looked grave and asked if they could have a copy of the Assessment Form to take home.

At the next regular session, they stated frankly that they now knew that their problems were more grievous than they had thought. They told that for one of the few times in their life together, they had been able to talk openly about their lives and their future, especially family functioning, values, and their children. Moreover, within the week, she had made some decisions. She had requested and received a long overdue extra maternity leave (for twins) and a leave of absence for 3 months. She planned to use the time "to straighten up their lives by changing their house into a home" and devoting extra attention to the children and their day care. He admitted openly that he had been "too passive" and that he would make an effort to redevelop their romance and for them to have at least one night each week away from the children in order to talk, go to dinner, or meet with friends, or go dancing -- for the first time in 4 to 5 years.

In view of her anxiety, she was started on a mild anti-anxiety medication. A supplemental antidepressant (Wellbutrin) was added to his maintenance antidepressant (Zoloft). They were scheduled for combined psychotherapy -- pharmocotherapy sessions 1&1/2 hours every two weeks. Two years since then, the general level of their family functioning and satisfaction with their daily lives have improved significantly. He has merged his growing law practice with a busy firm and is prospering. She has continued to work effectively and has received a promotion. Importantly, the 3 children are doing well. In addition, J and M and their children have become tied into their extended families and now tell that the big family activities have enriched their lives.

This presentation of an obviously therapeutic GLS Assessment reveals a number of significant points beyond those dealing explicitly with the functioning of the various essential subsystems.

First, J and M, as well as many couples and families, emphasized that the assessment gave them an overall view of their daily lives that has practical import.

Second, the emphasis on values and rules, as well as functioning, stimulates thoughts and questions about the meaning of daily living and its significance, especially for the children.

Third, as we have seen, in the case of J and M, the GLS Assessment provides many openings for psychodynamic and clinical interventions. For example, asking about the implications of their decision-making by default for the children was an "eye opener" for them. Such therapeutic interventions can be directed toward the difficulties and pathologies identified during the comprehensive assessment process.

Miller and Miller (1980) emphasize that GLST has immediate relevance to family psychiatry. It has applications to diagnosis, therapy, and prevention. They point out that the diagnostic strategy includes the identification of the subsystems and the measurement of critical variables over time, ascertains abnormalities, and can point toward a diagnosis. The subsequent therapy can be aimed toward changing the structure, process, and level of activity to relieve strains on critical subsystems. Inasmuch as prevention is the goal in family psychiatry, attempts need to be made to maintain the subsystem functioning relatively free of stress and strains. They conclude that, in therapy, "new insights are obtained from viewing a family as not simply a set of individual persons but as a system in itself made up of interacting human beings." Thus, GLST has explanatory and predictive as well as conceptual and descriptive value.

Suggested Modifications of the GLS Assessment Instrument

Our 10 years experience with the use of the GLS family assessment with families from the community, families with children in treatment, and those in private practice settings revealed some difficulties that can be rectified. The following are some of the major difficulties and suggested modifications of the assessment instrument.

First, both families and researchers agreed that the assessment was too time-consuming. Our analyses showed that of the 17 subsystems, 8 could differentially determine a family's level of functioning. An assessment of those 8 subsystems reveals many of the vital aspects of family life and functioning. The order of frequency (from greater to lesser) that those 8 caused problems for families was: the *Supporter, Reproducer, Decider, Boundary, Internal Transducer, Producer, Converter and Storage.* The first 3, the *Supporter* (referring to the adequacy of living space), the *Reproducer* (referring to the transmission of values and rules in the family), and the *Decider* (referring to decision-making in the family), cover a wide spectrum of family functioning and also showed the greatest differentiation between the 3 functioning groups. How the *Internal Transducer* subsystem functions (dealing with feelings and what goes on within the family) is especially important in studies of mental health/illness and, how the family deals with the *Storage* subsystem is important because this subsystem gave problems to almost all families. We think that families' problems with 3 other subsystems -- the *Boundary subsystem* (regulation of visitors, use of telephone and television), the *Producer* (upkeep of the home and yard), and the *Converter* (preparing the meals) -- are associated with the rapid rate of social and culture change. Families are being subjected to a plethora of stimuli and a large variety of influences (e.g. television and computer). Also, in many families both the father and mother now work outside the home full-time and rely on technological advances, even to take care of such a basic family function as cooking ("zap it in the microwave!").

Therefore, when reducing the amount of time is necessary, we suggest modifying the assessment instrument to include primarily those 8 subsystems. However, in certain circumstances, it may be desirable for the clinician or researcher to include the assessment of all 17 subsystems that we used.

Second, some of the questions about subsystem functioning required detailed explanations. For example, those about the *Distributer* subsystem, which focused on such family activities as who distributed food, clothing, and presents, that generally had been taken for granted, needed to be described. Our suggested change of the focus to "giving attention to family members" as well as to a few "activities distributing things" corrects this difficulty and places an added emphasis on family interactions. (See Appendix A modifications of Instrument.)

Third, the raters had some difficulties giving a single functional rating to a subsystem that involved 2 or 3 different activities. For example, the assessment of the important *Boundary* subsystem included questions about regulating visitors entering the home, the use of the telephone, and watching television. The regulation of one or more of them can vary widely depending on the stage of the family life cycle, the ages of the children, and other factors. Consequently a "single", or an "average" rating, might easily oversimplify the complexities of *Boundary* subsystem functioning. Therefore, we now advocate giving a separate rating for each of those activities as well as an overall subsystem rating when possible.

Fourth, family members often had difficulty answering questions about the specific amount of time spent carrying out a particular subsystem function. Therefore, we suggest that they should be asked whether the task takes too much time? the right amount? or very little?. Also, it may be meaningful to ask whether the time involved was burdensome? appropriate? or insufficient?

Fifth, inasmuch as the roles and activities of the wage-earners and also of the caregivers for children, the elderly, and/or ill family members are vital to family functioning, we recommend adding questions about them to the instrument. The questions about the wage earner(s) can be incorporated into those pertaining to the *Producer* subsystem, and questions about the primary caregiver(s) can be included in those pertaining to the *Internal Transducer* subsystem.

Sixth, in the evaluation of the *Producer* subsystem functioning, along with the questions about health care and health insurance, it may be helpful to include an emphasis on the importance of attention to exercise and nutrition in family life.

Seventh, to the GLS assessment, we advocate introducing questions about spirituality and religious practices (as appropriate) when discussing the *Reproducer* subsystem functioning. In our experiences, family functioning has too often been limited to discussions of stresses, pathologies, and fairly simplistic admonitions about self-fulfillment and "satisfaction." The inclusion of at least a brief discussion of spirituality, which can range from meditation to conventional religious practices, adds a fulfilling note of wholesomeness to a review of the more prosaic aspects of daily life.

Some Limitations of our Pilot Project

We recognize that although we completed a fairly complicated study of family functioning with 3 populations and tested the utility of a new assessment instrument tightly based on theory, our research was an exploratory Pilot Project. As such, it obviously had scientific limitations. One of the foremost was that even though we were able to report on 34 families in 3 populations, one of which was a true random sample from the community, the various groups contained too few families to allow us to carry out definitive statistical analyses. However, with the assistance of Professor David Teller, Ph.D. we completed some fairly straightforward statistical comparisons. In general, the major findings were that the combined HF and MF groups tended to be different from the LF group on many of the sociodemographic and family environment characteristics that we assessed as well as symptom status.

Perhaps a greater concern relates to the interrater reliability of the 3 investigators' ratings of the GLS family functioning videotapes. We developed a 100 percentage point scale on which there were 7 levels of agreement/disagreement: 1) all 3 raters agree; 2) 1 rater disagrees with a) a minimum of difference (5-9%), b) with a moderate difference (10-19%), and c) with a major difference (20% or plus); and 3) all 3 disagree with a) minimum difference (5-9%), b) with a moderate difference (10-19%), c) with a major difference (20% plus). (See Tables 8.1 and 8.2 this Chapter.)

In Study I, of the 320 ratings of the 17 subsystems by the 3 raters, there was complete agreement on the 100 point rating scale on 150 (47%) of the ratings, and 70% agreement when we included ratings with only minor (up to 9%) disagreement by one or more raters. There was major (20% or greater) disagreement by one or more raters on only 8% of the ratings. We were pleased with these results, but then found that the percentage of exact agreement in Study II was less. In Study II, of the 270 ratings, there was complete (100%) interrater agreement of 26%, and agreement of 48% when minor (up to 9%) disagreement of one or more raters was included. There was major (a difference of 20% or more) disagreement of one or more raters in 16% of the ratings.

Table 8.1 shows the number of times 1 rater disagreed with the other 2.

Table 8.1. Interrater Reliability

Freq. One rater differed from the other 2						
Degree of Difference	STUDY I			STUDY II		
	A	B	C	A	B	C
Min.	8%	11%	13%	8%	7%	22%
Mod.	7%	8%	11%	10%	15%	20%
Major	2%	1%	2%	3%	8%	5%
A, B, C, 3 Raters	Min. - Minimum difference 5 - 9%					
Freq. - % Time disagreed	Mod - Moderate difference 10 - 19%					
	Major Difference - 20% and over.					

In Study I, for the 3 raters, the percentages of minor disagreement were 8%, 11%, and 13%; for the moderate levels of disagreement, they were 7%, 8%, and 11%; and for major disagreement, they were 2%, 1%, and 2% respectively.

In Study II, the percentages of interrater disagreement were greater, for minor disagreement 6%, 7%, and 22%: for moderate disagreement, 10%, 15%, and 20%; and. for major disagreement 3%, 8%, and 5% respectively.

As to be anticipated, the level of agreement among the 3 raters was less on some subsystems than others. As shown in Table 8.2, in Study I, all 3 raters agreed most often on 5 subsystems -- the *Supporter, Extruder, Distributor, Ingestor,* and *Converter;* on those subsystems there were 2-4 minor disagreements. The most, 6-9 interrater disagreements at a minor level, were on the *Decider, Boundary, Motor, Storage, and Producer.* The most, 6-8 interrater disagreements at the moderate level, were with the *Internal Transducer, Memory, Storage and Producer.* All 3 raters most often disagreed at a major level on *Memory, (*3 families) and there were 2 major disagreements on the *Boundary, Decider, Encoder, and Reproducer.* There were no major disagreements on the *Ingestor, Extruder,* and the *Producer* subsystems ratings.

In Study II, all 3 raters agreed most often on the *Ingestor, and Extuder* subsystems. The most minor disagreements were on *the Encoder, Storage, Distributor, Decider and Output Transducer.* At the moderate level, the greatest number, 9, of interrater disagreements were on the: *Input Transducer, Producer* and the *Boundary* subsystems; also, there were 7-8 disagreements on the *Decider, Decoder, Output Transducer, and Reproducer* subsystems. The most, 7-4, major disagreements were on the *Internal Transducer, Memory, Encoder, Storage, and Supporter* subsystems. There were no major disagreements on the *Distributor, Motor, Extruder, Converter, and the Input Transducer* subsystems (see Table 8.2).

Table 8.2 Study I -- Study II Comparisons

INTERRATER RELIABILITY

Subsystem	Study I							Study II						
	Number of Ratings for 19 families							Number of Ratings for 16 families						
	All Agree	1 Rater Disagree			All Disagree			All Agree	1 Rater Disagree			All Disagree		
		Min	Mod	Major	Min	Mod	Major		Min	Mod	Major	Min	Mod	Major
Ingestor	11	3	2	0	1	2	0	13*	0	1	1	0	0	0
Converter	11	2	2	0	0	3	1	8	3	3	0	0	2	0
Extruder	13	0	2	0	2	2	0	10	3	1	0	0	2	0
Motor	7	7	1	0	0	3	1	7	4	2	0	0	3	0
Supporter	14	2	2	0	0	0	1	6	1	3	0	0	2	4
Storage	5	5	2	0	0	6	1	2	5	2	1	0	2	4
Producer	6	6	1	0	0	6	0	2	4	2	0	0	7	1
Distributor	12	2	2	2	0	1	0	5	5	5	0	0	0	0
Boundary	7	6	1	0	0	3	2	2	4	3	1	0	5	1
Input Trans	10	5	2	1	0	0	1	5	2	4	0	0	5	0
Int Trans6	6	4	3	1	1	3	1	0	2	2	2	0	5	5
Memory*	6	3	4	0	0	2	3	3	3	2	3	0	1	4
Decider	6	6	0	1	3	1	2	1	5	3	1	0	4	2
Decoder	10	2	3	0	1	1	1	2	4	4	1	0	3	2
Encoder	8	3	1	1	1	2	2	0	6	2	4	0	1	3
Output Trans	9	3	2	1	0	2	1	3	5	4	1	0	3	0
Reproducer	9	4	1	0	1	2	2	2	3	4	0	0	4	3

*One family no response

A--Agreement

Disagreement Level: Min - Minimum -- 5-9%
Mod - Moderate -- 10-19%
Major -- 20% and over

Furthermore, comparisons of the level of interrater agreement/disagreement showed that in both Study I and Study II there was complete agreement on the ratings of the *Ingestor* and the *Extruder* subsystems, and in Study I complete agreement also on the *Supporter, Distributor,* and *Converter.*

In both studies, there was only a minor level of interrater disagreement on the *Decider* and *Storage* subsystems and a moderate level of disagreement on the *Storage* and *Producer* subsystems. In both studies, there was major interrater disagreement on 2 subsystems, the *Internal Transducer* and *Memory.*

Overall, in Study I there was a minimum number of major disagreements, 26 (8%) of 343 ratings. In Study II, there were more, 44 (18%) of 245 ratings. The most disagreements in Study II were on the *Memory and Internal Transducer* subsystems.

We can only speculate about the reasons for differences in the levels of interrater agreement in the 2 studies. They are somewhat counterintuitive inasmuch as the raters were more experienced at Time 2 than at Time 1 and the economic level and the physical health levels in the two populations differed only moderately. Factors probably responsible for the differences include:

1) Differences in the composition of the 2 populations, specifically, the Study II population was more heterogeneous and contained larger families and, by design, more children than the Study I population.

2) We wondered whether the difference in the 2 populations' symptomatic status -- 11 (52%) asymptomatic and 8 (42%) symptomatic families in Study I, and in Study II, fewer, 6 (40%) asymptomatic and more, 9 (60%) symptomatic families -- influenced the ratings inasmuch as being symptomatic may have lessened the clarity of communication and contributed in other ways to the rating processes being complicated.

3) Bias undoubtedly was a factor contributing to the more frequent disagreements in the Study II population compared to the Study I population. The bias can stem for example, from such factors as the raters' "social distance" from most of the families and from their many years of clinical experience.

Our recommendations about the rating procedures are:

a) When working on such a complex subject as family functioning, even experienced raters need significant training that emphasizes limiting the rating to the specific factors about each subsystem that are distinctly observable.

b) The range of the rating scale should be limited to 5 and 10 point differences between various levels of functioning.

c) There is need to both specify and explicate the criteria more precisely than was done in this Pilot Study;

d) In addition to limiting the ratings specifically to the subsystems' functioning according to strict criteria, it may be helpful at the end of the rating session to give the rater an opportunity to offer a more general impression of the functioning of the subsystems and the family.

Despite the limitations of this Pilot Project, we have:

1) Devised a tightly theory-based model and assessment instrument that is pragmatic, neutral, and can be used with the whole family to evaluate family functioning. The model and assessment instrument deal specifically with the realities of day-to-day life and family function/dysfunction is not tautologically associated with health/illness. The model and the Instrument, therefore, can serve as an independent variable for a large variety of family studies in such fields as demography, economics, cultural anthropology, and in stress research as well as studies of mental and physical health and illness.

2) Tested the model and assessment instrument with 3 different research populations, including a small random sample from the community, a Clinic sample, and its neighborhood controls.

3) Used a variety of methodological approaches to enhance our understanding of the family and family functioning. For example, we determined the level of Husband:Wife agreement on the occurrence of SLE and also, used the Cantril "Ladder of Life" as an optimism/pessimism index, and then related those findings to family functioning and also to health/illness variables.

4) We gathered data on the community; for example, we specifically associated such census tract data as median family income with the research families' levels of functioning as a first step toward further evaluations of mesosystem variables associated with family functioning, health/illness, and the community. We think that such a comprehensive approach has the potential to increase researchers' abilities to base family studies on Engel's biopsychosocial model, on a 3-level family system -- individual-family-community--model and thus complete the biopsychosocial spectrum starting with behavioral genetics, then family self-report and observer-based data, and ending with such family-community research as Reiss and Oliveri's (1991) evaluations of the impact of SLE on individuals and families.

RECOMMENDATIONS

For comprehensive research Study on family functioning we now recommend using the following interviews and questionnaires.

1. Baseline Questionnaire that includes items concerning:
   a) Family composition, and for each member, age, sex, and roles of family members;

b)   Sociodemographic data, e.g. income, occupations, and educational level;
c)   Characteristics of the neighborhood;
d)   Physical health history and status;
e)   History of emotional difficulties/substance abuse problems;
f)   Marital history;
g)   Employment history;
h)   School history;
i)   Religious affiliation and level of participation;
j)   Stressful Life Events (SLE);
2.   The GLS Assessment Instrument;
3.   The Cantril "Ladder of Life";
4.   A Chronic Stressors Inventory and Rating Instrument;
5.   Coping Potential and availability of Family Resources.

REFERENCES

Bruce J., Lloyd C. R., Leonard A., (1995). *Families in focus: New perspectives on mother, father, and children*. The Population Council Report: New York, pp.13, 18, 20, 72-89, 98-100, 101-102.
Cantril, H., (1965). *The Pattern of Human Concerns*. New Brunswick: NJ, Rutgers University.
Engel G. L., (1997). *The need for a new medical model: A challenge for biomedicine.* Science, Vol. 196: pp. 126-136.
Miller, J. G., (1978). *Living System. New York: McGraw Hill Book Co.*
Miller J. G., & Miller J. L. (1980). The family as a system. In C. K. Hofling & J. M. Lewis (Eds.). *The family: Evaluations and treatment*. New York: Brunner/Mazel.
Reiss, D. & Oliveri, M. E., (1991).   The family's conception of accountability and competence; A new approach to the conceptualization and assessment of family stress. *Fam Process.*
Schwab, J. J., Stephenson, J., Ice, J. F., (1993). *Evaluating family mental health: History, epidemiology, and treatment issues. Vol. I of the Louisville Family Health Study.* New York: Plenum Press.

APPENDIXES

CRITERIA FOR ECONOMIC STATUS

Definition of Poverty according to the Federal Register.

Family Size	1985 Annual Income	Family Size	1995 Annual Income
1	$5,469	1	$7,470
2	6,998	2	10,030
3	8,573	3	12,590
4	10,989	4	15,150
5	13,007	5	17,710
6	14,696	6	20,270
7	16,656	7	22,830
8	18,512	8	25,290
9	22,083		

Our classification based on the 1985 figures was the following:

Poverty	Less than $3,000 per person, $5,484 for 2 persons, $14,400 for 5 persons
Poor	$3,000-$5,500 per person:
Fair	$6,000-$ 8,000 per person
Good	> $9,000 - < $12,000
Excellent	>$12,000 per person

CRITERIA FOR STRESS LEVELS

As part of the adult interview schedule, we asked the family member whether any of the following 30 life events occurred within the past year, and, if so, they were asked to rate the effect of the event as great, moderate or little; the children were asked independently to rate the effects of events.

Job Related:	A family member started to work for the first time or after a long period of not working; changed jobs; had troubles at work; stopped working.
Single events:	There was a major change in the financial status of the family; the family moved; a member had an outstanding personal achievement
School Related:	A family member started school; had an academic/school failure; suspended or expelled from school.
Changing Relationships	A family member became engaged, there was a marital separation; an addition to the family; a family member became pregnant; a divorce in the family; a family member got married; an increase or decrease in arguments in the family; family member was unfaithful to a spouse/significant other; family member broke up with a girl or boyfriend.
Traumatic events:	A family member had an accident, a major illness; was hospitalized; had an operation; death of a family member. Loss of a close friend through death or a move.
Legal Events:	A family member had a minor violation of the law, was involved with a lawsuit; was jailed; involved with drugs.

Additional events identified by the family.

The events were divided into positive or negative groups and were scored for their effects (great-3, moderate-2 and little-1). We obtained a score for each family by combining the number of events and their effects. The families were then ranked according to scores and placed into 3 groups: High, Mid and Low Stress.

CHRONIC STRESSFUL LIFE EVENTS RATING SCALE

The families were rated on a total of 28 events or situations on a 7-point scale by circling the appropriate number.

1. General Financial Circumstances
Good   Fair   Poor
1 ...... 2.......3 ...... 4.......5.......6 ...... 7................ Not Ratable

2. Occupational Roles are fulfilling or satisfying, to unsatisfying, or frustrating
Good   Fair   Poor
1 ...... 2.......3 ...... 4.......5.......6 ...... 7................ Not Ratable

3. Parenting (Chronic problems, burdens, frustrations, disappointment)
Good   Fair   Poor
1 ...... 2.......3 ...... 4.......5.......6 ...... 7................ Not Ratable

4. Quality of Housing:
Aesthetic   Unaesthetic
1 ...... 2.......3 ...... 4.......5.......6 ...... 7................ Not Ratable
Comfortable   Uncomfortable
1 ...... 2.......3 ...... 4.......5.......6 ...... 7................ Not Ratable
Adequate   Inadequate
1 ...... 2.......3 ...... 4.......5.......6 ...... 7................ Not Ratable
Well-kept   In need of repair
1 ...... 2.......3 ...... 4.......5.......6 ...... 7................ Not Ratable
Uncrowded   Crowded
1 ...... 2.......3 ...... 4.......5.......6 ...... 7................ Not Ratable

5. Marital or other Close Adult Relationship
Very Satisfying   Very Unsatisfying
1 ...... 2.......3 ...... 4.......5.......6 ...... 7................ Not Ratable

6. Chronic Health Problems and/or Disabilities in the Immediate Family
None   Few   Many
1 ...... 2.......3 ...... 4.......5.......6 ...... 7................ Not Ratable

7. Chronic Health Problems and/or Disabilities in Extended Family
   None   Few   Many
   1 ...... 2.......3 ...... 4 ....5.......6 ...... 7 .... Not Ratable

8. Involvement with Social Environment
   Overinvolved   Underinvolved
   1 ...... 2.......3 ...... 4 ....5.......6 ...... 7 .... Not Ratable

9. Level of Conflict in the Home
   None   Some   Excessive
   1 ...... 2.......3 ...... 4 ....5.......6 ...... 7 .... Not Ratable

10. Homemaking, Daily Living (insofar as the home is concerned)
    Non-stressful   Highly stressful
    1 ...... 2.......3 ...... 4 ....5.......6 ...... 7 .... Not Ratable

11. Financial Security
    Very Secure   Very Insecure
    1 ...... 2.......3 ...... 4 ....5.......6 ...... 7 .... Not Ratable

12. Family Problems
    None   Many
    1 ...... 2.......3 ...... 4 ....5.......6 ...... 7 .... Not Ratable

13. Possibly Dangerous Neighborhood which places Stress and Strain on
    Family Members
    Little   Much
    1 ...... 2.......3 ...... 4 ....5.......6 ...... 7 .... Not Ratable

14. Coping potential
    Very Poor   Moderate   Excellent
    1 ...... 2.......3 ...... 4 ....5.......6 ...... 7 .... Not Ratable

15. Family Resources (ties and relationships to other family members,
    friends, social supports, neighborhood, institutional)
    None   Some   Many
    1 ...... 2.......3 ...... 4 ....5.......6 ...... 7 .... Not Ratable

16. Characteristics of Family Environment
    Strict   Lax
    1 ...... 2.......3 ...... 4 ....5.......6 ...... 7 .... Not Ratable

Consistent   Inconsistent
1 ...... 2.......3 ...... 4.......5.......6 ...... 7................ Not Ratable
Mother's Availability
Little   Very much
1 ...... 2.......3 ...... 4.......5.......6 ...... 7................ Not Ratable
Father's Involvement
Little   Very much
1 ...... 2.......3 ...... 4.......5.......6 ...... 7................ Not Ratable
Parental Punishment of Children
Agreement   Disagreement
1 ...... 2.......3 ...... 4.......5.......6 ...... 7................ Not Ratable
Power Assertive
Low   Moderate   High
1 ...... 2.......3 ...... 4.......5.......6 ...... 7................ Not Ratable

17. Family Structure -- 1-2 Traditional, 2 parents available; 3-4, two parents
    or substitutes with less availability; 5-6, one parent with support; 7-8,
    child with unmarried mother and with no father or father substitute; 9-
    10, mother-child/children alone with little or no social support.
    1 ...... 2.......3 ...... 4.......5.......6 ...... 7.......8 ...... 9...... 10

18. Global Rating of Family Environment-Home Life
    Nonstressful   Very Stressful
    1 ...... 2.......3 ...... 4.......5.......6 ...... 7................ Not Ratable

19. Family Is Feeling Stress-Strain
    Little   Some   Excessive
    1 ...... 2.......3 ...... 4.......5.......6 ...... 7................ Not Ratable

ASSESSMENT SCALE FOR SUBSYSTEM FUNCTIONING

Percent	Criteria
100	Subsystem Functioning is Present Subsystem Functions without Interruption Subsystem Functioning Fulfills Its Purpose
81 - 99	Subsystem Functioning Present Interruption of Functioning only Transient Subsystem Functioning Fulfills Its Purpose
61 - 80	Subsystem Functioning Present Number of Reported Interruptions Below 5 Functioning is Interrupted for Less than 1 Week Functioning of Other Subsystems Not Adversely Affected
41 - 60	Subsystem Functioning Present Number of Interruptions Greater than 5, Less than 10 Functioning Reestablished within 1 Week to 1 Month a Slight Degree
21 - 40	Subsystem Functioning Partially Present Number of Interruptions Greater than 10, Less than 15 Functioning Interrupted for 1 to 3 Months Functioning is not Reestablished - or Fails to Fulfill Its Purpose During that Time Functioning of Other Subsystems Adversely Affected to a Moderate Degree
1 - 20	Subsystem Functioning Partially Present Number of Interruptions Greater than 15 Interruptions Chronic - More than 3 months Function Not Reestablished Subsystem Fails to Meet Its Purpose
1	Functioning of Other Subsystems Grossly Impaired
0	Subsystem Absent

CRITERIA FOR RATING SEVERITY OF PROBLEMS WITH SUBSYSTEM FUNCTIONING

Severity	Examples of Problems	Duration
1 - None	None i.e Budget Balanced	-------------
2 - Mild	Differ on Food Preference Can't Decide Who Cooks Conflict on What to Buy Overcrowded Living Quarters	Less than a week

3 - Moderate	Conflict on When to Go
	  Somewhere
	Member Forgets Responsibility
	Cook Gets Sick
	Members Forget to Give
	  Messages
	A Family Member Buys
	  Impulsively More than Once
	Child Expelled from School
		More than a week
		Less than a month

4 - Severe	Unemployment Poverty Serious Chronic Illness Residence in High Crime Neighborhood	More than a month

5 - Extreme	No transportation
	Natural Disaster
	Power Outages - More than 24
	  hours
	No Savings
	No Health Insurance
	No Communication of
	  Feelings
	Sexual or Physical Abuse	

FORM B-SCALE FOR OBSERVER'S RATINGS OF T-1 VIDEOTAPES

The 48 items referring to behaviors were rated as indicated by each observer, or as "Not applicable, or Not scorable".

1.	Did family members seem to be "listening" to each other?	Never	1
		Seldom	2
		Sometimes	3
		Often	4
		Very Often	5
		Not applicable	( )
		Not Scorable	( )
2.	Did family members talk for each other?	Never	1
		Seldom	2
		Sometimes	3
		Often	4
		Very Often	5
		Not applicable	( )
		Not Scorable	( )
3.	How often were messages sent directly to their appropriate targets?	Not at all	1
		Seldom	2
		Sometimes	3
		Often	4
		A lot	5
4.	How often were messages sent indirectly their appropriate targets?	Scale same as for item 3	
5.	How benign, supportive, or warm were their appropriate targets?	Scale same as for item 3	

6.	How neutral was the emotional tone of the conversation?	Scale same as for item 3	
7.	How hostile, critical, or malignant was the emotional tone of the conversations?	Scale same as for item 3	
8.	How much affect was present in the conversations?	None Little Some Much A lot	1 2 3 4 6
9.	Would you say the amount of affect was too little, just right, or too much?	Too little Just right Too much Not Ratable Not Applicable	1 2 3 ( ) ( )
10.	Each family member was also rated individually on item 9.		
11.	How often were "tension releasers" such as pauses, nervous laughter, joking, etc. present during the conversations?	Scale same as for item 3	
13.	How often were there angry outbursts to family members during the session?	None Few Some Many A lot	1 2 3 4 5
14.	How often was disruptive behavior present?	Scale same as for item 3	

15.	Would you say this behavior was Malicious? Neutral or Benign?	Malicious	1
		Neutral	2
		Benign	3

16.	How effectively was this behavior handled?	Not at all effective	1
		Seldom effective	2
		Somewhat effective	3
		Effective	4
		Very effective	5

| 17. | How often did one or more family members refuse to enter the discussion or show passive-aggressive behavior? | Scale same as for item 3 |

| 18. | How many family members exhibited this behavior? | Record actual no._____ |

| 19. | How often did family members verbally interrupt each other? | Scale same as for item 3 |

20.	How often did the discussion seem clear (not confused), and well-understood by family members?	Very confused	1
		Confused	2
		So-so	3
		Clear	4
		Very clear	5

| 21. | Draw a picture of this family's Channel and Net. | |

| 22. | How critical (malignant) were family members of one another? | Scale same as for item 3 |

| 23. | How considerate (benign) were family members of one another? | Scale same as for item 3 |

| 24. | How neutral (mixed) were family members toward one another? | Scale same as for item 3 |

| 25. | In terms of amount of conversation, how much conversation was generated by the family during the entire interview? | Scale same as for item 8 |

26. How many hand movements (gestures) did this family make? — Scale same as for item 13

27. Would you say the hand movements (gestures) that this family mad were more inward (body-focused) or more outward

More inward	1
Both inward and outward	2
More outward	3

28. Would you say this family's gestures tended to be hostile, neutral, or supportive?

Hostile	
Neutral	2
Supportive	

29. How congruent or matching were the of family members' postures during the session?

Not at all congruent	1
Seldom congruent	2
Sometimes congruent	3
Congruent	4
Very congruent	5

30. How much eye contact was there between family members and/or the interviewers? — Scale same as for item 8

31. How much benign, supportive, affectionate touching of body contact was shown by this family? — Scale same as for item 8

32. How much non-verbal communication was generated during the entire interview? — Scale same as for item 8

33. Was there one family member who seemed to take control during the session?

No	
Yes	

34. Specify who took control _____

35. How rigid did this family seem?

Not at all rigid	1
A little rigid	2
Somewhat rigid	3
Rigid	4
Very rigid	5

36.	How flexible did this family seem?	Not at all flexible	1
		A little flexible	2
		Somewhat flexible	3
		Flexible	4
		Very flexible	5

37.	How chaotic did this family seem?	Not at all chaotic	1
		A little chaotic	2
		Somewhat chaotic	3
		Chaotic	4
		Very chaotic	5

38. How often did people in the family have an equal say in the discussion?

Scale same as for item 3

39.	How defined were the individual family members boundaries?	Not at all defined	1
		A little defined	2
		Somewhat defined	3
		Firm	4
		Rigid	5

40. How defined were intergenerational boundaries?

Scale same as for item 39

41. To what extent were parent-child coalitions present?

Scale same as for item 13

42. Draw a picture of the coalitions in this family.

43.	How strong was the marital functional bond?	Very weak	1
		Weak	2
		So-so	3
		Strong	4
		Very strong	5

44. How strong was the marital affectional bond?

Scale same as for item 43

45. To what extent did each member participate verbally and also "functionally" as a presence? Scale same as for item 8

46. How often did family members speak up for themselves (express their wishes, wants, opinions) during the session? Scale same as for item 3

47. How often did family members go along with or agree with each other during the session? Scale same as for item 3

48. How autonomous/independent (of one another) are the members of the family? Scale same as for item 3

VIDEOTAPE SCRIPT

1. **Ingestor**
   A. How does your family go about buying food?
   B. Who buys food for the family?
   C. How is it decided who buys the food for your family?
   D. How much time does it take?
   E. What problems (issues) does your family have with food buying?
   F. How does your family deal with these problems (issues)?

2. **Converter**
   A. How does your family go about preparing meals?
   B. Who cooks for your family?
   C. How is it decided who cooks for your family?
   D. How much time does cooking for the family take?
   E. In one week there are 21 meals (3 meals a day for 7 days); in general, how many meals does your family eat together weekly?
      If there is an affirmative answer, then ask:
      1. How does your family go about handling seating arrangements at meals?
      2. Who handles this?
      3. How is it decided who sits where?
      4. How much time goes into handling seating arrangements?
      5. What problems does seating arrangements cause for your family?
      6. How does your family deal with these problems (issues)?

3. **Extruder**
   A. How are garbage and trash taken care of in your family?
   B. Who takes out the garbage and trash?
   C. How is it decided who takes out the garbage and trash?
   D. How much time is spent taking out garbage and trash?
   E. What kinds of problems (issues) does your family have in getting rid of garbage and trash?
   F. How does your family deal with these problems (issues)?

4. **Motor**
   A. How does your family get around, that is, travel from one place to another?
   B. Who takes the family members from place to place?

C. How is it decided who takes family members around?

D. How much time is spent taking family members from place to place?

E. What kind of transportation problems occur in your family?

F. How does your family deal with these problems?

5. Supporter

A. How does your family handle sleeping arrangements in this house?

B. Who handles the sleeping arrangements for your family?

C. How is it decided who handles the sleeping arrangements for your family?

D. How much time is spent in dealing with sleeping arrangements for your family?

E. What kinds of problems do sleeping arrangements cause for your family?

F. How does your family deal with these problems?

6. Storage

A. How does your family go about putting things away or storing things such as food, clothing, or outside tools?

B. Who does the storing?

C. How is it decided who stores or puts things away?

D. How much time is spent in storing or putting things away?

E. Is it easy to find things after they have been put away?

F. What kinds of problems does storing cause for your family?

G. How does your family deal with these problems?

7. Producer

I. House Repair and Upkeep

A. How does your family handle the repairs and upkeep of your house?

B. Who takes care of the repairs and upkeep of the house?

C. How does your family decide who takes care of the repair and upkeep?

D. How much time does it take?

E. What kinds of problems do house repair and upkeep cause for your family?

F. How does your family deal with these problems?

II Health Care

A. How does your family handle matters of health and illness?

B. Who takes care of health and illness matters in the family?

C. How is it decided who handles health and illness matters in your

family?
- D. How much time does this take?
- E. What problems does your family have in handling health and illness matters?
- F. How does your family deal with problems of handling health and illness matters?

III. Cleaning
- A. How does your family keep the house clean?
- B. Who cleans the house?
- C. How is it decided who cleans the house?
- D. How much time does it take?
- E. What problems does house cleaning cause your family?
- F. How does your family deal with these problems?

8. Distributor
- A. How is food, clothing, etc. distributed in your family?
- B. Who distributes things like food, clothing, toys, presents to members of your family?
- C. How is it decided who distributes things like food, clothing etc.
- D. How much time does this take?
- E. What problems does distribution cause for your family?
- F. How does your family deal with such problems?

9. Boundary
I People
- A. How does your family go about regulating who does and who does not come into your house?
- B. Who regulates who does or does not come into your house?
- C. How is it decided who regulates these things?
- D. How much time does this take?
- E. What problems (issues) does your family have concerning who does or does not come into your house?
- F. How does your family deal with these problems (issues)?

II Telephone
- A. How does your family go about regulating the use of the telephone?
- B. Who regulates the use of the telephone?
- C. How is it decided who regulates the use of the telephone?
- D. How much time does this take?
- E. What problems (issues) does your family have over the use of the telephone?
- F. How does your family deal with these problems (issues)?

III Television
   A. How does your family go about regulating what is watched on T.V.?
   B. Who regulates what is watched on T.V.?
   C. How is it decided who regulates what is watched on T.V.?
   D. How much time does this take?
   E. What problems (issues) does your family have with the T.V.?
   F. How does your family deal with these problems (issues)?

10. Input Transducer
   A. How does your family keep up with what is going on in the community and the world?
   B. Who in the family is involved in helping your family keep up with what is going on in the community and the world?
   C. How is it decided who helps your family keep up with what is going on in the outside world?
   D. How much time is spent on keeping up with the outside world?
   E. What kinds of problems does your family have in keeping up with what is going on in the outside world?
   F. How does your family deal with these problems?

11. Internal Transducer
   I Activities
   A. How does your family keep up to date with what is going on within the family?
   B. Who keeps up with what is going on within the family?
   C. How is it decided who keps up with what is going on within your family?
   D. How much time is spent keeping up to date with what is going on within the family?
   E. What problems does the family have concerning what is going on within the family?
   F. How does your family deal with these problems?

   II Feelings
   A. How does your family deal with feelings?
   B. Who keeps track of members' feelings in your family?
   C. How is it decided who keeps track of members' feelings?
   D. How much time is spent keeping track of members' feelings?
   E. What sorts of problems does your family have in keeping track of members' feelings?
   F. How does your family deal with these problems?

12. Channel and Net   (deals with communication; to be inferred and rated from videotape).

13. Memory
A. How does your family go about keeping records of its activities?
B. Who keeps records for the family?
C. How is it decided who keeps your family's records?
D. How much time is spent keeping records?
E. What problems over record-keeping does the family have?
F. How does your family deal with these problems?

14. Associator — Not specifically evaluated

15. Decider
I   *General*
A. How does your family go about making decisions?
B. Who makes decisions in your family?
C. How is it decided who makes the decisions?
D. How much time is spent in decision-making?
E. What kinds of problems over decision-making does your family have?
F. How does your family deal with these problems?

II   *Money*
A. How does your family go about deciding how money will be spent or saved?
B. Who decides how money is spent or saved?
C. How much time is devoted to money matters?
D. What kinds of problems over money matters does your family have?
E. How does your family deal with these problems?

16. Decoder
A. How does your family go about making things (e.g. events, activities, behaviors, situations, emotions) understandable to other family members?
B. Who in your family explains things to others?
C. How is it decided who makes things understandable?
D. How much time does this take?
E. What kinds of problems (issues) does your family have with explaining things to other family members?
F. How does your family deal with these problems (issues)?

17. Encoder

A. How does your family go about telling others about your family?
B. Who tells others about your family?
C. How is it decided who tells others about family matters?
D. How much time is spent doing this?
E. What kinds of problems (issues) does your family have over what is told to others about your family and what is kept within your family?
F. How does your family deal with such problems (issues)?

18. Output Transducer

A. How does your family handle family business such as paying bills, writing family letters, dealing with school, work, church, or law?
B. Who handles the business of the family?
C. How is it decided who handles the business of the family?
D. How much time does this take?
E. What problems does the family have concerning this activity?
F. How does your family deal with these problems?

19. Reproducer

I Values

A. How does your family go about teaching other members values and important ways of relating to one another?
B. Who in your family teaches the values of the family and ways of relating to one another?
C. How is it decided who teaches these things?
D. How much time does it take?
E. What kinds of problems does your family have with the teaching of values and ways of relating to one another?
F. How does your family deal with the problems?

II Discipline (ask only if there are children in the family)

A. How is discipline handled in your family?
B. Who does the disciplining in your family?
C. How is it decided who disciplines in your family?
D. How much time is spent disciplining?
E. What kinds of problems (issues) does your family have with discipline?
F. How does your family deal with those problems (issues)?

*III Rules (*ask only if there are children in the family)

A. How does your family go about making rules?
B. Who makes rules in your family?
C. How is it decided who makes rules in your family?

D. How much time does this take?

E. What kind of problems (issues) does your family have concerning rules?

F. How does your family deal with the problems (issues)?

VIDEOTAPE SCRIPT -- SUGGESTED MODIFICATIONS

1. For all of the subsystems, the third question (C) probably should be worded, "Does the task take too much time? the right amount? or very little?. Is the amount of time involved Burdensome? Appropriate? or Insufficient?.

2. The section on "Health Care" in the *Producer* subsystem needs to be moved to part 2 in the *Internal Transducer* subsystem.

3. Primary Care Givers -- A new section to be included under the subsystem *Internal Transducer*
   A. How does your family go about caring for the children?
   B. Who are the primary care-givers?
   C. How is it decided who is the primary caregiver?
   D. Do you find the amount of time spent in this activity is too much? The right amount? Very little?
   E. Is the amount of time Burdensome? Appropriate? Insufficient?.
   F. What kind of problems (issues) does your family have with care giving.
   G. How does your family deal with the problems.

4. The *Distributor* subsystem probably should be changed to include the distribution of "attention" as well as "things" to members of the family.
   A. How is time and attention divided among or given to members of your family?
   B. Who does it?
   C. How is it decided who does it?
   D. Is the amount of time spent on this activity too much? The right amount? Too little?
   E. Do you find the amount of time spent giving attention is Burdensome? Insufficient? Just right?
   F. What problems does this cause your family?
   G. How does your family deal with these problems?

5. Wage earners -- to be included in the *Producer* subsystem.
   A. How is your family supported financially?
   B. Who are the wage earners?
   C. How is it decided who the wage earners are?

D. Is the amount of time spent working too much? The right amount? Too little?.

E. Is the amount of time Burdensome? Appropriate? Insufficient?

F. What problems (issues) does your family have concerning work?

G. How does your family deal with these problems (issues)?

6. If desired, the overall videotaping script can be shortened to contain just the 8 subsystems -- *Supporter, Reproducer, Decider, Boundary, Internal Transducer, Producer, Converter, and Storage* -- that differentiated the functioning groups. But, to obtain a comprehensive view of family life, it is helpful to include all of the subsystems we described.

INDEX